Normal and Abnormal Swallowing
Second Edition

Springer
New York
Berlin
Heidelberg
Hong Kong
London
Milan
Paris
Tokyo

Bronwyn Jones, MD, FRACP, FRCR

Professor of Radiology, The Russell H. Morgan Department of
Radiology and Radiological Science, The Johns Hopkins
University School of Medicine, The Johns Hopkins Hospital,
and Director, The Johns Hopkins Swallowing Center,
Baltimore, Maryland, USA

Editor

Normal and Abnormal Swallowing
Imaging in Diagnosis and Therapy

Second Edition

With 164 Figures, 4 in Full Color

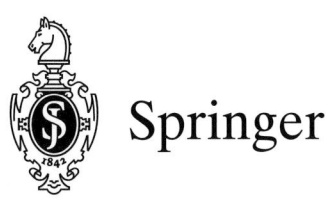

Bronwyn Jones, MD, FRACP, FRCR
Professor of Radiology
The Russell H. Morgan Department of Radiology and Radiological Science
The Johns Hopkins University School of Medicine
The Johns Hopkins Hospital
and
Director
The Johns Hopkins Swallowing Center
Baltimore, MD 21287
USA
bjones1@jhmi.edu

Cover illustration: On the left side: a single spot film in the frontal projection shows a translucent curved filling defect at the lower border of the pharynx representing a mucosal web. On the right side: a stop-frame print from a cinepharyngogram demonstrates an upright epiglottis, open larynx, laryngeal penetration, and aspiration along the anterior surface of the trachea. The bolus is passing past the open cricopharyngeus into the cervical esophagus.

Library of Congress Cataloging-in-Publication Data
Normal and abnormal swallowing : imaging in diagnosis and therapy / editor, Bronwyn Jones.—2nd ed.
    p.; cm.
  Includes bibliographical references and index.
  ISBN 0-387-95194-6 (alk. paper)
  1. Deglutition disorders—Imaging. 2. Swallowing. 3. Pharynx—Imaging. I. Jones, Bronwyn.
    [DNLM: 1. Deglutition. 2. Pharyngeal Diseases—diagnosis. 3. Deglutition Disorders—diagnosis. 4. Deglutition Disorders—therapy. 5. Diagnostic Imaging.
6. Pharynx. WV 400 N842 2002]
RC815.2 .N67 2002
616.3′1—dc21
                                        2001054923

ISBN 0-387-95194-6   Printed on acid-free paper.

© 2003, 1991 Springer-Verlag New York, Inc.
All rights reserved. This work may not be translated or copied in whole or in part without the written permission of the publisher (Springer-Verlag New York, Inc., 175 Fifth Avenue, New York, NY 10010, USA), except for brief excerpts in connection with reviews or scholarly analysis. Use in connection with any form of information storage and retrieval, electronic adaptation, computer software, or by similar or dissimilar methodology now known or hereafter developed is forbidden.
The use in this publication of trade names, trademarks, service marks, and similar terms, even if they are not identified as such, is not to be taken as an expression of opinion as to whether or not they are subject to proprietary rights.
While the advice and information in this book are believed to be true and accurate at the date of going to press, neither the authors nor the editors nor the publisher can accept any legal responsibility for any errors or omissions that may be made. The publisher makes no warranty, express or implied, with respect to the material contained herein.

Printed in the United States of America.

9 8 7 6 5 4 3 2 1   SPIN 10790013

www.springer-ny.com

Springer-Verlag   New York Berlin Heidelberg
A member of BertelsmannSpringer Science+Business Media GmbH

*To my mentor, the late Martin W. Donner, MD,
and the patients and colleagues of
The Johns Hopkins Swallowing Center*

Preface

It is now 11 years since the publication of the first edition of *Normal and Abnormal Swallowing: Imaging in Diagnosis and Therapy*. These 11 years have seen an enormous change in the specialty of the study of dysphagia. First, we have seen the tragic loss of two of the pioneering giants in the field: Wylie J. Dodds, MD, of the Medical College of Wisconsin, Milwaukee, and Martin W. Donner, MD, of The Johns Hopkins University School of Medicine, Baltimore, Maryland, a former coeditor of this book. Second, there has been a steady expansion in the number of professionals interested in and working in this specialty. The last 11 years have also seen the steady growth of the multidisciplinary journal *Dysphagia*, devoted to swallowing and its disorders, as well as the formation of the Dysphagia Research Society, which held its tenth annual meeting in October 2001. The dysphagia special interest division (SID 13) of the American Speech and Hearing Association (ASHA) now has some 3,000 members. At the same time, the world population is aging. Dysphagia will be an important health issue in this aging population.

Despite the high and increasing incidence of dysphagia, many physicians and allied health professionals are unfamiliar with the anatomy and physiology of the pharynx nor are they trained in the techniques used to examine dysphagic patients. An upper gastrointestinal series, for example, usually examines only the thoracic esophagus, neglecting the pharynx, unless symptoms suggest an oral or pharyngeal location. Even then, spot films only may be taken, with no dynamic imaging to evaluate the movement of the structures.

It is the intention of this book to familiarize the reader with imaging of the pharynx and with the spectrum of swallowing disorders. The text is intended not to be encyclopedic or exhaustive, but rather to present a practical approach to the role of imaging in the diagnosis and treatment of patients with dysphagia. An attempt has been made to define the role of the newer modalities such as ultrasound, computed tomography, and magnetic resonance imaging in the work-up of the dysphagic patient. It is felt that scintigraphy is outside the scope of this text; therefore, this technique has not been included.

Imaging has been illustrated with both spot films and still frames from either cinefluorographic studies or super-VHS studies. The reader is reminded that some resolution is lost when a dynamic study is frozen, and thus, a few of the illustrations are grainy.

The text concentrates on oral and pharyngeal disease but also emphasizes the interrelationships between pharynx and esophagus in health and disease.

A glossary is appended of some words and phrases commonly used in discussing dysphagia.

Baltimore, Maryland				Bronwyn Jones, MD, FRACP, FRCR

Acknowledgment

With deep appreciation to Fay R. Cromer, who (without grumbling) completely retyped those chapters authored by the editor.

Baltimore, Maryland						Bronwyn Jones, MD, FRACP, FRCR

Contents

Preface vii
Acknowledgment ix
Contributors xiii
Overview xvii

1. Radiation in Videorecorded Fluoroscopy 1
   MAHADEVAPPA MAHESH, BOB W. GAYLER, AND THOMAS J. BECK

2. Anatomical and Physiological Overview 11
   EMMETT T. CUNNINGHAM, JR., AND BRONWYN JONES

3. The Tailored Examination 35
   BRONWYN JONES

4. Interpreting the Study 55
   BRONWYN JONES

5. Adaptation, Compensation, and Decompensation 83
   BRONWYN JONES

6. Pharyngoesophageal Interrelationships and Reflexes
   Involved in Airway Protection 91
   BRONWYN JONES

7. Common Structural Lesions 103
   BRONWYN JONES

8. Ultrasound Imaging and Swallowing 119
   BARBARA C. SONIES, GLORIA CHI-FISHMAN, AND JERI L. MILLER

9. Cross-Sectional Imaging of Dysphagia 139
   STUART W. POINT, KAREN M. HORTON, R. NICK BRYAN,
   EMMETT T. CUNNINGHAM, JR., AND S. JAMES ZINREICH

10	Pharyngography in the Postoperative Patient	167
	STEPHEN E. RUBESIN, DAVID W. EISELE, AND BRONWYN JONES	
11	Swallowing in Children	205
	SANDRA S. KRAMER AND PEGGY S. EICHER	
12	Aging and Neurological Disease	227
	BRONWYN JONES	
13	Dysphagia in AIDS	243
	MAYA D. MEUX AND SUSAN D. WALL	
14	The Role of Radiology in Rehabilitation of Swallowing	261
	JEFFREY B. PALMER AND EILEEN A. CARDEN	

Conclusion: What Does the Future Hold? 275
BRONWYN JONES

Glossary 277

Index 279

Contributors

THOMAS J. BECK, ScD
Associate Professor of Radiology, The Russell H. Morgan Department of Radiology, The Johns Hopkins University School of Medicine, The Johns Hopkins Hospital, Baltimore, MD 21287, USA

R. NICK BRYAN, MD, PhD
Eugene P. Pendergrass Professor of Radiology, and Chairman, Department of Radiology, University of Pennsylvania School of Medicine, Philadelphia, PA 19104, USA

EILEEN A. CARDEN, MS
Speech Language Pathologist, Department of Rehabilitation Services, The Good Samaritan Hospital, Baltimore, MD 21239; and Consultant, The Johns Hopkins Swallowing Center, Baltimore, MD 21287, USA

GLORIA CHI-FISHMAN, PhD
Deputy Director, Oral Pharyngeal Function and Ultrasound Imaging Laboratory, Physical Disabilities Branch, Department of Rehabilitation Medicine, W.G. Magnuson Clinical Center, National Institutes of Health, Bethesda, MD 20892, USA

EMMETT T. CUNNINGHAM, JR., MD, PhD, MPH
Professor of Ophthalmology, and Director, The Uveitis Service, Department of Ophthalmology, New York University School of Medicine, New York, NY 10003; and Early Clinical Leader, Clinical Services, Pfizer, Inc., Groton, CT 06340, USA

PEGGY S. EICHER, MD
Medical Director, Center for Pediatric Feeding and Swallowing, St. Joseph's Hospital, Patterson, NJ 07503, USA

DAVID W. EISELE, MD
Professor and Chairman, Department of Otolaryngology—Head and Neck Surgery, University of California, San Francisco, San Francisco, CA 94121, USA

BOB W. GAYLER, MD
Associate Professor, The Russell H. Morgan Department of Radiology and Radiological Science, The Johns Hopkins University School of Medicine, The Johns Hopkins Hospital, Baltimore, MD 21287, USA

KAREN M. HORTON, MD
Assistant Professor, The Russell H. Morgan Department of Radiology and Radiological Science, The Johns Hopkins University School of Medicine, The Johns Hopkins Hospital, Baltimore, MD 21287, USA

BRONWYN JONES, MD, FRACP, FRCR
Professor of Radiology, The Russell H. Morgan Department of Radiology and Radiological Science, The Johns Hopkins University School of Medicine; and Director, The Johns Hopkins Swallowing Center, The Johns Hopkins Hospital, Baltimore, MD 21287, USA

SANDRA S. KRAMER, MD
Professor of Radiology, Department of Radiology, University of Pennsylvania School of Medicine; and Children's Hospital of Philadelphia, Philadelphia, PA 19104, USA

MAHADEVAPPA MAHESH, PhD
Chief Physicist, The Johns Hopkins Hospital, and Research Associate, The Russell H. Morgan Department of Radiology and Radiological Science, The Johns Hopkins University School of Medicine, Baltimore, MD 21287, USA

MAYA D. MEUX, MD
Assistant Clinical Professor of Radiology, University of California, San Francisco, San Francisco, CA 94121, USA

JERI L. MILLER, PhD
Physical Disabilities Branch, Department of Rehabilitation Medicine, W.G. Magnuson Clinical Center, National Institutes of Health, Bethesda, MD 20892, USA

JEFFREY B. PALMER, MD
Associate Professor of Rehabilitation Medicine, Department of Physical Medicine and Rehabilitation, and Department of Otolaryngology—Head and Neck Surgery, Good Samaritan Hospital, Baltimore, MD 21239; and Consultant, The Johns Hopkins Swallowing Center, The Johns Hopkins University, Baltimore, MD 21287, USA

STUART W. POINT, MD
Delaney Radiologists, Wilmington, NC 28409, USA

STEPHEN E. RUBESIN, MD
Professor of Radiology, Department of Radiology, Hospital of the University of Pennsylvania, Philadelphia, PA 19104, USA

Contributors

BARBARA C. SONIES, PhD
Chief, Oral Motor Function Section, and Director, Oral Pharyngeal Function and Ultrasound Imaging Laboratory, Physical Disabilities Branch, Department of Rehabilitation Medicine, W.G. Magnuson Clinical Center, National Institutes of Health, Bethesda, MD 20892, USA

SUSAN D. WALL, MD
Professor of Radiology, Department of Radiology, University of California, San Francisco; and Assistant Chief, Radiology, Veterans Administration Medical Center, San Francisco, CA 94121, USA

S. JAMES ZINREICH, MD
Professor of Radiology and Otolaryngology—Head and Neck Surgery, The Johns Hopkins University School of Medicine, The Johns Hopkins Hospital, Baltimore, MD 21287, USA

Overview

Dysphagia (difficulty in swallowing, implying difficulty of passage of bolus) is a surprisingly common symptom and, often, an extremely troublesome one. Dysphagia is a symptom that spans all ages, being common in the young and otherwise healthy, during the middle years, and in the elderly. It can be long-standing, frustrating, and all-consuming, and it can interfere with one of the most enjoyable social interactions, namely, eating. In addition, dysphagia is a symptom that may not be given due attention by friends or relatives, or may be dismissed as being of psychogenic or psychosomatic origin. The patient with unexplained pharyngeal dysphagia should not be dismissed as neurotic, nor should the condition be given the label "*globus hystericus*" or "dysphagia of psychogenic origin." A patient so dismissed or so labeled may never be re-evaluated, even if symptoms change.

The act of swallowing seems simple. It is something we do unconsciously, and once the voluntary oral phase has been completed, the remainder of the swallow is involuntary. However, the successful execution of a swallow requires the intricate coordination between several cranial nerves and 30 to 40 muscles of the face, mouth, pharynx, and esophagus. Neuromuscular diseases, head and neck surgery or trauma, local structural lesions, gastrointestinal disorders, cancer, and developmental disabilities can all produce problems with swallowing. The resulting impairment may range from mild discomfort to life-threatening disability.

Many patients adjust to slowly progressive disease by modification of their diet or speed of eating and may themselves be unaware of such compensatory behavior. Others may have lost sensory perception in the mouth, pharynx, or larynx resulting in dysphagia and may even aspirate without coughing (silent aspiration) or subjective awareness (silent dysphagia). Symptoms suggesting dysphagia may be subtle, absent, or referred; for example, respiratory diseases, such as asthma or laryngospasm, may in fact be due to an unsuspected problem with swallowing.

When all voluntary and involuntary compensatory mechanisms break down, massive aspiration or choking on food may dramatically demonstrate how advanced the underlying disorder has become. Estimates based on insurance statistics suggest that, in the United States alone, 8,000 to 10,000 individuals die from choking each year.

The scope of the problem of dysphagia is certainly significant and widespread. For example, studies in several medical institutions have revealed a surprisingly high incidence: 12 to 20% of patients in the general hospital population and 50 to 90% in the nursing-home environment. In the United States, esophageal carcinoma accounts for approximately 1% of all cancers and almost 10% of cancers of the gastrointestinal tract. Similarly, laryngeal and head and neck cancers cause a significant incidence of dysphagia both from the primary tumor and following surgical resection, chemotherapy, or radiation.

Our population is an aging one, with the potential for an increasing incidence of dysphagia related both to the aging process alone and to diseases that affect the elderly. More refined surgical techniques, improved life-support systems, and new and better medications also allow patients to survive longer even with debilitating disease.

The reason for the dysphagia may be obvious, such as prior radical head and neck surgery or obvious neuromuscular disease elsewhere, or the cause may be obscure. Imaging is essential for the evaluation of the dysphagic patient in both known and undiagnosed disease. Imaging is critical not only in the diagnosis of the cause of dysphagia but also in guiding therapeutic intervention.

1
Radiation in Videorecorded Fluoroscopy

MAHADEVAPPA MAHESH, BOB W. GAYLER, AND THOMAS J. BECK

The evaluation and management of patients with feeding and swallowing disorders frequently requires the use of specialized studies. There are a number of specialized methods currently available for evaluation of swallowing function. They include modified barium studies, ultrasonography, radionuclide imaging or scintigraphy, and endoscopy. Also a number of methods that use magnetic resonance imaging and ultrafast computed tomography have been developed. Swallowing specialists generally agree that modified barium studies with dynamically recorded fluoroscopic images have some advantages over other methods available. The technique defines the nature of a swallowing problem, documents the patient's response to the deficit, defines factors contributing to aspiration, and identifies therapeutic techniques and modifications that may enhance the swallowing function. Over the past decade, these modified barium studies have become the gold standard for the evaluation of swallowing function.

In the past, the dynamic recording method of choice for barium studies employed specialized cinefluorography systems. Now, dynamic fluoroscopic recording of noncardiac procedures is usually done with videocassette recorders, which can be easily connected to existing videofluoroscopy systems. Despite some loss of image quality compared to cine, videotape-recorded fluoroscopy or videofluorography (hereafter referred to as VTF) has many advantages over cinefluorography. For example, it does not require a specialized x-ray generator, cine camera, and cine film processing units or special projection equipment. Also, in terms of radiation exposure to the patient, cine exposure rates are 5 to 10 times higher than normal fluoroscopic exposure rates.

Videocassette recorders are available with a wide range of features and options. These range from low-end consumer products suitable for basic home use to high-end broadcast-quality equipment. The units chosen for medical recording will depend on the specific needs as well as the available budget. We believe that the following features are essential or at least highly desirable:

Super-VHS (S-VHS) formats. This provides better resolution with an overall cleaner effect than does conventional VHS. Resolution of conventional VHS format is approximately 240 lines, whereas for S-VHS format it can be as high as 400 lines.

Digital video formats. This is the latest technology with resolution higher than S-VHS and can provide 500 or more lines of resolution.

Recording triggered by a video signal. This avoids a situation in which an assistant is required to manually turn the recorder on and off during the procedure and either listen for verbal cues, which may be omitted, or watch the monitor, with delays in activating the cassette recorder.

Image annotation of date and time markers. This greatly facilitates locating individual studies.

Time indicator on the VCR control panel. This facilitates finding sequential studies on a tape when they are not being simultaneously observed on the monitor.

Modern fluoroscopic systems provide video signals at resolution as high as 1024 lines; however, the highest resolution of video recording devices currently available goes up to 500 lines (digital format). Therefore, there will be degradation in resolution no matter what type of recording device one uses. On the other hand, if the videorecording device is one of the basic types (most low-end VCRs), the resolution is further degraded. Hence by recording on S-VHS format (up to 400 lines) or in digital video format (up to 500 lines) at least one can try to achieve the best possible resolution in the recorded image.

Stationary fluoroscopic systems were initially used in the development of VTF swallowing procedures. Some users have recently begun to employ mobile C-arm fluoroscopes. With the advent of C-arm use, the system can be brought to the patient rather than the patient to the system. This has expanded the utilization of VTF swallowing studies into remote environments such as nursing homes and other extended-care facilities.

It is important to recognize that VTF involves radiation exposure to both patient and practitioner, and thus incorporates some risk. This chapter intends to cover basic principles of radiation exposure, risks for both patient and operator, and radiation safety issues.

Basic Radiation Considerations

Radiation Risk

X-rays and other ionizing radiation have been linked to tissue damage, cancer, and genetic injury. Most of what we know about these effects, however, has been obtained by observations of radiation doses higher than those normally encountered in VTF. Information on low-dose exposure has been extrapolated downward from high-dose data, and the risk of harm at doses normally seen with diagnostic x-ray procedures cannot be determined with certainty. In addition, we are all exposed to variable levels of natural environmental or background radiation; hence no "zero dose" level exists for comparison. Moreover, the effects associated with low radiation levels occur in the absence of significant radiation exposure. Nevertheless, the prudent clinician should undertake any x-ray examination with the intent of achieving the highest benefit at the least risk to both patient and operator.

Radiation Units

Radiation effects depend upon the amount of radiation energy absorbed, hence require the introduction of certain units of measure. *Radiation absorbed dose* is measured in Grays, where 1 Gray (Gy) results from the absorption of 1 Joule (J) of radiation energy in 1 kilogram of tissue [1 Gy = 100 rads, in older units]. Since the Gray is a relatively large unit, doses encountered in diagnostic radiology are typically measured in centigrays or milligrays (1 cGy = 1/100 Gy = 1 rad, 1 mGy = 1/1000 Gy = 100 mrad, 1 rad = 1 cGy = 10 mGy).

A second important unit is the Sievert (Sv), the unit of *dose equivalence* [1 Sv = 100 rem in older units]. Dose equivalence was introduced to account for the higher biological damage produced by neutrons, alpha particles, and other forms of ionizing radiation rarely used in medicine. For x-radiation, gamma, and beta radiation, the quantities of absorbed dose and dose equivalent are themselves equivalent; that is, 1 Sv $\simeq$ 1 Gy, 1 rem $\simeq$ 1 rad, and so forth.

Radiation Effects

In discussions of radiation effects, one encounters the term **stochastic** and **nonstochastic** (1). *Stochastic effects* are effects in which the likelihood of an outcome is dependent on the dose. In other words, higher doses make the harmful outcome more likely than lower doses. On the other hand, *nonstochastic effects* are not observed until radiation dose exceeds a certain threshold. Doses below the threshold will not produce the effect, but above the threshold the severity of the effect increases with dose. An example of a nonstochastic effect is early transient erythema. The threshold for erythema in the human is on the order of 2 Gy (200 rad) (2), provided the dose is delivered all at the same time to the same skin surface. Other examples of nonstochastic effects include the induction of lens cataracts, epilation, and acute life-threatening effects due to whole-body irradiation.

Generally, nonstochastic effects require doses in excess of 2 Gy (200 rad). These levels can be delivered to the patient with a diagnostic x-ray machine during prolonged fluoroscopic procedures. Currently, deleterious effects to the skin due to extended fluoroscopic procedures are of great concern (3). This is mainly because complex interventional procedures often involve prolonged fluoroscopy, and these procedures are becoming increasingly common. The resulting doses can easily exceed the minimum threshold required to cause skin damage. However, in VTF swallowing studies such high radiation doses to patients should occur only if there has been gross misadjustment of the x-ray machine or fluoroscopic studies of unconscionably long duration. At the lower dose levels normally encountered in diagnostic gastrointestinal examinations (0.1–100 mGy), the concern is primarily for the stochastic effects of radiation.

Stochastic effects differ from nonstochastic effects in three ways. First, the biological effect is *all or nothing*; that is, it either occurs or does not occur. Second, the *probability of the effect* but not the severity increases with *dose*. Third (at least theoretically), there is *no threshold dose level* below which the effect cannot occur. Other than radiation effects in pregnancy and high-dose fluoroscopy, the principal health risks of diagnostic levels of radiation are believed to be stochastic, namely, the induction of cancer and genetic mutations.

Possible Effects of Radiation

Induction of Cancer

Long-term studies of populations of individuals exposed to high levels of radiation, in particular the survivors of the atomic bombs dropped on Japan just before the end of World War II, have demonstrated increased rates of cancers and leukemia (4). The carcinogenic effect is delayed; cancers occur at higher rates in exposed populations years after exposure. Certain biological tissues, including thyroid, lung, active bone marrow, gastrointestinal tract, and female breasts, have been identified as particularly sensitive to radiation-induced cancers, while other tissues such as neurological tissues and skin are relatively insensitive.

Some extrapolated risk estimates are listed in Table 1.1, which gives the expected cancer mortality in a population of 1 million persons (5), together with the expected increase in mortality due to radiation-induced cancers resulting from a uniform 10 mSv (1 rem) radiation dose to each

TABLE 1.1. Estimated cancer mortality (5) and increased mortality due to radiation-induced cancers resulting from exposure to 10 mSv (1 rem) of ionizing radiation in a population of 1 million people (BIER V) (4).

Tissue exposed	Malignancy	Normal cancer mortality		Increased cancer mortality[a]	
		Male	Female	Male	Female
Lung	Lung cancer	365	273	190	150
Bone marrow	Leukemia	50	39	110	80
Thyroid	Thyroid cancer	2	3	[b]	[b]
Esophagus	Esophagus cancer	38	11	[b]	[b]
Breast	Breast cancer	2	174	[b]	70
All tissues	All cancers	1170	1094	770	810

[a] Normal cancer mortality rates are projected for 1999 including both races and sexes and are age adjusted to the 1990 U.S. standard population (5).
[b] Not estimated owing to the large uncertainties in these estimates.

member (4). To obtain a risk estimate at other dose levels, the values in Table 1.1 can be extrapolated. For example, a 50 mSv dose to the active bone marrow would result in an additional 550 male and 400 female deaths due to leukemia in 1 million individuals exposed at that level.

Note: It is relevant that in a typical VTF swallowing study the patient receives radiation exposure to all the high-risk tissues just named; moreover, the VTF operator may receive exposure to these tissues.

Induction of Genetic Mutations

Radiation exposure to the ovaries and testes can damage genetic material in the germ cells, possibly leading to mutations in future offspring of the exposed individual. The likelihood of a radiation-induced mutation depends on the numbers of persons with gonadal radiation exposure prior to procreation as well as the radiation dose they receive. Within this context, the major concern is for the *gene pool of the entire population*, rather than for the individual. Thus the relevant radiation dose is the average gonadal dose received by individuals prior to procreation, averaged over the entire procreating population. To reduce impact on the gene pool, technologists, radiologists, and other personnel should routinely use shields and other methods to minimize gonadal dose to both patient and operator. If these precautions are properly observed, gonadal doses to patients from VTF swallowing procedures should be negligible, since the x-ray beam is normally confined to the neck and upper thorax, remote from the gonadal tissues. A properly worn protective apron of 0.5 mm lead equivalence should keep the dose to these tissues in the operator at an inconsequential level.

Radiation Effects to the Unborn

It is well known that the developing embryo and fetus are particularly sensitive to the harmful effects of radiation. This is a pertinent concern for both female radiation workers and female patients who may be pregnant. Several kinds of effect have been observed in individuals who were exposed in utero, including prenatal death and congenital anomalies (1,4). These effects depend on the dose magnitude and the stage of fetal development at which the exposure occurred (1). Within the first 10 postconception days the principal radiation effect observed is failure of the embryo to implant on the uterine wall (i.e., spontaneous abortion). The period of organogenesis, from 10 to 40 days postconception, when the major organ systems are formed, is most sensitive for the induction of gross malformations. The period from 40 days to term is associated with skeletal damage, childhood cancer, and central nervous system anomalies (microcephaly and mental retardation).

There is a statistical link between radiation received by the mother during pregnancy and an increase in childhood cancers. Although the evidence is not universally accepted, it is conservatively assumed that the unborn child is some 1.5 to 2 times as sensitive as the adult to the induction of cancers as a result of in utero irradiation (1).

The heightened radiation risk in pregnancy has led workers in diagnostic radiology to be exceptionally cautious when either patient or operator is or may be pregnant. It is a good practice to determine the likelihood of pregnancy for all fertile women prior to x-ray examinations, particularly if irradiation of the pelvic region is involved. VTF swallowing studies should not, however, involve direct irradiation of the pelvis, and if properly done should deliver less than a few hundredths of a millisievert (a few millirem) to the fetus.

To put these values in perspective the National Council on Radiation Protection (NCRP) recommends that the radiation dose to the fetus carried by a radiation worker not exceed 5 mSv (500 mrem) over the entire gestation period, and not more than 0.5 mSv (50 mrem) in any one month (6). With proper precautions, the fetal radiation dose of the pregnant operator may easily be kept well within these limits.

Estimating Radiation Risk to Patients

Patient doses in diagnostic x-ray procedures, particularly those involving fluoroscopy, are in practice exceptionally variable. This is because dose is highly dependent on the operator, as well as on characteristics of both the machine and the patient. Thus, there is considerable uncertainty in estimating the radiation risk from VTF swallowing procedures. An additional complicating factor is that the tissues at significant risk for stochastic effects lie at some depth in the body, where one cannot easily measure the dose directly. Nevertheless one can still provide reasonable risk estimates for both nonstochastic and stochastic effects for patients undergoing VTF procedures.

Nonstochastic effects result when the radiation dose to a specific tissue exceeds a threshold value; thus risk is determined by assessing the maximum radiation dose received. In most x-ray procedures, the maximum radiation dose is at the point where the x-ray beam enters the patient, that is, at the skin surface.

Typical fluoroscopic times for VTF procedures range from 0.5 to 8 min (7,8). In our experience, using typical machine parameters on adult patients, this leads to a skin dose rate on the order of 11 mSv/min (1.1 rad/min) and thus a total skin entrance dose ranging from 6 to 88 mSv. This is usually an overestimate, since typical VTF swallowing procedures move the x-ray beam around, and thus no single region should get such a high dose. In many facilities the patient receives an additional skin dose from radiographic exposures taken during the swallowing study. In our experience, an average of 5 to 10 radiographic exposures is recorded during VTF procedures, resulting in an additional skin entrance dose of between 3 and 6 mSv. As in fluoroscopy, all radiographic exposures are not recorded in the same anatomical region. While there will be some overlapping of x-ray fields on the skin, summing the skin doses results in an overestimate of the actual skin dose. Even including radiographic exposures, the skin entrance dose should be on the order of 100 mSv or less. These doses are well below the threshold dose of 2 Sv (1 Sv = 1000 mSv) required to cause any significant skin injury (2); hence the risk of nonstochastic effects in the form of skin damage should be low for patients undergoing VTF procedures. Hence, the main radiation concern is for the potential risk of stochastic effects such as the induction of cancers or genetic mutations.

Assessing the risk of stochastic effects is somewhat more complicated because risk depends not only on the dose to particular tissues but also on the radiation sensitivity of that particular tissue. Estimating stochastic effects is further complicated by the fact that many tissues of concern lie at some depth from the skin surface and may be only partially irradiated. Stochastic risk is assessed by determining the *effective dose* from the procedure. An effective dose is the value of a uniform total-body exposure that will give the same level of statistical risk. Effective dose is computed by first determining the dose to each irradiated organ, multiplying the dose by the tissue weighting factor, and then summing these products. Tissue weighting factors are used to adjust the result for the differences in radiation sensitivity to stochastic effects of different tissues. Table 1.2 lists radiation doses to the sensitive organs, including lung, active bone marrow, esophagus, thyroid, and female breasts computed by the method of Rosenstein et al. (9). For these calculations we have used typical VTF x-ray machine settings. Organ doses are tabulated for specific imaging projections for an adult patient of average size. Here, the swallowing procedure is assumed to be divided into three regions, which view the upper, middle, and distal esophagus. For simplicity, each anatomical region is assumed as viewed in either an anteroposterior (AP) or a lateral projection. Since these projections involve some body rotation the AP was actually a right anterior oblique (RAO) projection, while the lateral was more properly described as a steep left posterior oblique (LPO).

To use Table 1.2, estimate the total duration of VTF time in each projection for each anatomical region of the procedure. This can be done with a stopwatch while viewing the video image in playback mode. Multiply time in minutes for each projection and the dose-per-minute value from Table 1.2, then sum over all projections. A simple example would be a procedure in which each projection of each region is exposed to a total of one minute. Summing the products of each table entry for the lung

TABLE 1.2. Estimated organ doses for VTF procedures.[a]

	Organ dose per minute of VTF (mSv/min)[b]				
Projection	Lung (0.12)[c]	Esophagus (0.05)[c]	Thyroid (0.01)[c]	Bone marrow (0.12)[c]	Breast (0.05)[c,d]
Upper esophagus					
Anteroposterior	0.13	0.42	6.39	0.10	0.03
Lateral	0.17	0.74	0.66	0.07	0.02
Middle esophagus					
Anteroposterior	0.32	0.32	0.10	0.09	0.40
Lateral	0.64	0.64	0.04	0.11	0.08
Lower esophagus					
Anteroposterior	0.33	0.29	0.01	0.09	0.66
Lateral	0.99	0.63	0.01	0.09	0.13

[a] Doses are listed per minute of fluoroscopy in each projection and assume a conventional undertable tube fluoroscope operated at 80 kVp on average adult. Total procedure dose for each organ is obtained by summing over all projections.
[b] Multiply by 100 for dose in millirem.
[c] Organ or tissue weighting factor (6).
[d] Computed for female breast only.

over one minute yields a total lung dose of 2.58 mSv (258 mrem). Similarly, the total doses for thyroid, esophagus, and active bone marrow would be 7.21 mSv (721 mrem), 3.05 mSv (305 mrem), and 0.55 mSv (55 mrem), respectively. When appropriate tissue weighting factors are used, the total effective dose for 1 minute of fluoroscopy is approximately 0.9 mSv (90 mrem). Higher dose-rate settings, larger patients, or electronic magnification can increase organ doses by as much as an order of magnitude above the listed values.

Modern systems often come with a dose-area product device, by which one can estimate the risk due to stochastic effect. Using such a device, Wright et al. (8) estimated the effective dose for a typical videofluoroscopy procedure on an average adult to be 0.4 mSv.

Protecting the Patient

Radiation workers are taught the triad of **time**, **distance**, and **shielding** as the mental litany to use in going about their daily tasks. Time should be minimized, distance maximized, and shielding should be used whenever and wherever appropriate for the exam. The following techniques can help to ensure that doses are kept at reasonable levels:

1. Limit the time that fluoroscopy is activated. The experienced fluoroscopist uses x-rays intermittently, rather than continuously. Always record the total fluoroscopic time for each patient from the control panel timer. Complete examinations of the pharynx and esophagus should require less than 5 min of fluoroscopic time.

2. Practice any difficult maneuvers with a patient first turning on the x-rays. This may include various head positions as well as specific swallowing maneuvers.

3. If the video system incorporates a digital "last image hold" feature, this can be used to minimize additional fluoroscopic time.

4. "Panning" or moving the image intensifier to follow the barium bolus should be minimized. Even though panning is necessary in the esophagus, it is not necessary in the pharynx region. It is usually better not to move the image intensifier so that anatomy movement and barium movement can be observed. Position the patient and fluoroscope before beginning fluoroscopy. If the fluoroscopic image indicates that recentering is necessary, discontinue fluoroscopy and move the image intensifier and recheck, rather than keeping the beam activated while the image intensifier is being moved. Minor movements can be done with the fluoroscope

activated, since this may in fact, save total time.

5. Think collimation. Frame the x-ray beam to the region of interest throughout the procedure. You should always see the collimator edges in the fluoroscopic frame.

6. Reviewing a just-recorded sequence may make it possible to avoid repeating a maneuver.

7. Make sure that the videorecording device is on and ready to operate before activating the fluoroscopic circuit.

8. Use high-dose and electronic magnification modes judiciously, only when conditions warrant their use, and for as short a time as possible.

9. Keep in mind that the x-rays are coming from the x-ray tube, and when possible, keep the most sensitive areas of the patient on the image intensifier side, away from the tube side. Some equipment permits the image intensifier and x-ray tube positions to be reversed. These options should be kept in mind when one is planning the routine sequencing of maneuvers.

10. Keep the x-ray tube as far away from the patient as possible, remembering the second word of the triad, "distance."

11. Shield the pelvic area of patients in the appropriate age range. With modern high-quality collimation, this adds only a small additional layer of radiation protection but is a good practice and helps provide peace of mind to the patient.

12. Many swallowing studies involve an assistant to give the patient the material to be ingested. A separate floor- or ceiling-mounted radiation shield can provide additional protection to the assistant's face and torso, since the lead apron may not be appropriately constructed for the position in which he or she will function. Remember that thyroid shields give neck coverage above the traditional lead apron.

13. Most of the modern fluoroscopy systems are digital. The advantage of digital systems over the conventional systems is that in digital systems, pulsed fluoroscopy can be utilized to further reduce radiation dose to the patients.

14. Ensure that the fluoroscopic system is working optimally and that dose limits and average dose levels are properly set by having the system checked by a qualified medical physicist annually.

Protecting the Operator

During the VTF procedure only a fraction of the x-ray beam passes through the patient to form the image; most of the x-rays are being either *absorbed* by the patient's tissues or *scattered* in different directions. Figure 1.1 depicts an upright fluoroscope viewed from above, showing primary x-rays emitted from the x-ray tube and x-rays scattered by the patient. Provided hands or other body parts are kept out of the beam, the main hazard to the operator is from x-rays scattered by the patient's tissues. Scattered x-rays are much less intense than the primary beam, but hazardous levels can occur from prolonged and repeated exposure. The following techniques can be used to provide adequate protection of the VTF operator.

1. Remember that the situations that result in a higher patient dose generally increase the dose to the operator as well. All the items involved in protecting the patient will have some effect on the dose to the operator.

2. Where possible, use distance to advantage. Dose rate falls off roughly as a square of the distance from the source, so doubling the distance from the patient and x-ray tube reduces the exposure rate to one fourth.

3. Employ shielding between the patient and operator. This will usually be a lead apron, but a ceiling- or floor-mounted shield can also be used for additional protection to the face and neck area. Pregnant female operators should employ a wraparound 0.5mm lead equivalence apron. In addition, they should wear two radiation-monitoring devices (radiation badges), one outside the apron (near collar) and other underneath the apron at waist level. In accordance with regulations, the total radiation dose to the fetus for the entire gestation period should not exceed 5mSv (500mrem) and not

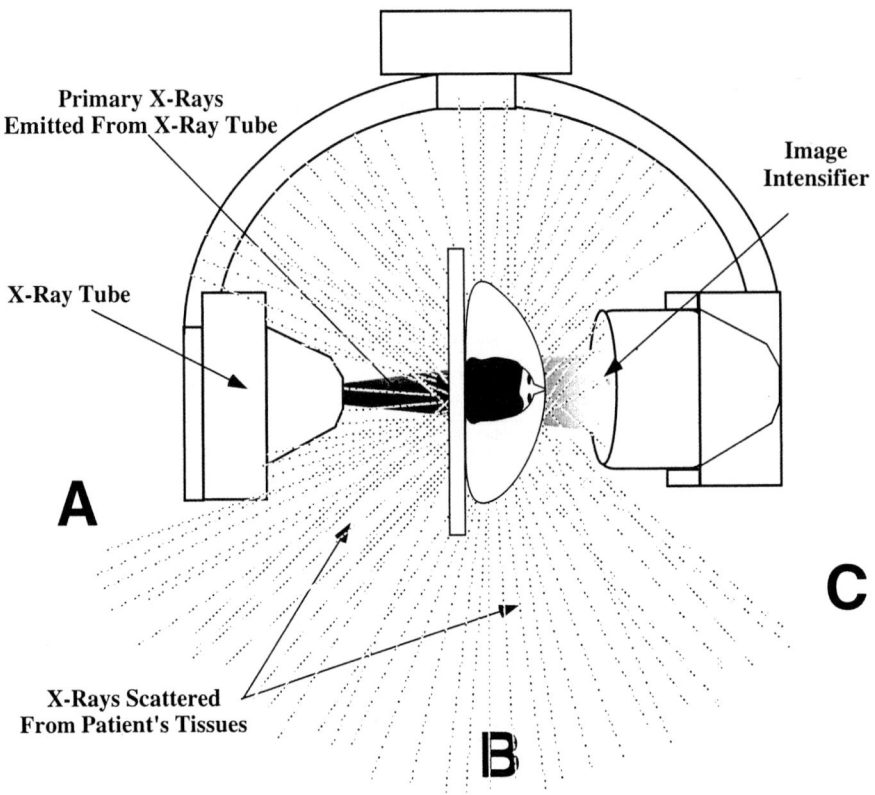

FIGURE 1.1. An upright fluoroscope viewed from above, depicting primary x-rays emitted from the x-ray tube and x-rays scattered from the tissues of the patient within the x-ray beam. A, B, and C indicate possible personnel locations.

more than 0.5 mSv (50 mrem) in any one month (6).

4. Some fluoroscopists use lead glasses to protect the lens of the eye. Lead glasses and thyroid shields are encouraged for those who do fluoroscopy daily but are not typically necessary in the practice of one or two fluoroscopic sessions a week. The record of film badges worn at the collar may be used to guide practice in this area.

5. When placement of the hands in or near the direct x-ray field cannot be avoided, thick leaded gloves (but not lead-lined thin surgical gloves) should be worn.

6. Use position to advantage. In Figure 1.1, note that positions A, B, and C are roughly equal in distance from the patient. Moving toward C affords the fluoroscopist greater protection behind the fluoroscopic carriage. If the x-ray table is constructed without a shielded base, position A should be avoided, since scatter is more intense in that direction.

7. Use a radiation monitor badge to measure the levels received. This badge should be worn at the collar outside the lead apron. When pregnant fluoroscopists or assistants are in the room, they should wear an additional badge beneath the apron at waist level to monitor dose to the abdomen over the location of the fetus. The benefit of a radiation badge exists as long as it is returned for analysis at required time intervals.

In summary, knowledge about radiation, attention to detail, and properly functioning equipment will keep radiation levels to the patient and to operating personnel to a minimum.

References

1. Hall EJ. *Radiobiology for the Radiologist*. 4th ed. Philadelphia: JB Lippincott; 1994.
2. Food and Drug Administration. *Avoidance of Serious X-ray-Induced Skin Injuries to Patients During Fluoroscopically Guided Procedures*. Rockville, MD: US Center for Devices and Radiological Health; September 30, 1994. Public Health Advisory.
3. Wagner LK, Eifel PJ, Geise RA. Potential biological effects following high x-ray dose interventional procedures. *J Vasc Interven Radiol* 1994; 5:71–84.
4. Committee on the Biological Effects of Ionizing Radiation. *Health Effects of Exposure to Low Levels of Ionizing Radiation: BEIR V Report*. Washington DC: National Academy Press; 1990.
5. Landis SH, Murray T, Bolden S, Wingo PA. Cancer statistics, 1999. *CA Cancer J Clin* 1999; 49(1):8–31.
6. National Council on Radiation Protection and Measurements. *Limitation of Exposure to Ionizing Radiation*. Washington DC: NCRP; 1993. Report 116.
7. Leiobovic SJ, Caldicott WJH. Gastrointestinal fluoroscopy: patient dose and methods for its reduction. *Br J Radiol* 1998;56:715–719.
8. Wright RER, Boyd CS, Workman A. Radiation doses to patients during pharyngeal videofluoroscopy. *Dysphagia* 1998;13:113–115.
9. Rosenstein M, Suleiman OH, Burkhart RL, Stern SH, Williams G. *Handbook of Selected Tissue Doses for the Upper Gastrointestinal Fluoroscopic Examination*. Rockville, MD: US Center for Devices and Radiological Health, FDA; 1992.

2
Anatomical and Physiological Overview

EMMETT T. CUNNINGHAM, JR., AND BRONWYN JONES

The seemingly effortless act of swallowing is, in reality, quite complex, involving approximately 50 paired muscles and virtually all levels of the central nervous system. For historical reasons, and as a matter of convenience, swallowing has been divided into three anatomically and temporally distinct stages, or phases. The first, or oral phase, is primarily preparatory, and is that period during which foodstuffs are chewed and mixed with saliva to produce the proper texture and consistency for smooth transit through the pharynx and esophagus. The second, or pharyngeal phase, begins when the bolus passes the faucial pillars to enter the upper pharynx and ends when it crosses the pharyngoesophageal sphincter. The third, or esophageal phase, covers that period during which the bolus is transported from the pharynx to the stomach via the esophagus.

Numerous authors have reviewed various aspects of the anatomy (1–31), physiology (9,10,14,21,32 60), and neurobiology (9,10, 51,61–80) of swallowing, and it is not our intention to re-cover this ground in great detail. Rather, we present an overview of swallowing, covering only the most salient points, to provide a proper reference for later chapters. The anatomy, physiology, and central neural control of each of the three phases of swallowing will be considered in turn.

Oral Phase

The oral phase is almost entirely voluntary, and involves ingestion and mechanical formation of the bolus. Many of the facial muscles, the muscles of mastication, and the intrinsic and extrinsic muscles of the tongue are recruited during this stage (Table 2.1; Figure 2.1). These include the following:

1. Perioral muscles, which are important in grasping and sucking, and act to seal the oral cavity.
2. The platysma and lateral pterygoid muscles, which act to open the jaw.
3. The temporalis, masseter, and medial pterygoid muscles, which act to close the jaw and grind food.
4. All the foregoing muscles acting in concert with the buccinator and intrinsic and extrinsic tongue muscles, which form and control the bolus.

Equally important are the supporting bones and cartilage (Table 2.1), which provide a scaffolding for these muscles, and the salivary glands, which provide for proper bolus formation, consistency, and transport (81,82).

Some authors have considered the procurement and masticatory aspects of swallowing to

TABLE 2.1. Muscles contributing to the oral phase of swallowing.

Muscle	Origin	Insertion	Innervation Nerve	Innervation Nucleus	Primary action during deglutition
Levator labii superioris	Upper lip	Upper lip	Buccal n.	VII	Elevate upper lip
Levator labii superioris alaque nasi	Maxilla, frontal process	Upper lip and alar cartilage	Buccal n.	VII	Elevate upper lip
Levator anguli oris	Maxilla, canine fossa	Corner of mouth	Buccal n.	VII	Elevate corner of mouth
Zygomaticus major	Zygoma, temporal process	Corner of mouth	Buccal n.	VII	Elevate corner of mouth
Zygomaticus minor	Zygoma, maxillary process	Upper lip	Buccal n.	VII	Elevate upper lip
Risorius	Masseteric fascia	Corner of mouth	Buccal, mandibular nn.	VII	Laterally displace corner of mouth
Depressor labii inferioris	Mandible, oblique line	Lower lip	Buccal, mandibular nn.	VII	Depress lower lip
Depressor anguli oris	Mandible, oblique line	Corner of mouth	Buccal, mandibular nn.	VII	Depress corner of mouth
Mentalis	Mandible, incisive fossa	Dermis of skin	Buccal, mandibular nn.	VII	Protrude lower lip, depress jaw
Orbicularis oris	Nearby muscle, maxilla, alveolar arches of mandible and maxilla	Dermis of lips; nearby muscles	Buccal, mandibular nn.	VII	Close and purse lips
Buccinator	Pterygomandibular raphe, alveolar arches of mandible and maxilla	Muscles of mouth	Buccal n.	VII	Flatten cheeks
Platysma	Pectoral and deltoid fascia	Inferior mandible; skin	Cervical n.	VII	Depress mandible and lower lips
Temporalis	Temporal bone, inferior line and fossa	Mandible, coronoid process and anterior ramus	Anterior and posterior deep temporal nn.	V_m	Elevate and retract jaw
Masseter	Zygomatic arch	Anterior ramus of mandible	Masseteric n.	V_m	Elevate jaw
Medial pterygoid	Pterygoid fossa and plate	Medial ramus of mandible	Medial pterygoid n.	V_m	Elevate jaw
Lateral pterygoid	Pterygoid plate and sphenoid bone	Neck of mandible and articular capsule of TMJ[a]	Lateral pterygoid n.	V_m	Depress and medially displace jaw
Intrinsic muscles of the tongue (longitudinal, transverse, vertical)	—	—	Hypoglossal n.	XII	Shape tongue
Genioglossus	Hyoid; superior mental spine of mandible	Inferior surface of tongue	Hypoglossal n.	XII	Protrude and depress tongue
Styloglossus	Styloid process; stylomandibular ligament	Tongue muscles	Hypoglossal n.	XII	Retract and elevate tongue
Hyoglossus	Hyoid	Tongue muscles	Hypoglossal n.	XII	Depress tongue

[a] Temporomandibular joint.

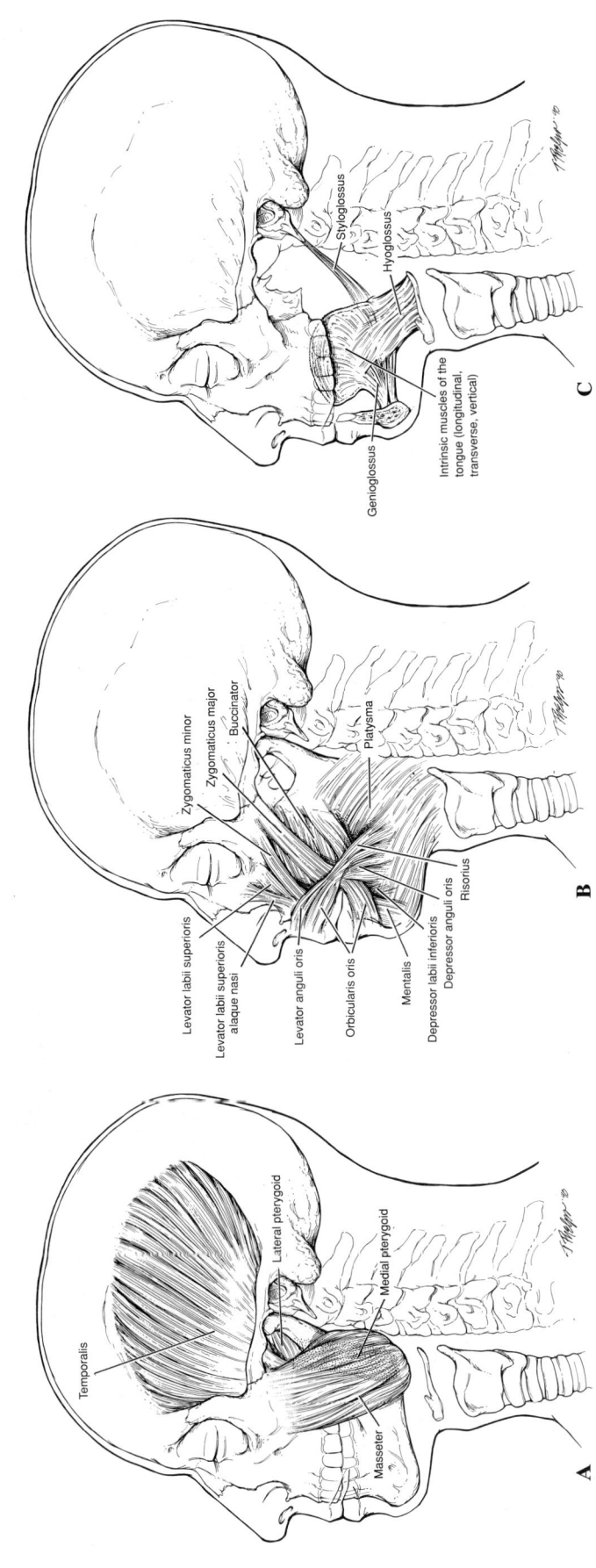

FIGURE 2.1. Illustration of the anatomical relationship of the muscles contributing to the oral phase of swallowing. These muscles are controlled by discrete groups of motor neurons in the fifth (A), seventh (B), and twelfth (C) cranial motor nuclei (see Table 2.1).

TABLE 2.2. Muscles contributing to the pharyngeal phase of swallowing.

Muscle	Origin	Insertion	Innervation Nerve	Innervation Nucleus	Primary action during deglutition
Mylohyoid	Mandible, mylohyoid line	Hyoid	Mylohyoid n.	V_m	Elevate and anteriorly displace hyoid and larynx; propel bolus
Anterior digastric	Mandible, digastric fossa	Hyoid	Mylohyoid n.	V_m	Elevate and anteriorly displace hyoid and larynx; propel bolus
Tensor veli palatini	Scaphoid fossa; spine of sphenoid; auditory tube	Palatal aponeurosis	Pharyngeal plexus	V_m	Elevate soft palate to seal nasopharynx
Geniohyoid	Mandible, inferior mental spine	Hyoid	Hypoglossal n.	XII	Elevate and anteriorly displace hyoid and larynx; propel bolus
Hyoglossus	Hyoid	Tongue muscles	Hypoglossal n.	XII	Elevate and anteriorly displace hyoid and larynx; propel bolus
Styloglossus	Styloid process	Tongue muscles	Hypoglossal n.	XII	Seal pharyngeal inlet
Pterygopharyngeus	Pterygoid plate; mandible; tongue	Pharyngeal raphe	Pharyngeal plexus	NA	Seal pharyngeal inlet
Palatoglossus	Soft palate	Tongue	Pharyngeal plexus	NA	Seal pharyngeal inlet
Palatopharyngeus	Soft palate	Thyroid cartilage and muscular pharynx	Pharyngeal plexus	NA	Seal pharyngeal inlet
Stylopharyngeus	Styloid process	Muscular pharynx and thyroid cartilage	Pharyngeal plexus	NA	Seal pharyngeal inlet
Salpingopharyngeus	Auditory tube	Muscular pharynx	Pharyngeal plexus	NA	Seal pharyngeal inlet
Levator veli palatini	Temporal bone; auditory tube	Palatal aponeurosis	Pharyngeal plexus	NA	Elevate soft palate to seal nasopharynx
Musculus uvulae	Palatal bone and aponeurosis	Uvula	Pharyngeal plexus	NA	Elevate soft palate to seal nasopharynx
Stylohyoid	Styloid process	Hyoid	Facial n.	VII	Seal pharyngeal inlet
Posterior digastric	Temporal bone, mastoid notch	Hyoid	Facial n.	VII	Seal pharyngeal inlet
Superior constrictor	Pterygoid hamulus and plate; mandible, mylohyoid line; tongue	Pharyngeal raphe	Pharyngeal plexus	NA	Seal pharyngeal inlet

Muscle	Origin	Insertion	Innervation	Spinal	Action
Thyrohyoid	Thyroid cartilage	Hyoid	Hypoglossal n.	C1	Depress and posteriorly displace hyoid and larynx
Sternohyoid	Sternoclavicular joint	Hyoid	Ansa cervicalis	C1-3	Depress and posteriorly displace hyoid and larynx
Sternothyroid	Manubrium	Thyroid cartilage	Ansa cervicalis	C1-3	Depress and posteriorly displace hyoid and larynx
Omohyoid	Superior scapula	Hyoid	Ansa cervicalis	C1-3	Depress and posteriorly displace hyoid and larynx
Hypopharyngeus (middle constrictor)	Hyoid; stylohyoid ligament	Pharyngeal raphe	Pharyngeal plexus	NA	Clear bolus
Thyropharyngeus (inferior constrictor)	Thyroid cartilage	Pharyngeal raphe	Pharyngeal plexus	NA	Clear bolus
Cricopharyngeus (inferior constrictor)	Cricoid cartilage	Pharyngeal raphe	Pharyngeal plexus	NA	Clear bolus
Aryepiglottic	Arytenoid cartilage	Epiglottis	Inferior laryngeal n.	NA	Adduct vocal cords to protect airway
Lateral cricoarytenoid	Cricoid cartilage	Arytenoid cartilage	Inferior laryngeal n.	NA	Adduct vocal cords to protect airway
Transverse arytenoid	Arytenoid cartilage	Arytenoid cartilage	Inferior laryngeal n.	NA	Adduct vocal cords to protect airway
Oblique arytenoid	Arytenoid cartilage	Arytenoid cartilage	Inferior laryngeal n.	NA	Adduct vocal cords to protect airway
Thyroarytenoid	Cricothyroid ligament	Arytenoid cartilage	Inferior laryngeal n.	NA	Adduct vocal cords to protect airway
Cricothyroid	Cricoid cartilage	Thyroid cartilage	Superior laryngeal n.	NA	Adduct vocal cords to protect airway

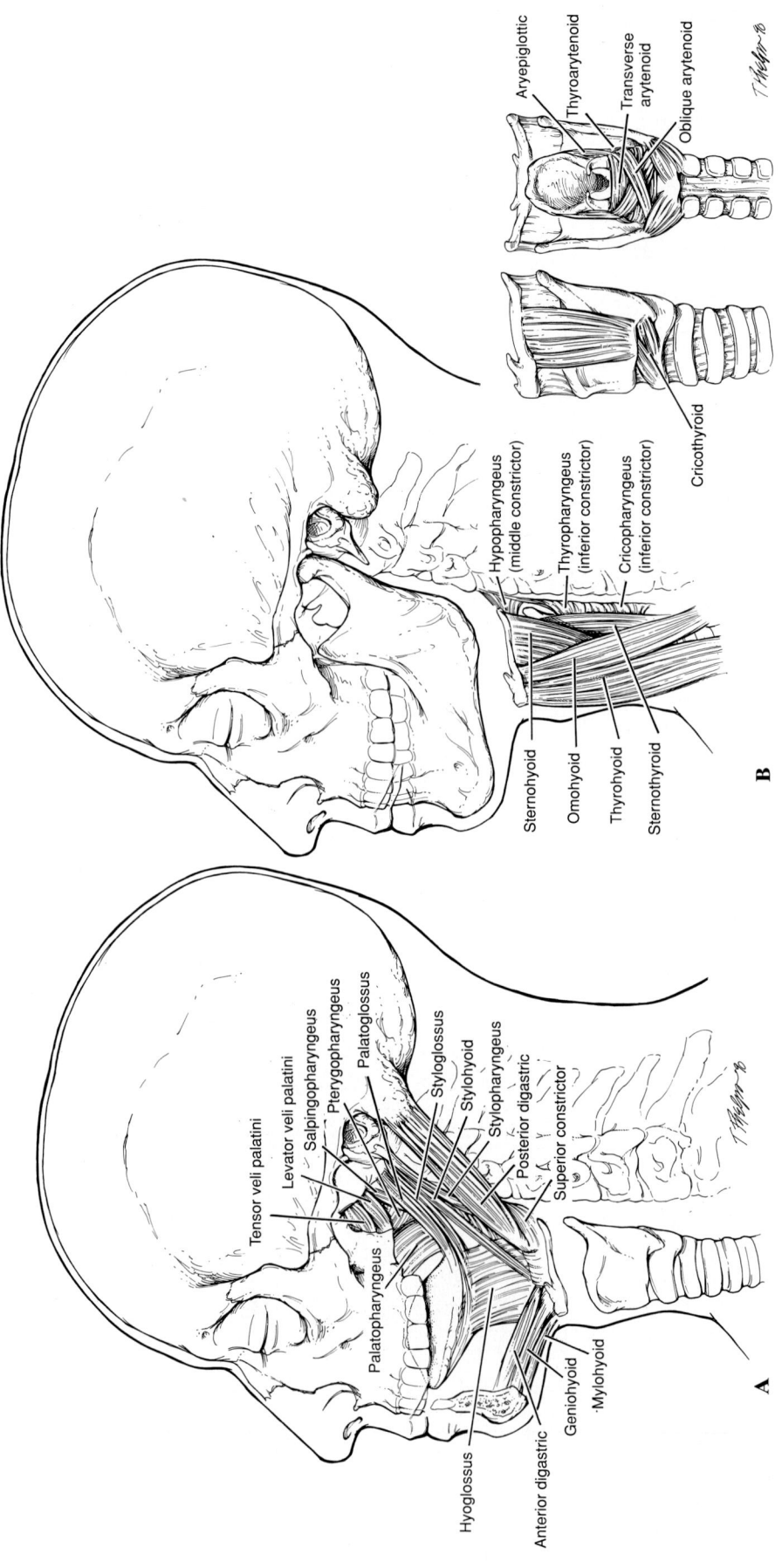

FIGURE 2.2. Illustration of the anatomical relationship of the muscles contributing to the pharyngeal phase of swallowing. These muscles are controlled by discrete groups of motor neurons in the fifth, seventh, ninth, and twelfth cranial motor nuclei, as well as by motor neurons in cervical portions of the spinal cord (see Table 2.2). Functionally, these muscles may be thought of as acting either early (A) or late (B) in the pharyngeal stage. The intrinsic and extrinsic laryngeal muscles are also shown (B).

2. Anatomical and Physiological Overview

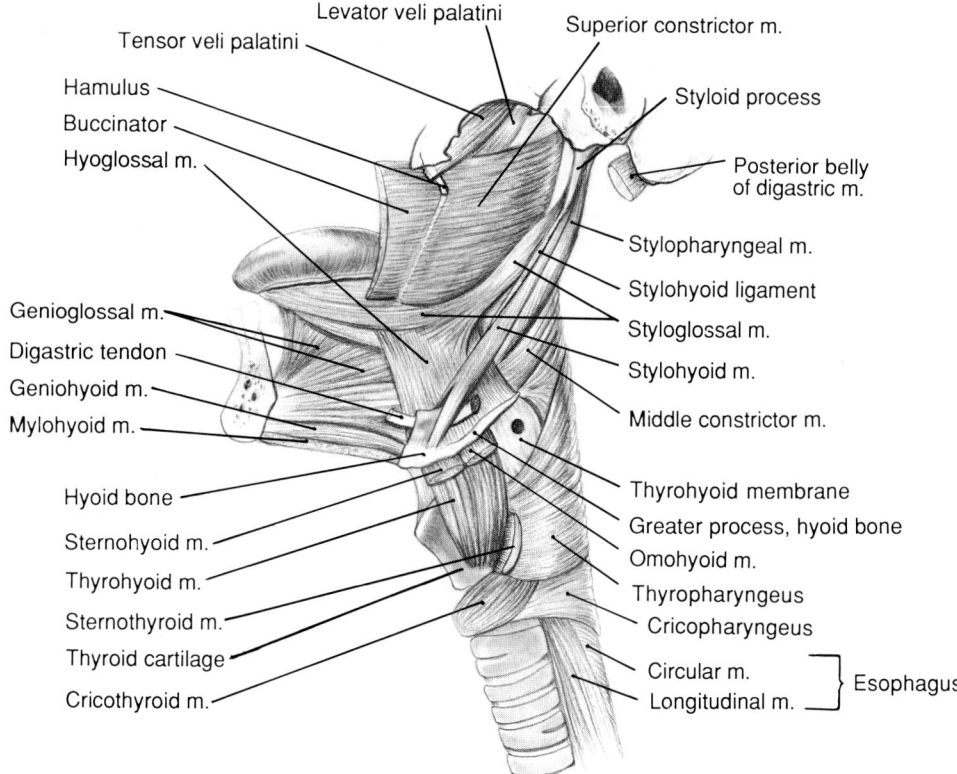

FIGURE 2.3. Lateral view of the pharyngeal and extrinsic laryngeal musculature. (Reprinted with permission from Bosma JF, Donner MW, Tanaka E, Robertson D. Anatomy of the pharynx, pertinent to swallowing. *Dysphagia* 1986;1:23–33.)

constitute the so-called oral preparatory phase, thus distinguishing it from the more restricted oral phase of swallowing, or swallow initiation. In this view, the oral phase of swallowing consists of placement of the tip of the tongue against the posterior surface of the maxillary incisors, depression of the midline tongue, and transport of the formed bolus along the dorsum of the tongue to the pharyngeal inlet, much of which seems to depend on highly patterned, bilateral peristaltic contractions of intrinsic and extrinsic tongue muscles (1,2,14,43,51,60,83–87). In fact, given the sheer complexity and relative autonomy of mastication (65,88–90), distinction between the oral preparatory phase and the oral phase of swallowing is probably warranted.

Neural Control of the Oral Phase

The basic neural control of mastication appears to reside in the lower pons and upper medulla, and to involve an ill-defined pattern generator located in the reticular formation. The masticatory pattern generator is thought to project to, and thereby orchestrate the activity of, motor neurons in the fifth, seventh, and twelfth cranial nerves. These motor neurons, in turn, elicit patterned chewing movements (51,65,88–90). Information from the oral cavity reaches the medulla via sensory branches of the fifth, seventh, and ninth cranial nerves, all of which send afferents to the nucleus of the solitary tract (NTS) and the spinal trigeminal nucleus (51,91). Somatosensory information conveyed by the fifth nerve seems to be most important for coordinating mastication.

Once in the NTS and the spinal trigeminal nucleus, sensory information is presumed to influence the masticatory program by direct projections to the pattern generator (51,92,93). In addition, much of the activity of the oral phase is regulated by higher, forebrain centers (9,51,66,73–77). This arrangement seems logical

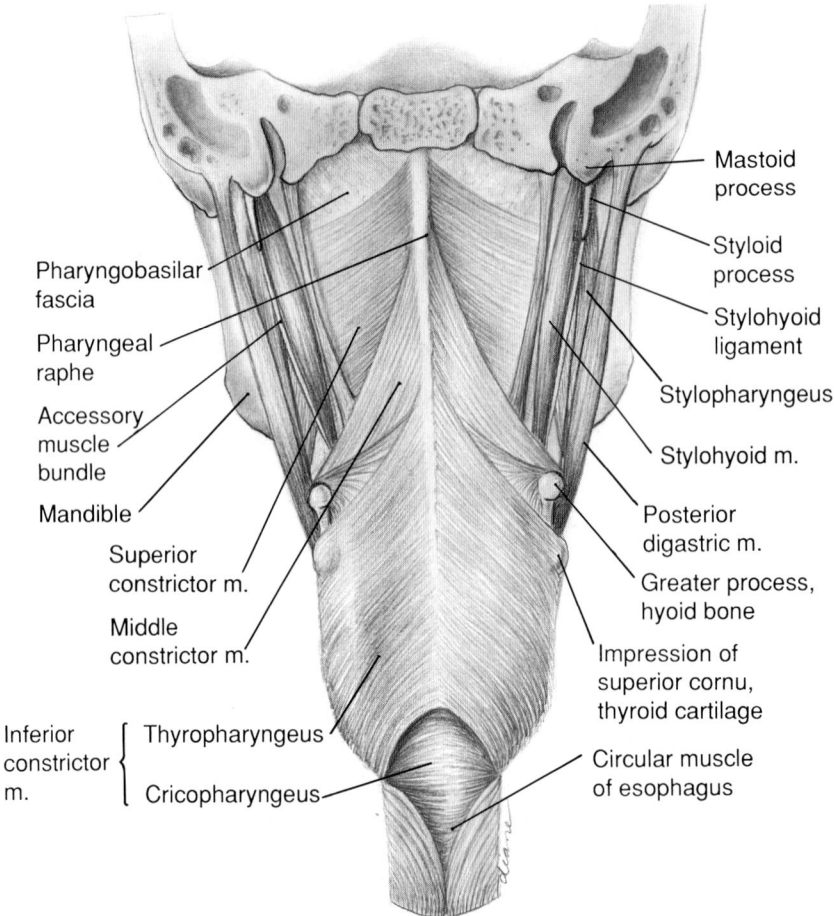

FIGURE 2.4. Posterior view of the pharyngeal musculature. (Reprinted with permission from Bosma JF, Donner MW, Tanaka E, Robertson D. Anatomy of the pharynx, pertinent to swallowing. *Dysphagia* 1986;1:23–33.)

given the relative control one has over the facial, lingual, and masticatory muscles and is actually borne out by neurological studies of patients with pathological lesions of the cortical hemispheres and descending corticobulbar pathways, many of whom have difficulty with chewing and with swallow initiation (9,73–77). It is also supported by studies in experimental animals, which have demonstrated facilitatory effects of stimulation of the cortex, amygdala, and lateral hypothalamus on both mastication and swallowing (9,66). Hence, while many of the patterned movements of mastication appear to be "hardwired" in the brain stem, most of the movements constituting bolus procurement and formation are actually quite "plastic," owing in large part to descending inputs from the forebrain.

Pharyngeal Phase

Although more patterned than much of the oral phase, the pharyngeal phase is exceedingly complex, largely as a result of the intricate anatomical relationships and close temporal activation of the more than two dozen muscles that must function together to transport a bolus effectively from the mouth to the esophagus (Table 2.2; Figures 2.2–2.7).

Events during the pharyngeal phase may be thought of as occurring either early or late (Figure 2.7). The early part of the pharyngeal phase consists of the following activities:

1. Sealing of the nasopharynx by contraction of the tensor veli palatini, the levator veli palatini, and the musculus uvulae.

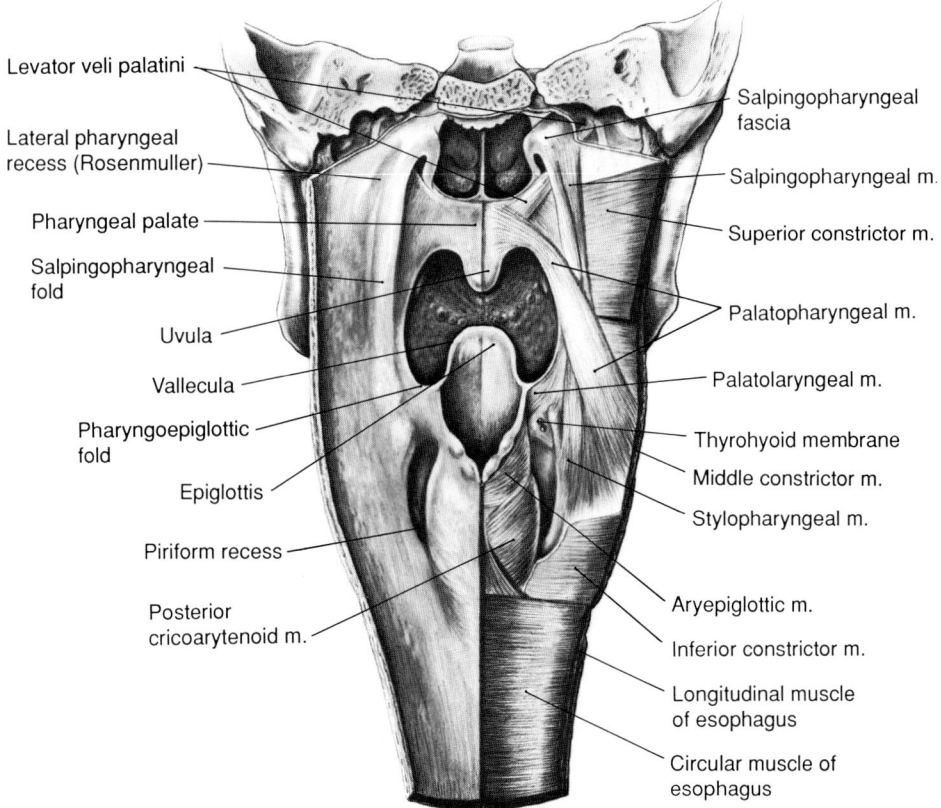

FIGURE 2.5. Posterior view of the internal pharyngeal musculature and recesses. The mucosa has been stripped from the left half of the preparation to better demonstrate the musculature. (Reprinted with permission from Bosma JF, Donner MW, Tanaka E, Robertson D. Anatomy of the pharynx, pertinent to swallowing. *Dysphagia* 1986;1:23–33.)

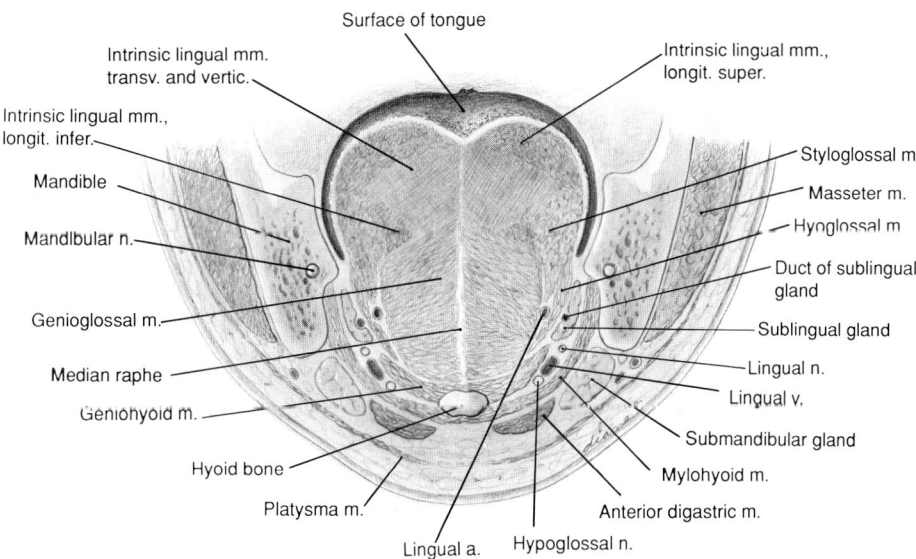

FIGURE 2.6. Coronal section through the tongue and sublingual area. (Reprinted with permission from Bosma JF, Donner MW, Tanaka E, Robertson D. Anatomy of the pharynx, pertinent to swallowing. *Dysphagia* 1986;1:23–33.)

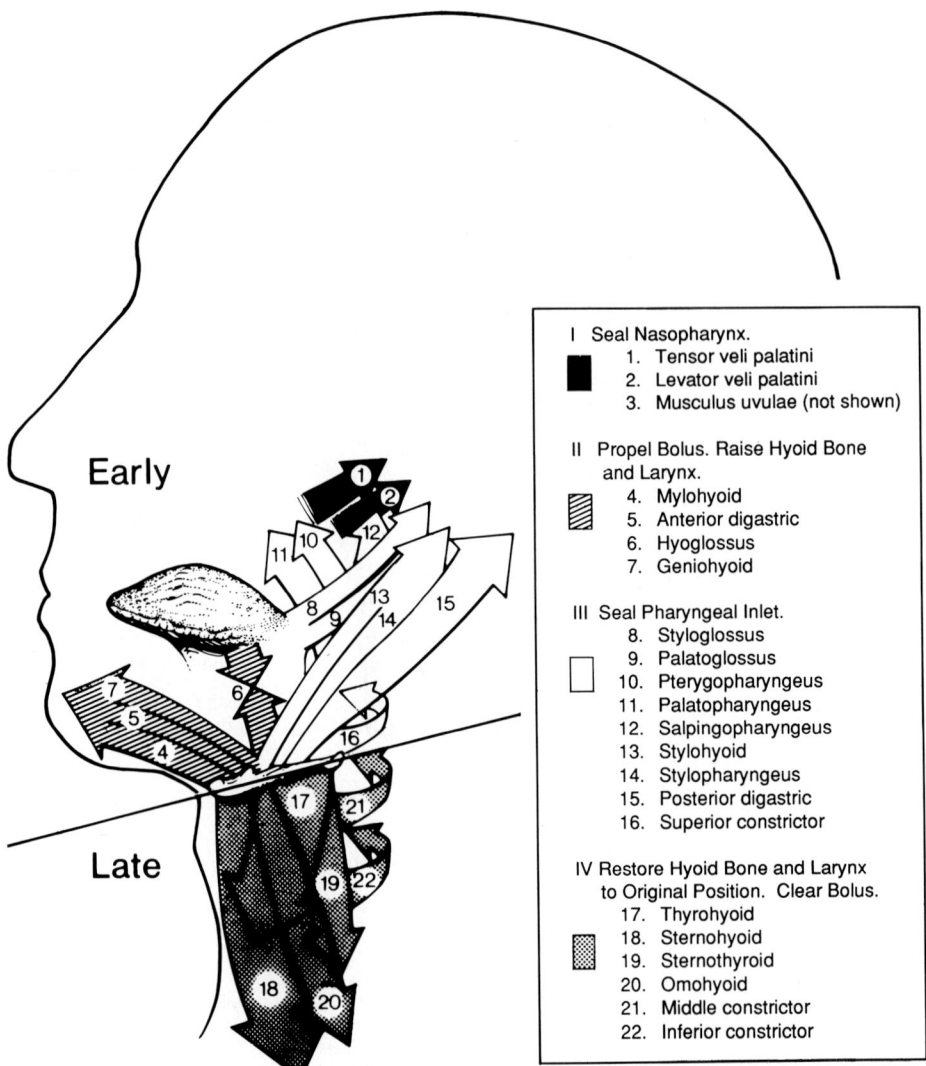

FIGURE 2.7. Schematic summary of muscular activity during the early and late parts of the pharyngeal stage.

2. Contraction of the mylohyoid, anterior digastric, hyoglossus, and geniohyoid muscles to propel the bolus, and to anteriorly and superiorly displace the hyoid bone and larynx, thereby protecting the airway. A number of other factors also contribute to airway protection, including epiglottic tilt and compression against the laryngeal aditus; reflex inhibition of respiration; contraction of the intrinsic laryngeal muscles, which act to appose the arytenoids, close the false cords, and thicken and adduct the vocal cords; and cough (11,12,94–104).

3. Contraction of the superior pharyngeal constrictor, styloglossus, palatoglossus, pterygopharyngeus, palatopharyngeus, stylopharyngeus, salpingopharyngeus, stylohyoid, and posterior digastric muscles, which act to seal the pharyngeal inlet, thus preventing regurgitation of the bolus into the oral cavity.

By contrast, the late part of the pharyngeal stage consists of the following activities:

1. Contraction of the thyrohyoid, sternohyoid, sternothyroid, and omohyoid muscles, the so-called strap muscles, in concert with the middle and inferior pharyngeal constrictors, all of which act to clear the bolus from the pharynx and to restore the hyoid bone and larynx to their original position.

2. Opening of the upper esophageal sphincter, which involves both inhibition of tonic contraction and passive opening by the upward movement of the larynx (105–107).

The temporal sequence and strength of muscular contractions in the pharyngeal phase of swallowing have been studied with a number of techniques, including manometry (108–119), electromyography (120–123), cineradiography (99,108,124–140), videofluorography (106,141–144), and pressure recording techniques in combination with either electromyography (145) or videofluorography (146–154). Of these, electromyographic studies have provided the most precise information on the activity of individual muscles.

Figure 2.8 shows a summary figure from the classical electromyographic study of Doty and Bosma (120) on the temporal activation of the muscles of deglutition in the dog. While this study did not examine all the muscles constituting the pharyngeal phase (Table 2.2), it did investigate many of them. Thus, of the four muscles that act to propel the bolus (Table 2.2; Figures 2.2–2.7), only the mylohyoid, geniohyoid, and "posterior tongue" are shown; of the numerous muscles that act to seal the pharyngeal inlet, only the palatopharyngeus is shown; and of the muscles that act to clear the bolus from the pharynx, only the superior, middle, and inferior constrictors are shown. The muscles of the soft palate and the strap muscles are not illustrated. From the muscles that are shown, however, a few important generalizations may be gleaned. First, the pharyngeal stage is exceptionally rapid, requiring just over a second from beginning to end (151,155,156). Second, there is considerable overlap in the temporal activation of the muscles constituting the early part of the pharyngeal phase, presumably providing for tight closure of the pharyngeal inlet in the immediate wake of the bolus. Third, the entire sequence occurs during expiration, or decreased diaphragmatic activity. This last point has been supported by a number of studies demonstrating that the majority of swallows occur at the end of inspiration (157–159), or at the beginning of expiration, presumably providing a negative suction force on the bolus as it enters the esophagus. Of note, Cerenko and colleagues employed combined videofluoroscopy and manometry to demonstrate the presence of a negative suction force on the bolus late in the pharyngeal phase. These authors (153) also demonstrated that during normal wet swallows the greatest impetus to bolus transit comes from the initial tongue thrust, while the pharyngeal constrictors appear to have more of a clearing function (Figure 2.9). This supports a similar suggestion made by Ekberg and colleagues (160), who showed that the speed of a given tongue thrust increases with increasing bolus size, whereas the speed of the pharyngeal clearing wave remains constant.

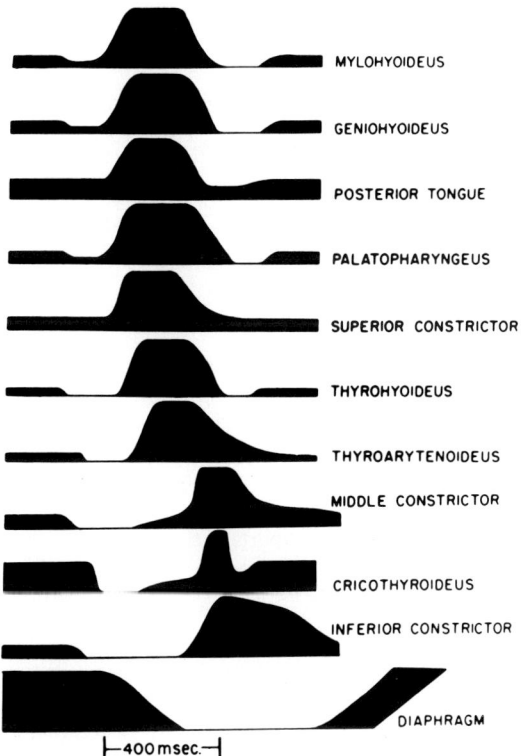

FIGURE 2.8. Schematic summary of the electromyographic activity of many of the muscles of deglutition. Note that deglutition begins with the decreased diaphragmatic activity of expiration. Note also that the entire swallow is completed in under 1 s. (Reprinted with permission from Doty RW, Bosma JF. An electromyographic analysis of reflex deglutition. *J Neurophysiol* 1956;19:44–60; kindly provided by Dr. Bosma.)

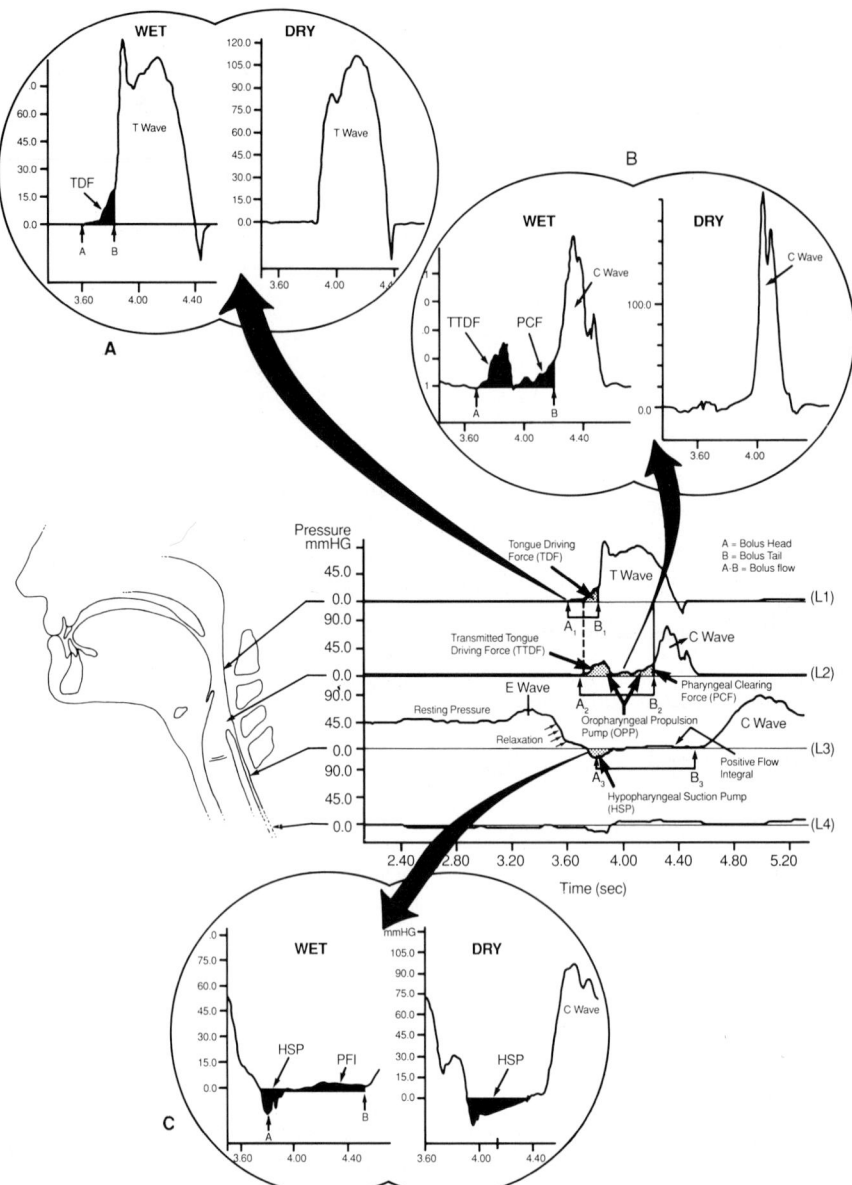

FIGURE 2.9. Schematic summary of manofluoroscopic data illustrating the various forces acting on a bolus along its path through the pharynx. The relative contributions from tongue thrust (A), the pharyngeal constrictors (B), and the so-called hypopharyngeal suction pump (C) are each shown for wet and dry swallows. Note that during normal wet swallows the tongue driving force and its continuation, the so-called transmitted tongue driving force, act most to move the bolus, followed in turn by the hypopharyngeal suction pump and the pharyngeal clearing wave. *PFI*, positive flow integral. (Amended with permission from Cerenko D, McConnel FMS, Jackson RT. Quantitative assessment of pharyngeal bolus driving forces. *Otolaryngol Head Neck Surg* 1989;100:57–63; kindly provided by Drs. Cerenko, McConnel, and Jackson.)

Radiographic techniques, particularly cineradiography and videofluorography, provide a uniquely dynamic and functional view of swallowing (139). Figure 2.10 shows a series of still frames taken from a cineradiogram of a normal swallow, with accompanying schematics to

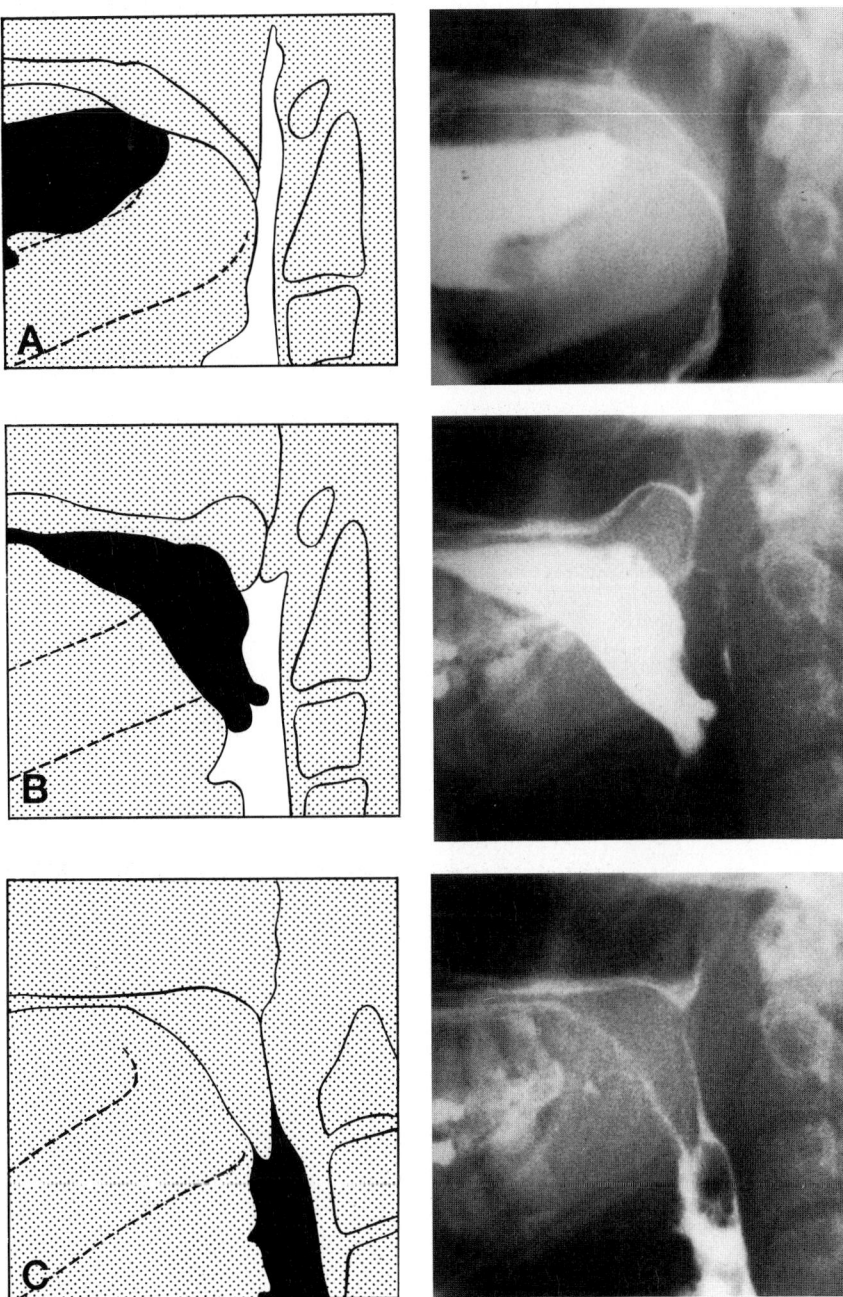

FIGURE 2.10. Six selected stop frames from a cinepharyngoesophagogram demonstrating various components of the oropharyngeal phase. (A) The bolus is first held in the mouth, where leakage is prevented by apposition of the soft palate to the back of the tongue, the latter of which is coated from prior swallows. (B) The bolus then passes through the fauces to enter the oropharynx. The soft palate is elevated by approximately 90° and is apposed to Passavant's cushion, a focal converging segment of the posterior pharyngeal wall. Note that contrast has also been introduced via the nose and is therefore coating the nasal surface of the soft and hard palates. (C–F) Passavant's cushion remains apposed to the soft palate while the peristaltic wave of the pharyngeal constrictors clears the bolus from the pharynx. Note that the epiglottis does not begin to return to its original position and that the larynx does not begin to open until the bolus has entered the esophagus.

(Continued)

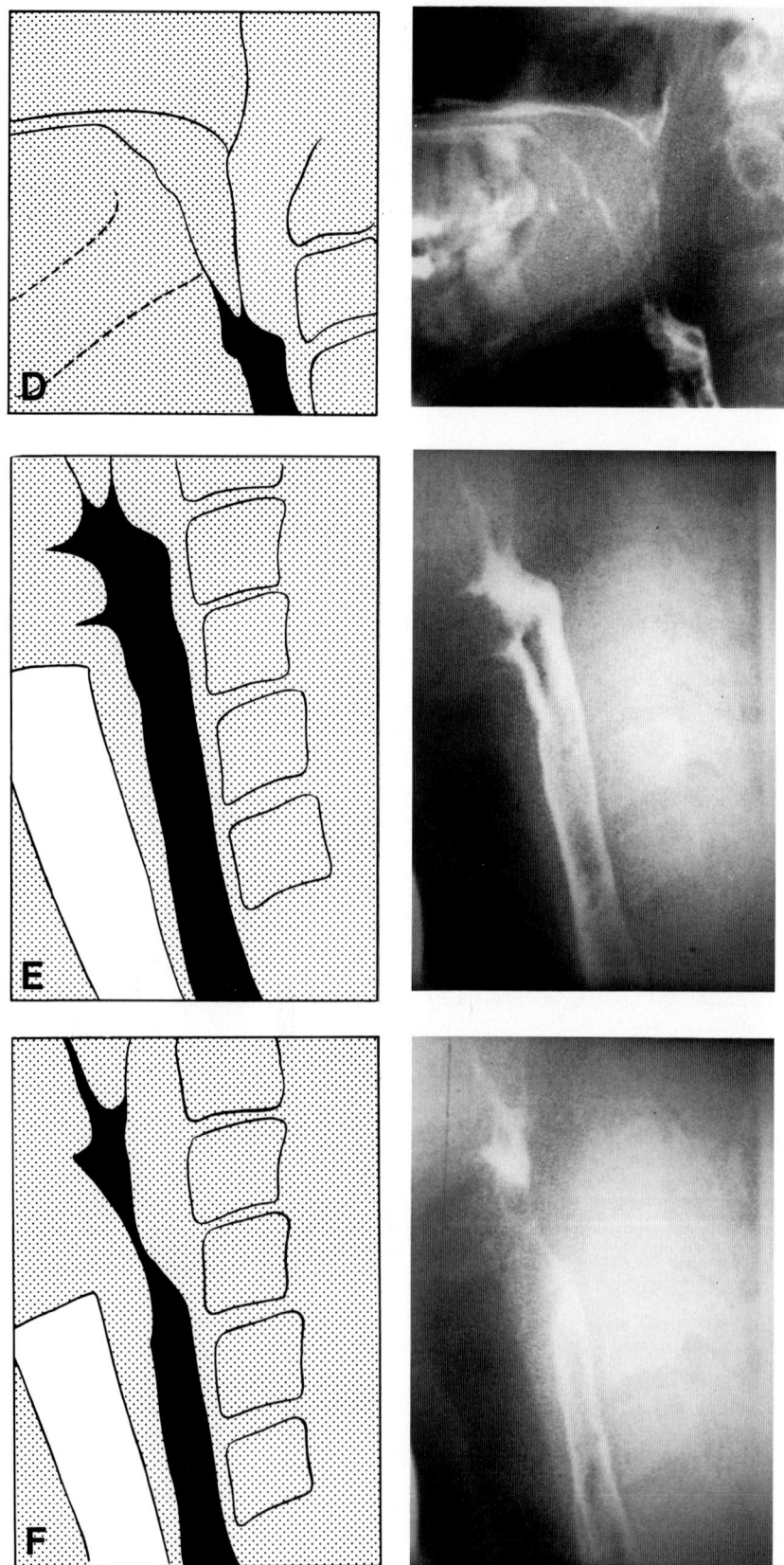

FIGURE 2.10. *Continued*

illustrate the relevant anatomy. Initially, the bolus is held in a midline depression in the dorsal surface of the tongue and is retained there by contact of the edges of the tongue with the overlying palate (in this "midsagittal" view, only the midline contact between the posterior tongue and the soft palate is visible). As the bolus is propelled into the pharynx, the soft palate elevates to seal the nasopharynx and prevent regurgitation. While the nasopharynx remains closed, the posterior aspect of the tongue is quickly retracted and the hyoid bone and larynx are elevated by the action of the mylohyoid, anterior digastric, hyoglossus, and geniohyoid muscles. At about the same time, the numerous slinglike muscles that straddle the pharyngeal inlet contract, thus forming an airtight seal and preventing regurgitation into the oral cavity. The clearing wave of the pharyngeal constrictors is also visible. Excursion of the larynx, in conjunction with momentary neural inhibition, causes maximal opening of the upper esophageal sphincter, thus giving a columnlike appearance to the radiopaque bolus as it passes the sphincter. Once the bolus has passed into the cervical esophagus, the tongue, hyoid bone, and larynx return to their original position, the vestibule opens, and the upper esophageal sphincter closes (see also Figures 2.7 and 2.11).

As mentioned, the motion of the lower pharynx during swallowing is very important because it provides for optimal opening of the neurally inhibited upper esophageal sphincter. Kramer and associates (161) and Palmer and colleagues (143) have studied the range of motion of the pharyngoesophageal segment with the aid of radiopaque markers placed on

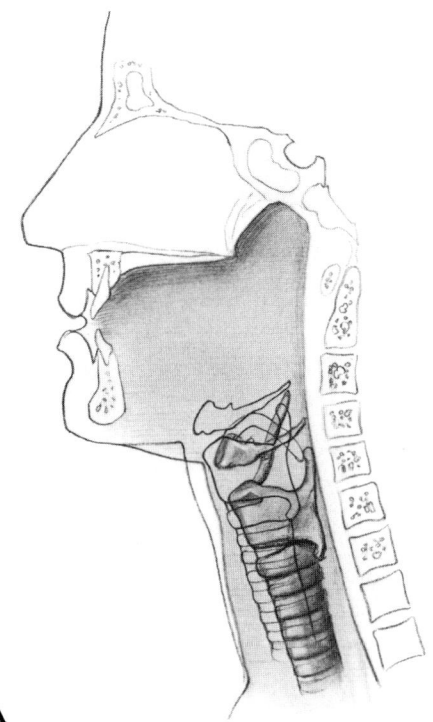
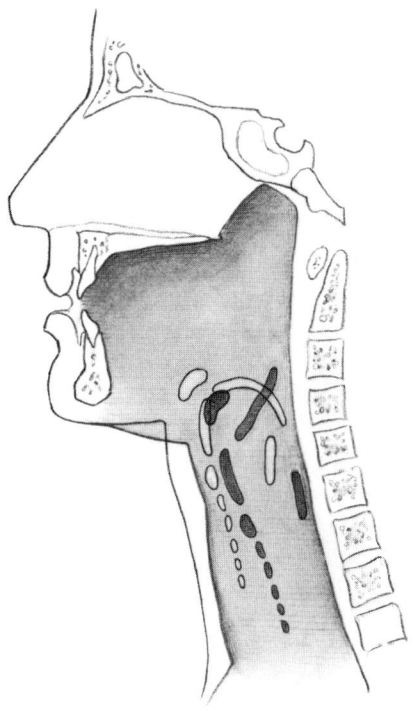

FIGURE 2.11. Schematic lateral (A) and midsaggital (B) views of the movement of the hyoid bone, the larynx, and the tracheal cartilage during a normal swallow. Note the anterior and superior displacement of these structures, as well as the epiglottic tilt. (Reprinted with permission from Zerhouni EA, Bosma JF, Donner MW. Relationship of cervical spine disorders to dysphagia. *Dysphagia* 1987;1: 129–144.)

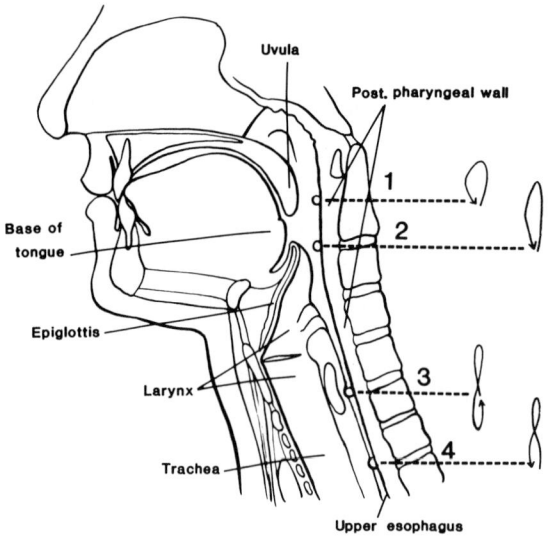

FIGURE 2.12. Schematic representation of the movement of the posterior pharyngeal wall during a normal swallow. Note the decreased relative mobility of the upper (1 and 2) as compared to the lower (3 and 4) posterior wall. (Reprinted with permission from Palmer JB, Tanaka E, Siebens AA. Motions of the posterior pharyngeal wall in swallowing. *Laryngoscope* 1988;98(4):414–417; kindly provided by Dr. Palmer.)

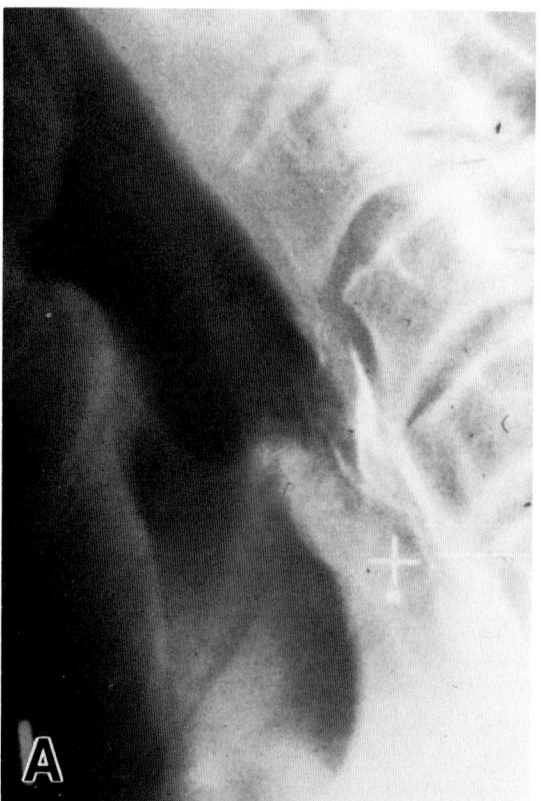
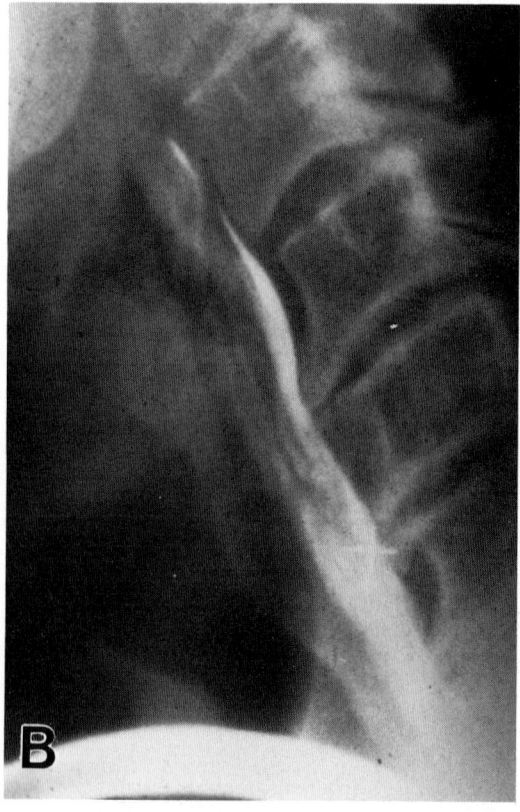

FIGURE 2.13. Two stop frames from a cineradiogram to illustrate the cephalad movement of the posterior pharynx during deglutition. Note the position of barium trapped in the retropharyngeal space at rest (A) and at midswallow (B).

the posterior pharyngeal wall (144) (Figure 2.12). A similar point is made in Figure 2.13, where we show cineradiograms of this region taken on a patient who had a barium swallow to evaluate a penetrating wound to the neck, and in whom some residual barium was retained in the retropharyngeal space. Both Figures 2.12 and 2.13 demonstrate the considerable mobility normally present in the posterior pharyngeal wall, an issue highlighted by the occurrence of swallowing disorders in patients suffering from a relative immobility of this region (162).

Neural Control of the Pharyngeal Phase

The coordinated musculature contractions that occur during the pharyngeal stage are controlled by a relatively discrete set of neural connections in the caudal medulla. These pathways have been well-characterized in the rat (172) (Figure 2.14) and are assumed to be similar in humans. Important differences between the pharyngeal reflexes and the masticatory reflexes summarized in the preceding section include the following.

1. Most of the sensory information important to eliciting a swallow is conveyed from the posterior tongue, faucial pillars, and pharynx (9,10) through the ninth and tenth cranial nerves, as opposed to the fifth cranial nerve, which seems to be more involved with feedback control of mastication (51,91).

2. The main pattern generator for the pharyngeal phase of swallowing appears to be located within and immediately ventral to the NTS (51,93).

Otherwise, just as the masticatory pattern generator in the more rostral reticular formation projects to specific motor nuclei innervating the muscles of mastication, so too does the pharyngeal pattern generator in and near the NTS project to motor nuclei innervating the muscles involved in the pharyngeal phase of swallowing. The pharyngeal pattern generator is also similar to the masticatory pattern generator in that it receives fairly heavy descending inputs from the forebrain. These descending inputs appear to be largely excitatory, and they seem to facilitate the initiation of reflex mastication and swallowing (51,66).

Esophageal Phase

Compared with the bewildering complexity of the oral and pharyngeal phases of swallowing, the esophageal phase consists of the ostensibly simple task of transporting the bolus from the pharynx to the stomach. By far the most effective stimulus for eliciting esophageal peristalsis is esophageal distension (163). This is especially true during swallowing, where the combined effect of a negative intrathoracic pressure at the end of inspiration, and the physical distension caused by the bolus itself, act in concert to elicit reflex peristalsis.

Regarding the control of peristalsis per se, considerable controversy exists over the relative roles of the vagus nerve and the central nervous system versus intrinsic esophageal neurons and nerve plexuses (51–59,63,64,67–70,80). In short, most believe that for the upper third of the esophagus, where striated muscle predominates, esophageal peristalsis is largely dependent upon the vagus nerve and an intact medullary reflex (51,80). By contrast, for the lower, smooth muscle portion of the esophagus, the vagus seems to have more of a modulatory role, acting to facilitate a fairly autonomous intrinsic peristaltic mechanism (51,64). Vagal innervation of the esophagus is also important for eliciting reflex relaxation during swallowing, so-called deglutitive inhibition, and in response to increased gastric pressure, as occurs during belching and reflux (80). Moreover, it may be that vagal sensory information from the esophagus can elicit paradoxical changes in cardiac and/or respiratory rhythm, in a manner very similar to the way in which pain fibers innervating the esophagus have been suggested to produce referred angina-like chest pain during spasm or reflux (164–166). Such "referred reflexes" might thus explain the numerous reports of swallowing and reflux-induced change in cardiorespiratory patterns, including tachycardia (167–171), bradycardia associated with syncope and, less frequently, seizures (167,172–175), apnea (167,176–180), and exacerbation of asthmatic attacks (181,182).

Neural Control of the Esophageal Phase

Medullary pathways controlling esophageal peristalsis follow the same general pattern outlined for other swallowing reflexes (Figure 2.14). Specifically, sensory fibers travel in the vagus nerve and end centrally in a discrete portion of the nucleus of the solitary tract. The nucleus of the solitary tract, in turn, projects to esophageal motor neurons, which complete the loop by innervating the esophagus. Noteworthy, however, is that motor neurons innervating the striated portion of the esophagus are in the ventrolateral medulla, in the nucleus ambiguus (NA), whereas motor neurons innervating the smooth muscle portion and the lower esophageal sphincter reside in the dorsal motor

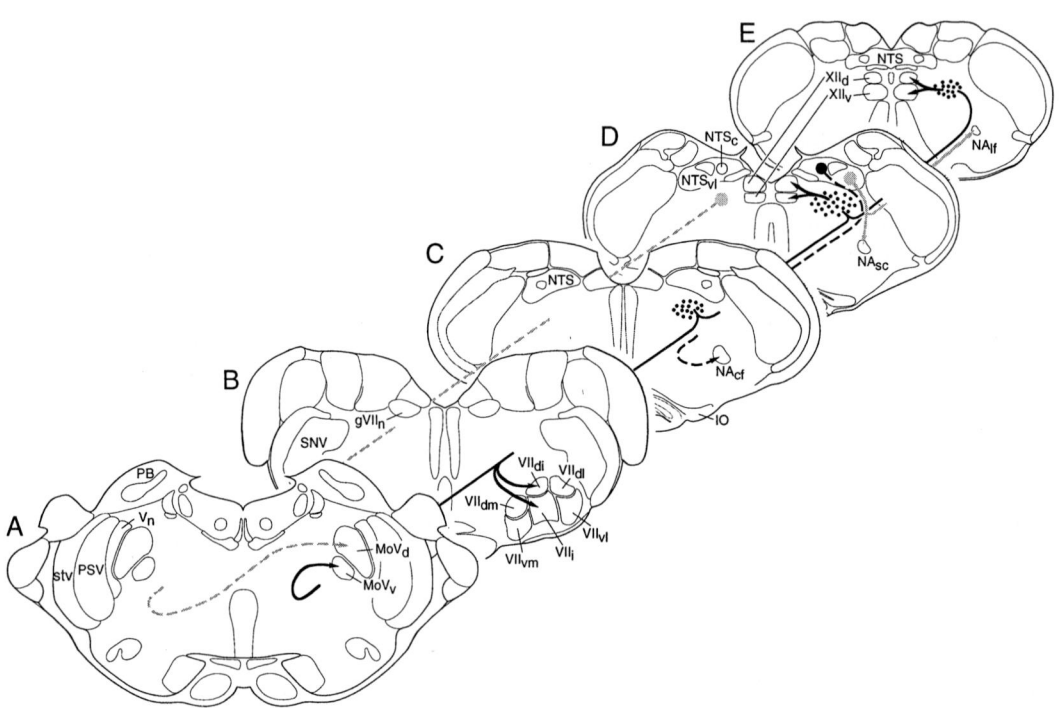

FIGURE 2.14. Schematic summary of the dorsal medullary pathways involved in the control of the pharyngeal and esophageal phases of swallowing in the rat. Projections are shown from the dorsomedial reticular column (DMRC) and nucleus of the solitary tract (NTS) to the fifth (MoV, A), seventh (VII, B), tenth (nucleus ambiguus, NA; C–E), and twelfth (XII; D,E) cranial nerve nuclei. Projections from the DMRC are distributed preferentially to the ventral subdivision of MoV, to the dorsal and intermediate subdivisions of VII, and to both the dorsal and ventral subdivisions of XII, which together trigger swallow initiation and coordinate the early pharyngeal phase of swallowing. Although this aspect is not illustrated, the pathways are largely bilateral. By contrast, dorsal medullary inputs to the NA arise primarily from the NTS, are primarily unilateral, and are organized such that the ventrolateral, intermediate, and interstitial subdivisions of the NTS project to the region of the loose (larynx) and semicompact (pharynx) formations within the NA, whereas the central subdivision of the NTS provides input to the compact (esophagus) formation. These pathways thus control the late pharyngeal and esophageal phases, respectively. Swallow initiation, laryngeal closure and pharyngeal transit, and esophageal transit each appears to be subserved by independent medullary reflexes. (Reproduced with permission from Cunningham ET Jr, Sawchenko PE. Dorsal medullary pathways subserving oromotor reflex function in the rat: implications for the central neural control of swallowing. J Comp Neurol 2000;417: 448–466.)

nucleus of the vagus nerve, immediately ventral to the NTS itself (80).

Summary

The complex oromotor behavior of ingestion is best understood when considered in three partially overlapping phases: the oral phase, the pharyngeal phase, and the esophageal phase. Each phase is temporally and functionally distinct, yet when triggered in turn the seemingly effortless act of swallowing results.

References

1. Pernkopf E. *Atlas der topographischen Anatomie des Menschen*. 1 Band. Munich: Urban and Schwarzenberg; 1963.
2. Williams PL, Warwick R. *Gray's Anatomy*. 37th ed. Philadelphia: WB Saunders; 1989.
3. Murakami Y, Fukuda H, Kirchner JA. The cricopharyngeus muscle. *Acta Otolaryngol (suppl) (Stockh)* 1972;311:5–19.
4. Dickson DR. Anatomy of the normal velopharyngeal mechanism. *Clin Plast Surg* 1975;2:235–248.
5. Archer CR, Friedman W II, Yeager VL, et al. Computer tomography of the larynx. *J Comput Assist Tomogr* 1978;2:404–411.
6. Netter FR. *The CIBA Collection of Medical Illustrations*. Summit, NJ: CIBA; 1983. *Nervous System*; Vol 1. *Anatomy and Physiology*; part 1.
7. Netter FH. *The CIBA Collection of Medical Illustrations*. Summit, NJ: CIBA; 1978. *Digestive System*; Vol 3. *Upper Digestive Tract*; part 1.
8. Bosma IF, Donner MW, Tanako E, Robertson D. Anatomy of the pharynx, pertinent to swallowing. *Dysphagia* 1986;1:23–33.
9. Miller AJ. Deglutition. *Physiol Rev* 1982;62:129–184.
10. Miller AJ. Neurophysiological basis of swallowing. *Dysphagia* 1986;1:91–100.
11. Curtis DJ. Laryngeal dynamics. *CRC Crit Rev Diagn Imaging* 1982;18:29–80.
12. Curtis DJ. Radiology of the laryngopharynx. In: English GM, ed. *Otolaryngology*. New York: Harper & Row; 1985:65–130.
13. Curtis DI. Radiographic anatomy of the pharynx. *Dysphagia* 1986;1:51–62.
14. Logemann I. Anatomy and physiology of normal deglutition. In: Logemann J, ed. *Evaluation and Treatment of Swallowing Disorders*. San Diego: College Hill Press; 1983:9–36.
15. Lufkin R, Larson S, Hanafee W. NMR anatomy of the larynx and tongue base. *Radiology* 1983;148:173–175.
16. Lufkin RB, Hanafee WN, Wortham D, Hoover L. MRI of the larynx and hypopharynx using surface coils. *Radiology* 1986;158:747–754.
17. Lulkin R, Hanafee W. Surface coil MRI of the larynx and hypopharynx. *Am J Nucl Radiol* 1985;6:491–497.
18. Hill BJ. Radiology of the larynx. *Otolaryngol Clin North Am* 1973;6:549–561.
19. Silver AJ, Sane P, Hilal SK. CT of the nasopharyngeal region: normal and pathologic anatomy. *Radiol Clin North Am* 1984;22:161–176.
20. Hollinshead WH. Anatomy of the pharynx and esophagus. In: English GM, ed. *Otolaryngology*. New York: Harper & Row; 1985:1–21.
21. Donner MW, Bosma JF, Robertson DL. Anatomy and physiology of the pharynx. *Gastrointest Radiol* 1985;10:19–212.
22. McMyn JK. The anatomy of the salpingopharyngeus muscle. *J Laryngol Otol* 1940;55:1–22.
23. Hoover LA, Wortham DG, Kaiser MC, et al. Magnetic resonance imaging of the larynx and tongue base: clinical applications. *Otolaryngol Head Neck Surg* 1987;97:245–256.
24. Rubesin SE, Rabischong P, Bilaniuk LT, Laufer I, Levine MS. Contrast examination of the soft palate with cross sectional correlation. *RadioGraphics* 1988;8:641–665.
25. Rubesin SE, Jones B, Donner MW. Radiology of the adult soft palate. *Dysphagia* 1987;2:8–17.
26. Rubesin SE, Jessurun J, Robertson D, Jones B, Donner MW. Lines of the pharynx. *RadioGraphics* 1987;7:217–237.
27. Christianson R, Lufkin R, Hanafee W. Normal magnetic resonance imaging anatomy of the tongue, oropharynx, hypopharynx, and larynx. *Dysphagia* 1987;1:119–127.
28. Sasaki CT, Isaacson G. Functional anatomy of the larynx. *Otolaryngol Clin North Am* 1988;21:595–612.
29. Mafee MF, Campos M, Faju S, Samett E, Mahamadi H, Sadighi S, Heffex L, Friedman M, Chow JM. Head and neck: high field magnetic resonance imaging versus computed tomography. *Otolaryngol Clin North Am* 1988;21:513–546.
30. Gritzmann N, Fruhwald F. Sonographic anatomy of tongue and floor of the mouth. *Dysphagia* 1988;2:196–202.
31. Jones B, Gayler BW, Donner MW. Pharynx and cervical esophagus. In: Levine MS, ed.

Radiology of the Esophagus. Philadelphia: WB Saunders; 1989:311–336.
32. Cannon WB. *The Mechanical Factors of Digestion.* New York: Longmans, Green; 1911.
33. Negus VE. The second stage of swallowing. *Acta Otolaryngol (suppl) (Stockh)* 1948–49;78:79–82.
34. Negus VE. The mechanism of swallowing. *J Laryngol Otol* 1943;58:46–59.
35. Ardan G, Kemp F. The mechanism of swallowing. *Proc R Soc Med* 1951;44:103–1040.
36. Bosma J. A correlated study of the anatomy and motor activity of the upper pharynx by cadaver dissection and by cinematic study of patients after maxillofacial surgery. *Ann Otol Rhinol Laryngol* 1953;62:51–72.
37. Bosma J. Deglutition: pharyngeal stage. *Physiol Rev* 1957;37:275–300.
38. Bosma J. Physiology of the mouth, pharynx, and esophagus. In: Paparella M, Shumrick D, eds. *Otolaryngology.* Vol 1. *Basic Sciences and Related Disciplines.* Philadelphia: WB Saunders; 1973:356–370.
39. Ingelfinger FJ. Esophageal motility. *Physiol Rev* 1958;38:533–584.
40. Bosma J, Fletcher SG. The upper pharynx: a review, II: physiology. *Ann Otol Rhinol Laryngol* 1962;71:134–157.
41. Kawamura Y. Recent concepts of the physiology of mastication. *Adv Oral Biol* 1964;1:77–109.
42. Code CF, Schlegel JF. Motor action of the esophagus and its sphincters. In: Heidel D, exec ed. Code, CF, sect ed. *Handbook of Physiology.* Sec 6, *Alimentary Canal.* Vol 4; *Motility.* Bethesda, MD: American Physiological Society; 1968:1821–1839.
43. Lowe A. The neural regulation of tongue movement. *Prog Neurobiol* 1981;15:295–344.
44. Dellow P. The general physiological background of chewing and swallowing. In: Sessle B, Hannan A, eds. *Mastication and Swallowing.* Toronto: University of Toronto Press; 1976:6–21.
45. Bosma JF, Donner MW. Physiology of the pharynx. In: Paparella MM, Shumrick DA, eds. *Otolaryngology.* Philadelphia: WB Saunders; 1980:332–345.
46. Hendrix TR. The motility of the alimentary canal. In: Mountcastle VB, ed. *Medical Physiology.* 14th ed. St. Louis, MO: CV Mosby; 1980: 1320–1347.
47. Goyal RK, Cobb BW. Motility of the pharynx, esophagus, and esophageal sphincters. In: Johnson LR, ed. *Physiology of the Gastrointestinal Tract.* New York: Raven Press; 1981: 359–391.
48. Logemann JA. Swallowing physiology and pathophysiology. *Otolaryngol Clin North Am* 1988;21:613–623.
49. Curtis DI, Cruess DF, Dachman AM. Normal swallowing: normal function incidence of variation. *Invest Radiol* 1985;20:717–720.
50. Kennedy JG, Kent RD. Physiological substrates of normal deglutition. *Dysphagia* 1988;3:2–37.
51. Miller AJ. *The Neuroscientific Principles of Swallowing and Dysphagia.* San Diego: Singular Publishing Group; 1999.
52. Miller AJ. Swallowing: neurophysiologic control of the esophageal phase. *Dysphagia* 1987; 2:72–82.
53. Diamant NE. Physiology of the esophagus. In: Sleisenger M, Fordtran IS, eds. *Gastrointestinal Disease: Pathophysiology, Diagnosis, Management.* 4th ed. Philadelphia: WB Saunders; 1989: 548–559.
54. Diamant NE. Normal esophageal physiology. In: Cohen S, Soloway RD, eds. *Diseases of the Esophagus.* New York: Churchill Livingstone; 1982:1–33.
55. Diamant NE. Physiology of esophageal motor function. *Gastroenterol Clin North Am* 1989; 18(2):179–194.
56. Christensen I. Motor functions of the pharynx and esophagus. In: Johnson LR, ed. *Physiology of the Gastrointestinal Tract.* 2nd ed. New York: Raven Press; 1987:595–612.
57. Christensen I. The esophagus. In: Christensen J, Wingate D, eds. *A Guide to Gastrointestinal Motility.* Bristol, England: John Wright; 1982: 75–100.
58. Gidda IS. Control of esophageal peristalsis. *Viewpoints Dig Dis* 1985;17:13–16.
59. Goyal RK, Crist JR. Neurology of the gut. In: Sleisenger M, Fordtran IS, eds. *Gastrointestinal Disease: Pathophysiology, Diagnosis, Management.* 4th ed. Philadelphia: WB Saunders; 1989: 21–52.
60. Dodds W. The physiology of swallowing. *Dysphagia* 1989;3:171–178.
61. Sumi T. Neuronal mechanisms in swallowing. *Pflugers Arch* 1964;278:467–477.
62. Doty RW. Neural organization of deglutition. In: Heidel D, exec ed; Code EF, sect ed. *Handbook of Physiology.* Sect 6; *Alimentary Canal.* Vol 4; *Motility.* Bethesda, MD: American Physiological Society; 1968:1861–1902.
63. Weisbrodt NW. Neuromuscular organization of esophageal and pharyngeal motility. *Arch Intern Med* 1976;136:524–531.

64. Diamant NE, El-Sharkawy TY. Neural control of esophageal peristalsis. A conceptual analysis. *Gastroenterology* 1977;72:546–556.
65. Dubner R, Sessle BJ, Storey AT. *The Neural Basis of Oral and Facial Function.* New York: Plenum Press; 1978.
66. Hockman CH, Bieger D, Weerasuriya A. Supranuclear pathways of swallowing. *Prog Neurobiol* 1978;12:15–32.
67. Roman C, Gonella J. Extrinsic control of digestive tract motility. In: Johnson LR, ed. *Physiology of the Gastrointestinal Tract.* New York: Raven Press; 1981:223–278.
68. Roman C, Gonella J. Extrinsic control of digestive tract motility. In: Johnson LR, ed. *Physiology of the Gastrointestinal Tract*, 2nd ed. New York: Raven Press; 1987:507–553.
69. Roman C. Contrôle nerveux de la déglutition et la motricité oesophagienne chez les mammifères. *J Physiol (Paris)* 1986;81:118–131.
70. Roman C. Nervous control of esophageal and gastric motility. In: Bertaccini G, ed. *Handbook of Experimental Pharmacology.* Vol 59. Berlin: Springer-Verlag; 1982:223–278.
71. Jean A. Control of the central swallowing program by inputs from the peripheral receptors. A review. *J Auton Nerv Syst* 1984;10:225–233.
72. Jean A. Brainstem organization of the swallowing network. *Brain Behav Evol* 1984;25:109–116.
73. Morrell RM. The neurology of swallowing. In: Groher ME, ed. *Dysphagia: Diagnosis and Management.* Boston: Butterworth; 1984:3–35.
74. Morrell RM. Neurologic disorders of swallowing. In: Groher ME, ed. *Dysphagia: Diagnosis and Management.* Boston: Butterworth; 1984:37–59.
75. Buchholz D. Neurologic causes of dysphagia. *Dysphagia* 1987;1:152–156.
76. Buchholz D. Neurologic evaluation of dysphagia. *Dysphagia* 1987;1:187–193.
77. Kirshner HS. Causes of neurogenic dysphagia. *Dysphagia* 1989;3:184–188.
78. Sessle BJ, Henry IL. Neural mechanisms of swallowing: neurophysiological and neurochemical studies on brain stem neurons in the solitary tract region. *Dysphagia* 1989;4:61–75.
79. Carpenter DO. Central nervous system mechanisms in deglutition and emesis. In: Wood ID, exec ed; Schultz SG, sect ed. *Handbook of Physiology*, Vol 4; *Gastrointestinal Motility and Circulation.* Bethesda, MD: American Physiological Society; 1989:685–714.
80. Cunningham ET Jr, Sawchenko PE. Central neural control of esophageal motility: a review. *Dysphagia* 1990;5:35–51.
81. Hughes CV, Baum BJ, Fox PC, Marmary Y, Yeh C-K, Sonies BC. Oral-pharyngeal dysphagia: a common sequela of salivary gland dysfunction. *Dysphagia* 1987;1:173–177.
82. Kapila YV, Dodds WJ, Helm JF, Hogan WJ. Relationship between swallow rate and salivary flow. *Dig Dis Sci* 1984;29:528–533.
83. Tomura Y, Ide Y, Kamijo Y. Studies on the morphological changes of the tongue movements during mastication by x-ray TV cinematography. In: Kawamura Y, Dubner R, eds. *Oral Sensory and Motor Functions.* Tokyo: Quintessence; 1931:45–52.
84. Thexton AJ. Oral reflexes elicited by mechanical stimulation of palatal mucosa in the cat. *Arch Oral Biol* 1973;18:971–980.
85. Cook IJ, Dodds WJ, Dantas RO, Kern MK, Massey BT, Shaker R, Hogan WJ. Timing of videofluoroscopic, manometric events, and bolus transit during the oral and pharyngeal phases of swallowing. *Dysphagia* 1989;4:8–15.
86. Hamlet S, Stone M, Shawker TH. Posterior tongue grooving in deglutition and speech: preliminary observations. *Dysphagia* 1988;3:65–68.
87. Shaker R, Cook IJS, Dodds WJ, Hogan WJ. Pressure-flow dynamics of the oral phase of swallowing. *Dysphagia* 1988;3:79–84.
88. Moller E. The chewing apparatus. *Acta Physiol Scand* 1966;69:1–229.
89. Anderson D. Mastication. In: Heidel D, exec ed; Code EF, sect ed. *Handbook of Physiology.* Sect 6; *Alimentary Canal.* Vol 4: *Motility.* Bethesda, MD: American Physiological Society; 1968:1811–1820.
90. Sessle B, Hannan A, eds. *Mastication and Swallowing.* Toronto: University of Toronto Press; 1976.
91. Norgren R. Central neural control mechanisms of taste. In: Geigers R, exec ed. Mountcastle VB, sect ed. Bloom E, vol ed. *Handbook of Physiology.* Sect 1; *The Nervous System.* Vol III; *Sensory Processes, Part 2.* Bethesda, MD: American Physiological Society; 1984:1087–1124.
92. Loewy AD, Burton H. Nuclei of the solitary tract: efferent projections to the lower brain stem and spinal cord of the cat. *J Comp Neurol* 1978;181:421–450.
93. Cunningham ET Jr, Sawchenko PE. Dorsal medullary pathways subserving oromotor reflex function in the rat: implications for

neural control of swallowing. *J Comp Neurol* 2000;417:448–466.
94. Negus V. The function of the epiglottis. *J Anat* 1927;62:1–8.
95. Ardran GM, Kemp FH. The protection of the laryngeal airway during swallowing. *Br J Radiol* 1952;25:406–416.
96. Pressman JJ, Kelemen G. Physiology of the larynx. *Physiol Rev* 1955;35:506–554.
97. Ardran GM, Kemp FH. Closure and opening of the larynx during swallowing. *Br J Radiol* 1956;29:205–208.
98. Shelton RL, Bosma JF, Sheets BV. Tongue, hyoid and larynx displacement in swallow and phonation. *J Appl Physiol* 1960;15:283–288.
99. Ardran FM, Kemp FH. The mechanism of the larynx, II: the epiglottis and closure of the larynx. *Br J Radiol* 1967;40:372–389.
100. Ekberg O, Sigurjonsson SV. Movement of the epiglottis during deglutition. A cineradiographic study. *Gastrointest Radiol* 1982;7:101–107.
101. Laitman J, Crelin E, Conlogue F. The function of the epiglottis in monkey and man. *Yale J Biol Med* 1977;50:43–48.
102. Ekberg O. Defective closure of the laryngeal vestibule during deglutition. *Acta Otolaryngol (Stockh)* 1982;93:309–317.
103. Curtis DJ, Sepulveda GU. Epiglottic motion: video recording of muscular dysfunction. *Radiology* 1983;148:473–477.
104. Curtis DJ, Hudson T. Laryngotracheal aspiration: analysis of specific neuromuscular factors. *Radiology* 1983;149:517–522.
105. Kahrilas PJ, Dodds WJ, Dent J, Logemann JA, Shaker R. Upper esophageal sphincter function during deglutition. *Gastroenterology* 1988;95:52–62.
106. Cook IJ, Dodds WJ, Dantas RO, Massey B, Kern MK, Lang IM, Brasseur JG, Hogan WJ. Opening mechanisms of the human upper esophageal sphincter. *Am J Physiol* 1989;257:G748–G759.
107. Nilsson ME, Isacsson G, Isberg A. The mobility of the upper esophageal sphincter in relation to the cervical spine—a morphological study. *Dysphagia* 1989;3:161–170.
108. Fyke FE, Code CF. Resting and deglutition pressure in the pharyngoesophageal region. *Gastroenterology* 1955;29:24–34.
109. Fyke FE, Code CF, Schlegel JC. The gastroesophageal sphincter in healthy human beings. *Gastroenterologia* 1956;86:135–150.
110. Atkinson M, Kramer P, Wyman SM, Ingelfinger FJ. The dynamics of swallowing, I: normal pharyngeal mechanisms. *J Clin Invest* 1957;36:581–588.
111. Sokol E, Heitmann P, Wolf B, Cohen B. Simultaneous cineradiographic and manometric study of the pharynx, hypopharynx, and cervical esophagus. *Gastroenterology* 1966;51:660–674.
112. Dodds WJ, Hogan WJ, Lydon SB, Stewart ET, Stef JJ, Arndorfer RC. Quantification of pharyngeal motor function in normal human subjects. *J Appl Physiol* 1975;39:692–696.
113. Berlin BP, Tedesco F, Fierstein JT, Ogura JH. Manometric studies of the upper esophageal sphincter. *Ann Otol Rhinol Laryngol* 1977;86:598–602.
114. Asoh R, Goyal RK. Manometry and electromyography of the upper esophageal sphincter in the opossum. *Gastroenterology* 1978;74:514–520.
115. Newman A. Manometry in the evaluation of esophageal function. *Otolaryngol Clin North Am* 1978;11:405–417.
116. Orlowski J, Dodds WJ, Linehan JH, Dent J, Hogan WJ, Arndorfer RC. Requirements for accurate manometric recording of pharyngeal and esophageal peristaltic pressure waves. *Invest Radiol* 1982;17:567–572.
117. Welch RW, Luckman K, Ricks PM, Drake ST, Gates GA. Manometry of the normal upper esophageal sphincter and its alterations in laryngectomy. *J Clin Invest* 1979;63:1036–1041.
118. Dodds WJ, Kahrilas PJ, Dent J, Hogan WJ. Considerations about pharyngeal manometry. *Dysphagia* 1987;1:209–214.
119. Kahrilas PJ, Dent J, Dodds WJ, Hogan WJ, Arndorfer RC. A method for continuous monitoring of upper esophageal sphincter pressure. *Dig Dis Sci* 1987;32:121–128.
120. Doty RW, Bosma JF. An electromyographic analysis of reflex deglutition. *J Neurophysiol* 1956;19:44–60.
121. Faaborg-Anderson K. Electromyographic investigation of intrinsic laryngeal muscles in humans. *Acta Physiol Scand (suppl)* 1957;140:1–149.
122. Basmajian JV, Cutta CR. Electromyography of pharyngeal constrictors and levator palatini in man. *Anat Rec* 1961;139:561–563.
123. Kawasaki M, Ogura JH, Takenouchi S. Neurophysiologic observations of normal deglutition, I: its relationship to the respiratory cycle. *Laryngoscope* 1965;74:1747–1765.
124. Johnstone AS. A radiological study of deglutition. *J Anat* 1942;77:97–100.

125. Rushmer RF, Hendron JA. The act of deglutition: a cinefluorographic study. *J Appl Physiol* 1951;3:622–630.
126. Saunders JB, De CM, Davis C, Miller ER. The mechanism of deglutition (second stage) as revealed by cine-radiography. *Ann Otol Rhinol Laryngol* 1951;60:897–916.
127. Ramsey GH, Watson JS, Gramiak R, Weinberg SA. Cinefluorographic analysis of the mechanism of swallowing. *Radiology* 1955;64:498–518.
128. Shedd DP, Scatliff JH, Kirchner JA. The buccopharyngeal propulsive mechanism in human deglutition. *Surgery* 1960;48:846–853.
129. Shedd DP, Kirchner JA. Oral and pharyngeal components of deglutition. *Arch Surg* 1961;82:373–380.
130. Sloan RF, Brummett SW, Westover JL. Recent cinefluorographic advances in palatopharyngeal roentgenography. *Am J Roentgenol Radium Ther Nucl Med* 1964;92:977–985.
131. Cleall JF. Deglutition: A study of form and function. *Am J Orthodont* 1965;51:566–594.
132. Moll KL. A cinefluorographic study of velopharyngeal function in normals during various activities. *Cleft Palate J* 1965;2:112–122.
133. Hedges RB, McLean CD, Thompson FA. A cinefluorographic study of tongue patterns in function. *Angle Orthod* 1965;35:253–268.
134. Donner MW, Silbiger ML. Cinefluorographic analysis of pharyngeal swallowing in neuromuscular disorders. *Am J Med Sci* 1966;251:600–616.
135. Sokol E, Heitmann P, Wolf B, Cohen B. Simultaneous cineradiographic and manometric study of the pharynx, hypopharynx and cervical esophagus. *Gastroenterology* 1966;51:660–674.
136. Perry HT Jr. Muscle contraction patterns in swallowing. *Angle Orthod* 1972;42:66–80.
137. Flowers CR, Morris HL. Oral-pharyngeal movements during swallowing and speech. *Cleft Palate J* 1973;10:181–191.
138. Ekberg O, Nylander G. Cineradiography of the pharyngeal stage of deglutition in 150 individuals without dysphagia. *Br J Radiol* 1982;55:253–277.
139. Jones B, Kramer SS, Donner MW. Dynamic imaging of the pharynx. *Gastrointest Radiol* 185;10:213–224.
140. Birch-Iensen M, Borgstrom PS, Ekberg O. Cineradiography in closed and open pharyngeal swallow. *Acta Radiol* 1988;29:407–410.
141. Curtis DJ, Cruess DF. Pharyngoesophageal swallowing: a review of 618 videorecorded cases. *Milit Med* 1984;149:545–549.
142. Curtis DJ, Cruess DF, Berg T. The cricopharyngeal muscle: a videorecording review. *Am J Roentgenol* 1984;142:497–500.
143. Palmer JB, Tanaka E, Siebens AA. Motions of the posterior pharyngeal wall in swallowing. *Laryngoscope* 1988;98:414–417.
144. Hamlet SL, Muz J, Patterson R, Jones L. Pharyngeal transit time: assessment with videofluoroscopic and scintigraphic techniques. *Dysphagia* 1989;4:4–7.
145. van Overbeek JJM, Wit HP, Paping RHL, Segenhout HM. Simultaneous manometry and electromyography in the pharyngoesophageal segment. *Laryngoscope* 1985;95:582–584.
146. Cohen BR, Wolf BS. Cineradiographic and intraluminal pressure correlations in the pharynx and esophagus. In: Heidel D, exec ed. Code CF, sect ed. *Handbook of Physiology*. Sect 6; *Alimentary Canal*. Vol 4; *Motility*. Bethesda, MD: American Physiological Society; 1968:1841–1860.
147. Isberg A, Nilsson ME, Schiratzki J. Movement of the upper esophageal sphincter and a manometric device during deglutition. *Acta Radiol (Diagn)* 1985;26:381–388.
148. Isberg A, Nilsson ME, Schiratzki J. The upper esophageal sphincter during normal deglutition. *Acta Radiol (Diagn)* 1985;26:563–568.
149. McConnel FMS. Analysis of pressure generation and bolus transit during pharyngeal swallowing. *Laryngoscope* 1988;98:71–78.
150. McConnel FMS, Cerenko D, Hersh T, Weil U. Evaluation of pharyngeal dysphagia with manofluorography. *Dysphagia* 1988;2:187–195.
151. McConnel FMS, Cerenko D, Jackson RT, Hersh T. Clinical application of manofluorogram. *Laryngoscope* 1988;98:705–711.
152. McConnel FMS, Cerenko D, Jackson RT, Guffin TN Jr. Timing of major events of pharyngeal swallowing. *Arch Otolaryngol Head Neck Surg* 1988;114:1413–1418.
153. Cerenko D, McConnel FMS, Jackson RT. Quantitative assessment of pharyngeal bolus driving forces. *Otolaryngol Head Neck Surg* 1989;100:57–63.
154. Nilsson ME, Isberg A, Schiratzki H. The location of the upper esophageal sphincter and its behavior during bolus propagation—a simultaneous cineradiographic and manometric investigation. *Acta Otolaryngol* 1988;106:314–320.

155. Borgstrom PS, Ekberg O. Speed of peristalsis in pharyngeal constrictor musculature: correlation to age. *Dysphagia* 1988;2:140–144.
156. Sonies BC, Parent U, Morrish K, Baum BJ. Durational aspects of the oral-pharyngeal phase of swallow in normal adults. *Dysphagia* 1988;3:1–10.
157. Clark GA. Deglutition apnoea. *J Physiol (Lond)* 1920;54:lix.
158. Nishino T, Yonezawa T, Honda Y. Effects of swallowing on the pattern of continuous respiration in human adults. *Am Rev Respir Dis* 1985;132:1219–1222.
159. Selley WG, Flack FC, Ellis RE, Brooks WA. Respiratory patterns associated with swallowing, I: the normal adult pattern and changes with age. *Age Ageing* 1989;18:168–172.
160. Ekberg O, Olsson R, Sundgren-Borgstrom P. Relation of bolus size and pharyngeal swallow. *Dysphagia* 1988;3:69–72.
161. Kramer SS, Anderson JH, Strandberg JD, Donner MW. A permanent radiopaque marker technique for the study of pharyngeal swallowing in dogs. *Dysphagia* 1987;1:163–167.
162. Zerhouni EA, Bosma JF, Donner MW. Relationship of cervical spine disorders to dysphagia. *Dysphagia* 1987;1:129–144.
163. Paterson WG, Rattan S, Goyal RK. Experimental induction of isolated lower esophageal sphincter relaxation in anesthetized opossums. *J Clin Invest* 1986;77:1187–1193.
164. Cunningham ET Jr, Ravich WJ, Jones B, Donner MW. Vagal reflexes referred from the upper aerodigestive tract: an infrequently recognized cause of common cardiorespiratory responses. *Ann Intern Med* 1992;116(7):575–582.
165. Rothstein RD, Ouyang A. Chest pain of esophageal origin. *Gastroenterol Clin North Am* 1989;18(2):257–273.
166. Richter JE, Bradley LA, Castell DO. Esophageal chest pain: current controversies in pathogenesis, diagnosis, and therapy. *Ann Intern Med* 1989;110:66–78.
167. Palmer ED. The abnormal upper gastrointestinal vagovagal reflexes that affect the heart. *Am J Gastroenterol* 1976;66(6):513–522.
168. Greenspon AJ, Volosin KJ. Swallowing induced tachycardia: electrophysiologic and pharmacologic observations. *PACE Pacing Clin Electrophysiol* 1988;11:1566–1570.
169. Matsubara K, Jnoue D, Moridawa Y, Shirayama T, Omori I, Katsume H, Nakagawa M. Swallowing-induced arrhythmia. *Clin Cardiol* 1988;11:798–800.
170. Khan QA, Khan B. Swallowing-induced tachycardia. *J Tenn Med Assoc* 1988;81(3):141–143.
171. Ransbottom JC, Mirro MI. Refractory swallowing-induced paroxysmal supraventricular tachycardia. *Clin Cardiol* 1988;11:51–52.
172. Levin B, Posner JB. Swallow syncope: report of a case and review of the literature. *Neurology* 1972;22:1086–1093.
173. Armstrong PW, McMillan DG, Simon JB. Swallow syncope. *Can Med Assoc J* 1985;132:1281–1284.
174. Kalloo AN, Lewis JH, Maher K, Benjamin SB. Swallowing: an unusual cause of syncope. *Dig Dis Sci* 1989;34(7):1117–1120.
175. Elam MP, Laird JR, Johnson S, Stratton JR. Swallow syncope associated with complete atrioventricular block: a case report and review of the literature. *Milit Med* 1989;9:465–466.
176. Bellgaumkar TK, Scott KE. Apnea in premature infants: recording by arterial catheter. *Ear J Pediatr* 1976;123:301–305.
177. Wilson SL, Thach BT, Broulliette RT, Abu-Osba YK. Swallowing associated with respiratory pauses in infants (abstract). *Pediatr Res* 1980;14:653.
178. Menon A, Scheift G, Thach BT. Frequency and significance of swallowing during prolonged apnea in infants. *Am Rev Respir Dis* 1984;130:969–973.
179. Roberts JL, Mathew OP, Thach BT. Observations made on severe apneic spells in two infants at risk for sudden death. *Early Hum Dev* 1985;10:261–271.
180. Pickens DL, Schefft G, Thach BT. Prolonged apnea associated with upper airway protective reflexes in apnea of prematurity. *Am Rev Respir Dis* 1988;137:113–118.
181. Pope CE II. Respiratory complications of gastro-oesophageal reflux. *Scand J Gastroenterol (suppl)* 1989;168:67–72.
182. Goldman IM, Bennett JR. Gastro-oesophageal reflux and asthma; a common association, but of what clinical importance? *Gut* 1990;31:1–3.

3
The Tailored Examination

BRONWYN JONES

Each Patient with Dysphagia Is Different

Each patient with dysphagia is different, for the underlying causes for the symptom, dysphagia, are many and diverse and include both structural and functional causes. Structural lesions include benign lesions such as rings, webs, and strictures and malignant lesions such as cancer and lymphoma. Many neuromuscular conditions can cause dysphagia including cerebrovascular accident, amyotrophic lateral sclerosis (ALS, motor neuron disease), Parkinson's disease, multiple sclerosis, myopathies, and myasthenia gravis (see Chapter 12 for discussion in more depth). Many systemic disorders can produce dysphagia such as dermatomyositis and scleroderma (1). Medications can produce or exacerbate swallowing function either by producing drug-induced pharyngitis or esophagitis or by affecting neuromuscular transmission of peristalsis (1,2).

It is useful to think of patients with dysphagia in several different categories, namely:

1. Initial evaluation and no known underlying explanation for the symptom: the examination will be directed at evaluation of structure and function of all structures involved in transport of liquid and solid from mouth to stomach.

2. Onset of symptoms with onset of a known disease (e.g., cerebrovascular accident resulting in hemiparesis and dysphagia): the symptom is assumed to be caused by the known disease.

3. Patient has a disease that can produce dysphagia (e.g., Parkinson's disease): is the dysphagia caused by the known disease, or is there another cause for the symptom (i.e., an unrelated structural or functional abnormality)?

Remember that dysphagia can be multifactorial, and just because the patient has a disease that *can* cause dysphagia, it does not mean that it *is* causing dysphagia (3).

In cases 2 and 3 the study will often be performed jointly by a team of radiologist and an allied health professional such as a speech-language pathologist, who will have performed a clinical evaluation of the patient prior to the study.

Time should be spent with the patient prior to the actual radiographic examination, taking a brief, relevant history (see Table 3.1). Points in the history then are used to guide and tailor the examination to the individual patient.

Principles of Examination

Tailor the Examination to Each Patient (Table 3.2)

Although there is a "routine" examination, as with any radiological technique, studies of patients with swallowing problems lend themselves to tailoring. The basic routine is then modified in an attempt to reproduce symptoms and detect an abnormal swallow by provocative tests (Table 3.3) (4–6). The routine examination is also modified by the clinical condition of the

TABLE 3.1. Important history data.

Onset of symptoms
Subtlety of dysphagia
Position
Sleep, snore, drool
Speech
Variability, comprehensibility
Feeding time (beginning to end of meal)
Dysphagia for liquids, solids, or both
Cough, choking
Weight loss
Fatigue
Medications
Cardiac-respiratory symptoms (e.g., asthma or fainting)
Systemic disease

TABLE 3.2. Tailor the examination.

Initial patient position, centering, and initial contrast
Vary the bolus consistency
Chill, heat, or acidify the barium
Solid bolus if solid food dysphagia

patient: the sicker the patient, the less routine and more tailored the examination. The examination is also varied depending on whether it is the initial diagnostic procedure or a "therapeutic" study directed at the effect of various bolus consistencies or maneuvers on aspiration or retention (see Chapter 14).

The Initial Swallow: Centering

The initial swallow should be taken with the patient in the lateral, frontal, or left posterior oblique position depending on the information volunteered by the patient during the history taking. For example, if aspiration is suspected (cough/choke episodes, pneumonia), the first swallow should be centered over the larynx in the lateral position. If asymmetry or displacement is suspected (thyroid disease, neck surgery, pharyngeal or laryngeal tumor), the first swallow should be observed in the frontal position centered over the pharynx. With suspected esophageal pathology (food sticking in chest, chest pain, regurgitation, heartburn), the erect left posterior oblique position should be chosen for that initial swallow.

Depending on what is observed at that first swallow, the decision can be made to stay in that position (if abnormality is seen) or to move on to another position. For example, if aspiration is seen, it may be decided to characterize the aspiration and/or try different consistencies or maneuvers in an attempt to decrease or abolish the aspiration.

The Initial Swallow: Consistency

In general it is best to begin with what is felt to be safest (this information may be volunteered by the patient or may be decided upon by the speech-language pathologist following the clinical evaluation).

For example, if the clinical evaluation suggests that the patient chokes on liquids, it may be wise to begin with a small volume of purée or a small volume of thin liquid rather than a large volume of high-density barium. The clinical suspicion of an obstruction in pharynx or esophagus may indicate a small volume of thin liquid and the need to "see what one is dealing with."

Radiographic Evaluation of Patients with Dysphagia Must Include All Structures Involved in Swallowing

As already stressed, the examination should begin by centering over the symptomatic area. All structures involved in swallowing, however, must be evaluated: lips, tongue, palate, pharynx, larynx, and esophagus.

It used to be thought and taught that the level of an obstructing lesion could be accurately localized by the patient. However, studies have shown that this is incorrect, and many patients with a distal obstructing lesion localize the symp-

TABLE 3.3. Stress the patient.

Extend the head
Supine position (nasopharyngeal regurgitation)
Prone position (tongue or pharyngeal constrictors)
Acidify or chill the barium
Solid bolus

TABLE 3.4. Examine the entire swallowing chain.

Poor localization of symptoms
Multiple lesions
Esophageal disease may result in pharyngeal disease

3. The Tailored Examination   37

toms to upper chest or even neck [see Chapter 6 on pharyngoesophageal (PE) interrelationships and Figure 6.1, which gives a pictorial table of the results of one study by Edwards (7)].

Remember also that more than one lesion may be found, and any such lesion could produce the symptom, dysphagia (Figure 3.1) (3).

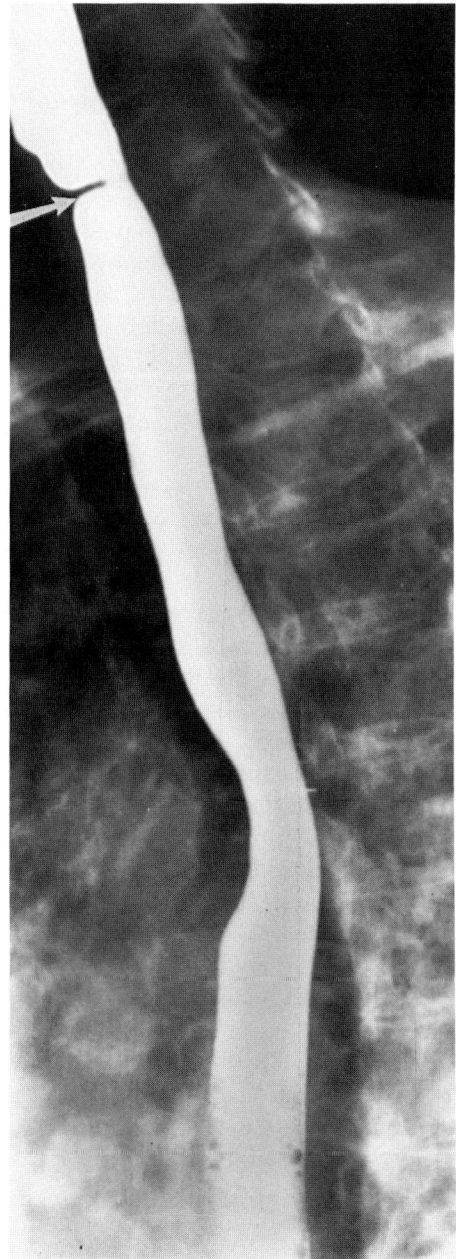

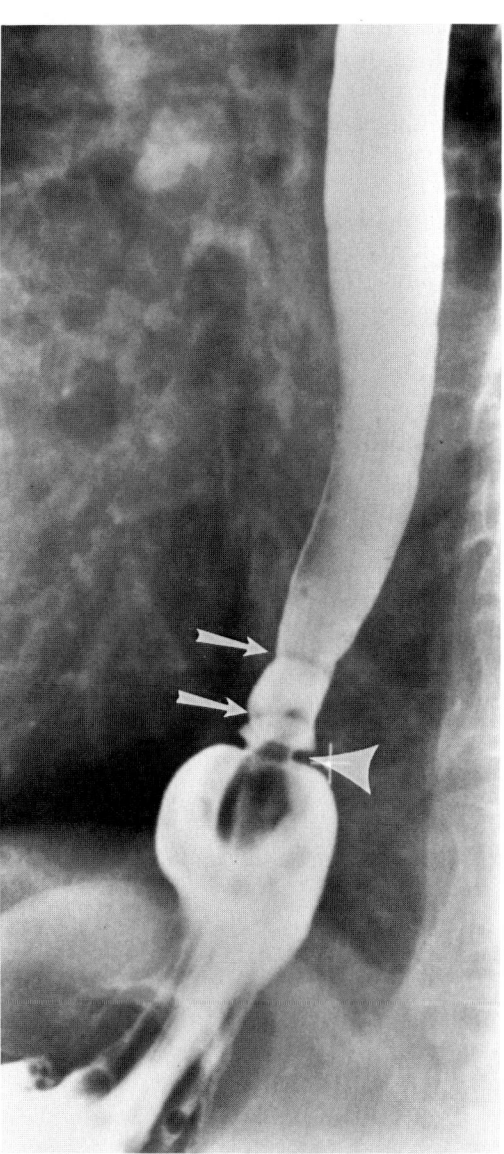

FIGURE 3.1. Double lesions. Two prone oblique drinking esophagus views of a 40-year-old woman with pharyngeal dysphagia. There is a high-grade obstructing web on the anterior wall of the cervical esophagus (A) (arrow); in the distal esophagus (B), there are two more nonobstructing webs (arrows), a stenotic Schatzki's ring measuring less than 1 cm in luminal diameter (arrowhead), and a small sliding hiatal hernia. Symptoms responded to dilatation of both the pharyngeal and esophageal narrowing.

Each Patient Should Be Examined in Both the Erect and Recumbent Position (If at All Possible)

The pharynx is best evaluated in the upright lateral and frontal positions with the patient either standing or sitting. Special chairs are available that can be wheeled in front of the fluoroscopic table for examining incapacitated patients in the position in which they normally eat, or are fed. Smaller adult patients and pediatric patients can sit on the footrest of the fluoroscopic table.

Some fluoroscopic units allow rotation of the fluoroscopic tube rather than the patient. In these units, supine or semisupine views (obtained with a cross-table tube, if possible) can be performed if the patient is unable to stand. The patient may be strapped onto the fluoroscopic table for security. Be sure to flex the head slightly if the patient will be swallowing in the horizontal position, as swallowing with the head extended narrows the PE segment and may precipitate decompensations such as aspiration.

If the patient is examined in a special chair, it is important to subject the esophagus to fluoroscopy at some time, either at the same "sitting" or subsequently. The patient may have to be transferred from the chair onto the fluoroscopic table, since most chairs will not allow evaluation of the esophagus and most fluoroscopic units do not move down far enough to permit viewing of the entire esophagus with the patient in the chair.

Motility of the esophagus (i.e., peristalsis) can be assessed in the horizontal position only. In the erect position, the esophagus empties by gravity, not peristalsis. In the erect position, even an atonic esophagus (such as in scleroderma) will empty of barium by gravity unless there is a stricture or increased tone in the lower esophageal sphincter (such as achalasia). Other abnormalities in the esophagus (such as Schatzki's ring), may be evident only when the esophagus above and the hiatal hernia below it are distended in the right anterior oblique position with the patient prone over a bolster and continuous drinking (Figure 3.2) (8,9). For comparison of erect and horizontal findings in these conditions, see later: Table 3.9.

If Possible, the Examination Should Be Biphasic

A biphasic examination includes both dynamic recording (videofluorography on super-VHS tapes) for evaluation of function and double-contrast examination for mucosal detail (10,11). This type of study can really be performed only if the patient can safely swallow high-density barium and swallow rapidly. Thus it is contraindicated if the patient is found to have pharyngeal decompensations that preclude repetitive swallows (such as aspiration, retention from pharyngeal paresis). Under such circumstances more attention might be given to which consistencies and volumes of bolus the patient can safely swallow and which maneuvers (chin tuck, head rotation or tilt, supraglottic swallow, Mendelsohn maneuver, etc.) improve the safety of the swallow.

If the biphasic study is possible, the double-contrast technique may show mucosal lesions not suspected on a single contrast swallow. Also, it has been shown that the double-contrast technique is easier to perform than the single-contrast technique and is both more sensitive and more accurate than the combination of single-contrast radiography and videofluorography in the diagnosis of pharyngeal tumors (10). The double-contrast technique is recommended for lesions of the base of the tongue (11).

Dynamic recording allows the frame-by-frame analysis necessary to evaluate a motility disturbance (Table 3.5). This is easily accomplished by hooking up a link between the fluoroscopic foot pedal or hand switch and an S-VHS recorder such that when the fluoroscope is on, the VCR automatically records the fluoroscopic image. This represents recording at 30 frames/s, which allows optimal visualization and allows slow frame-by-frame analysis as well as backup and reverse analysis.

The 100 or 105 mm spot film camera with maximum frame rates of 6 to 8 frames/s is unfortunately inadequate in the evaluation of many patients with swallowing disorders. In many cases a lesion may be seen only briefly; for example, a lesion such as a web, or a cleft

3. The Tailored Examination

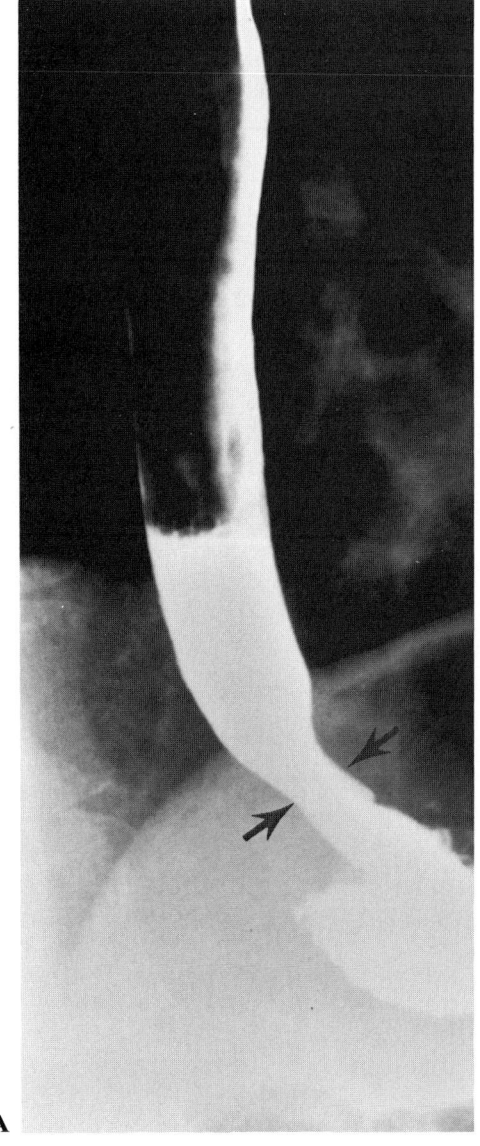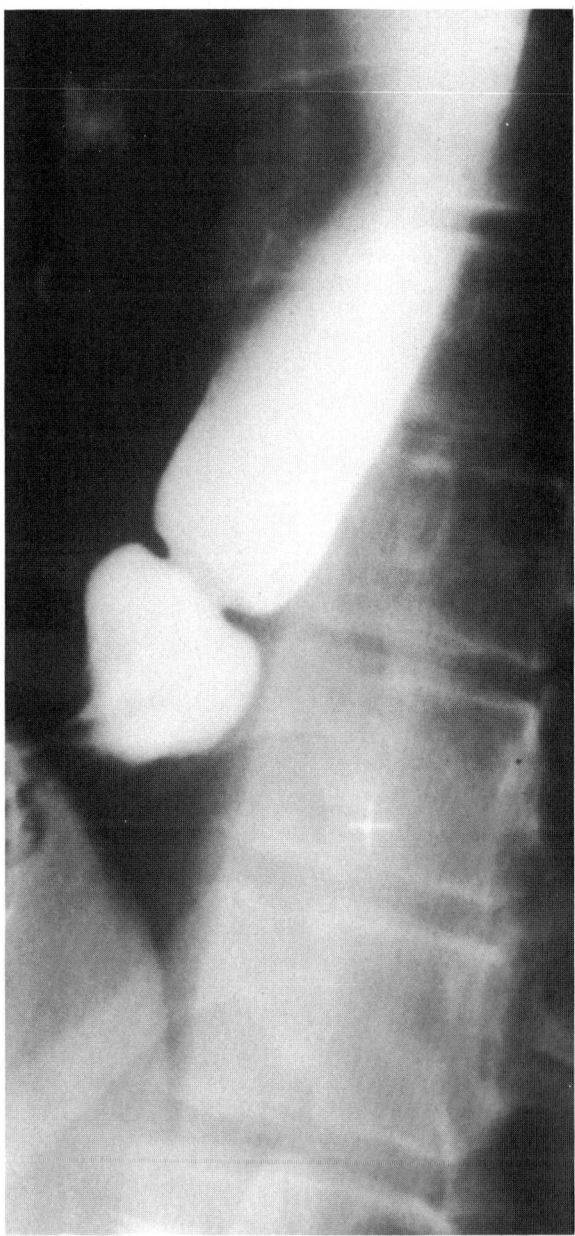

FIGURE 3.2. Schatzki's ring. (A) The erect left posterior oblique view, with the patient gulping barium following gas powder, shows no evidence of luminal narrowing or a ring in either the distal esophagus or the submerged segment of the esophagus (arrows). (B) In the prone oblique view, with the patient over a bolster, there is an obvious Schatzki's ring above a small sliding hiatal hernia. The ring measured a maximal luminal diameter of 12 mm and was clinically significant.

(Figure 3.3), may be present on only one or two frames of a continuous sequence. The continuous movement of the individual structures cannot be perceived at a rate of 6 to 8 frames/s. See Table 3.6 for common reasons for failure of diagnosis.

TABLE 3.5. The value of dynamic imaging.

Allows assessment of individual structures in real time, slow motion, backup mode, and frame by frame
Abnormality (e.g., web) may be visible only transiently
Subtle (but clinically significant) aspiration may be missed on fluoroscopy

TABLE 3.6. Reasons for failure of diagnosis.

Restricting examination to symptomatic area
Failure to use dynamic imaging
Failure to reassess if symptoms change

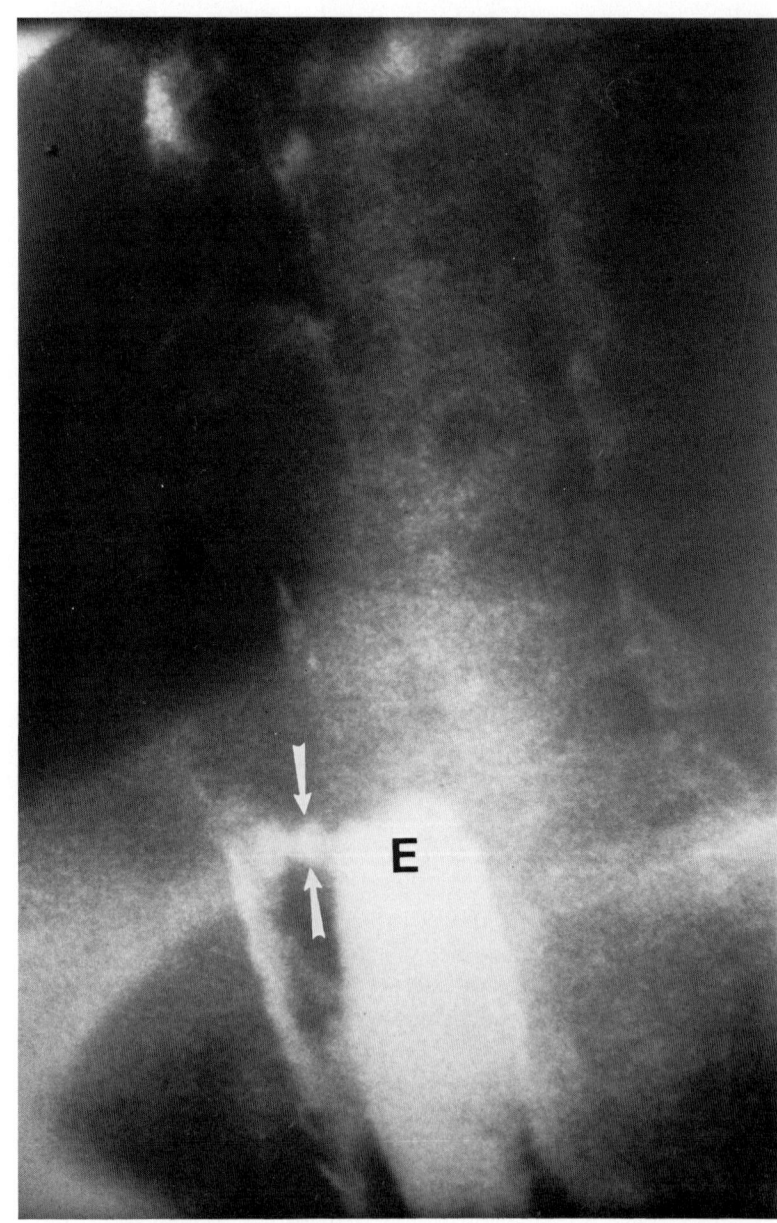

FIGURE 3.3. Tracheo-esophageal fistula. A stop-frame print from a 16mm movie demonstrates a whiff of contrast passing from the proximal thoracic esophagus (E) into the trachea (arrows). This was visible only on a few frames and would undoubtedly have been missed with spot filming. It was only evident when the film was reviewed in slow motion.

If a biphasic study is possible, the following "routine" is suggested by the author.

Suggested Routine

1. *Erect lateral* (with high-density barium unless contraindicated by history or clinical evaluation).

   a. *Movement of the soft palate and tongue* is observed while the patient enunciates the word "candy" and the letter "e." The superior surface of the soft palate can be coated for better visualization by intranasal instillation of barium through a small catheter while the patient sniffs.

   b. One swallow is recorded, centered high for evaluation of tongue, soft palate, and proximal pharyngeal structure and function.

   c. A second swallow is recorded, centered lower down to include the larynx, the distal pharynx, and the cervical esophagus.

   d. An optional oblique view during swallowing may be useful in stocky, broad-shouldered individuals to permit visualization of the cricopharyngeus and the cervical esophagus.

   e. Spot films are made of the barium-coated pharynx at rest and during phonation of a prolonged "eee" (Figure 3.4; see also later: Figures 3.8–3.10) (12).

2. *Upright frontal* (high-density barium) (pharynx).

   a. *Vocal cord movement*: say "ee" for adduction, sniff for retraction.

   b. Two swallows are recorded to distend the pharynx.

   c. Spot films are made of the barium-coated, air-filled pharynx, one at rest and one during a Valsalva maneuver (blowing up a balloon or saying "oooo") (Figures 3.5 and 3.6).

3. *Upright LPO* (left posterior oblique with high-density barium). Double-contrast views of the esophagus. Gulp barium rapidly, or gulp barium rapidly immediately following gas powder, washed down with a few milliliters of water.

4. *Prone oblique* RAO (right anterior oblique with thin barium) for:

   a. One or two single swallows to assess esophageal peristalsis.

   b. Continuous drinking of large mouthfuls for distended single-contrast views of the esophagus (over a bolster). Remember that some lesions (such as a Schatzki's ring) may be evident only during continuous drinking and straining (8,9) (Figure 3.3). An additional spot film can be made of the collapsed, coated esophagus; this mucosal relief view is excellent for demonstrating esophagitis and varices (although smaller varices may be better seen when the esophagus is empty but relaxed) (13).

   c. Check for gastroesophageal reflux. Significant reflux may be seen after the patient has turned from the prone to the supine position. Or turn the patient onto the right side, cough or perform Valsalva maneuver, and return to the supine position.

   If the history strongly suggests gastroesophageal reflux and this has not been demonstrated, a water siphon test can be performed (14–16).

5. *Stomach* (upright LPO).

   a. For air-distended fundus. However, fluoroscopy of the entire stomach is important with additional views of the stomach if any abnormality is seen. For example, Halpert et al. reported three patients with gastric carcinoma involving the antrum who presented with dysphagia as their predominant symptom (17).

   b. Check for delayed gastric emptying. Patients with gastric atony or outlet obstruction may present with reflux refractory to treatment. Delay in gastric emptying may make the treatment of gastroesophageal reflux more difficult.

See Table 3.7 for important technical factors and Chapter 1 for estimated radiation dosages from these swallowing studies.

Tailoring the Examination

Stress the Patient to Demonstrate Subtle Abnormalities

Vary the Head or Body Position

1. The **supine** position (ideally with cross-table fluoroscopy) may demonstrate previously unsuspected *premature leakage* into the oropharynx prior to swallowing (by stressing the tongue-palate seal) or *nasal regurgitation* (by stressing the soft palate–Passavant's cushion seal).

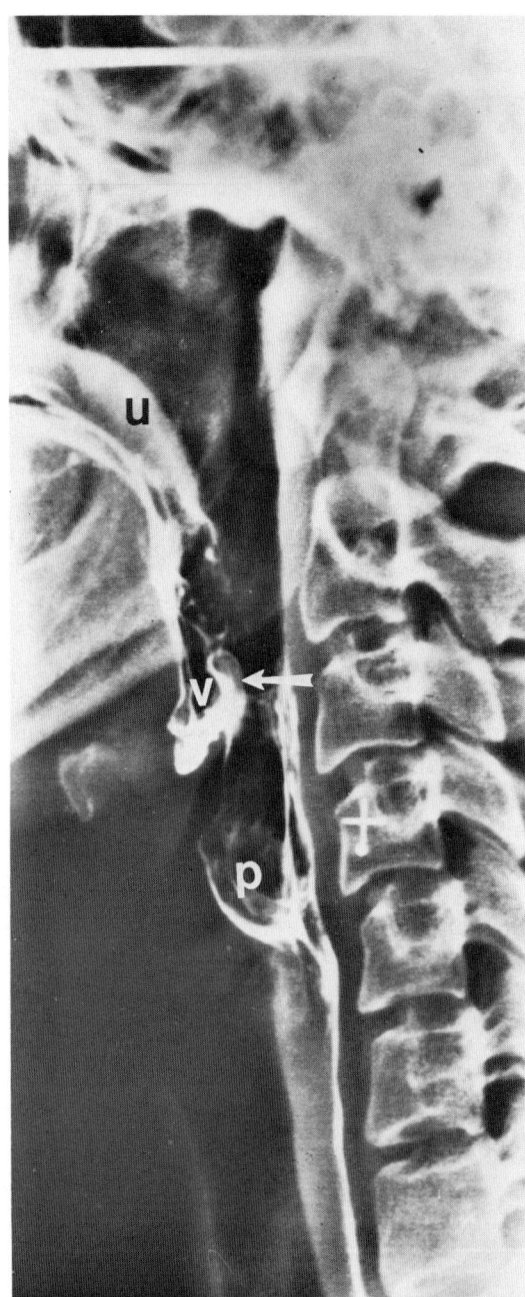
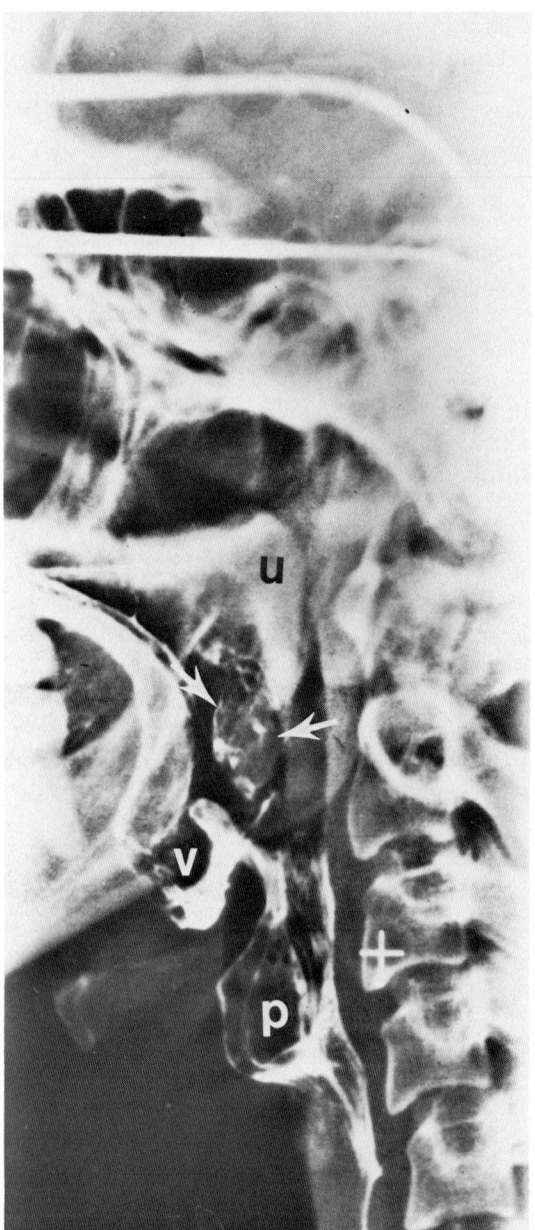

FIGURE 3.4. Lateral spot films at rest and during phonation. (A) The barium-coated pharynx at rest is not distended, and it is difficult to appreciate mucosal detail. The epiglottis (arrow) is seen clearly but the valleculae (v) and piriform sinus (p) are not well distended. The soft palate (u) abuts the tongue. (B) During phonation of a prolonged "eee," the tongue base moves forward, opening the valleculae (v) and expanding the piriform sinus (p). The soft palate (u) elevates to a right angle, revealing the tonsillar fossa; the tonsil is outlined (arrows).

3. The Tailored Examination

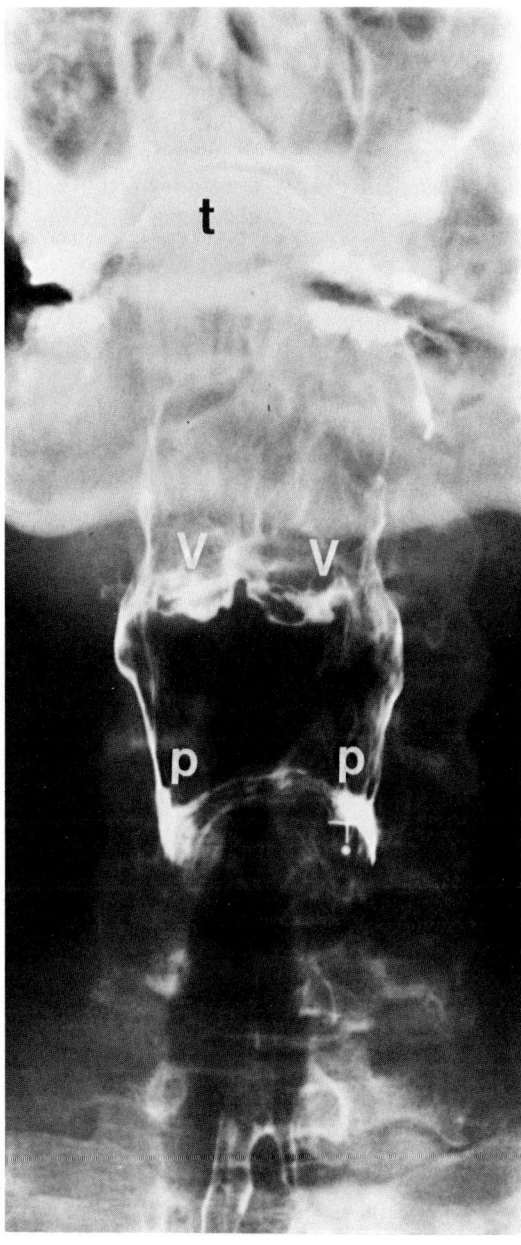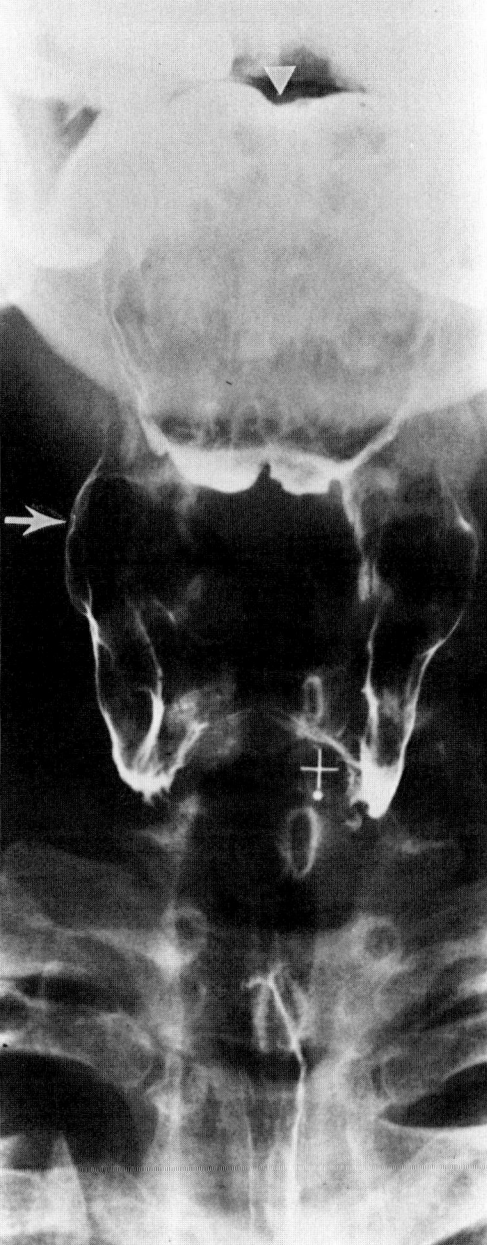

FIGURE 3.5. Anteroposterior pharynx at rest and during Valsalva manuever. (A) The barium-coated pharynx at rest shows the valleculae (V) and the piriform sinuses (p). The epiglottis cannot be clearly defined. The tongue (t) can also be seen outlined by contrast. (B) In the Valsalva maneuver the walls of the piriform sinus bulge out laterally in a symmetrical fashion. The area above the support of the thyroid cartilage bulges out slightly more (arrow). Note the midline groove in the tongue during the Valsalva maneuver (arrowhead). (Reproduced with permission from Jones B, Gayler BW, Donner MW. The pharynx and cervical esophagus. In: Levine MS, ed. *Radiology of the Esophagus*. Philadelphia: WB Saunders: 1989.)

2. The **semisupine** position may assist in swallowing in certain instances. If the patient's head rests against the machine, neck muscles usually involved in the maintenance of head and neck posture may be recruited into helping laryngeal and pharyngeal elevation, thus enabling a more effective swallow.

3. The **prone-oblique** position may demonstrate subtle tongue or pharyngeal constrictor weakness by pitting these muscles against gravity. Remember that if there is weakness of pharyngeal constrictors identified in the erect position it may be dangerous to put the patient into the prone horizontal position. If the beneficial effect of gravity is removed, the patient may decompensate and a weak but compen-

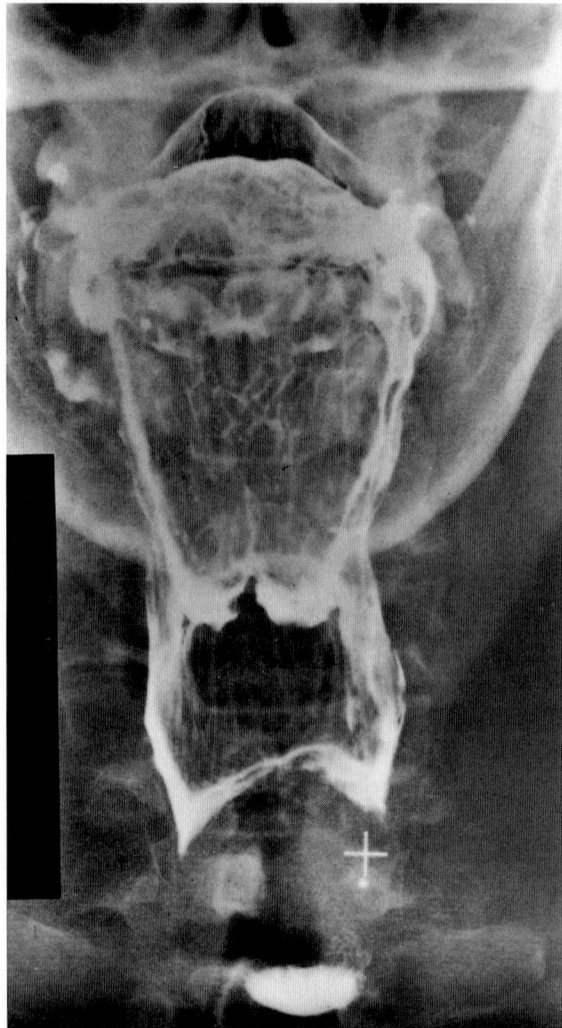 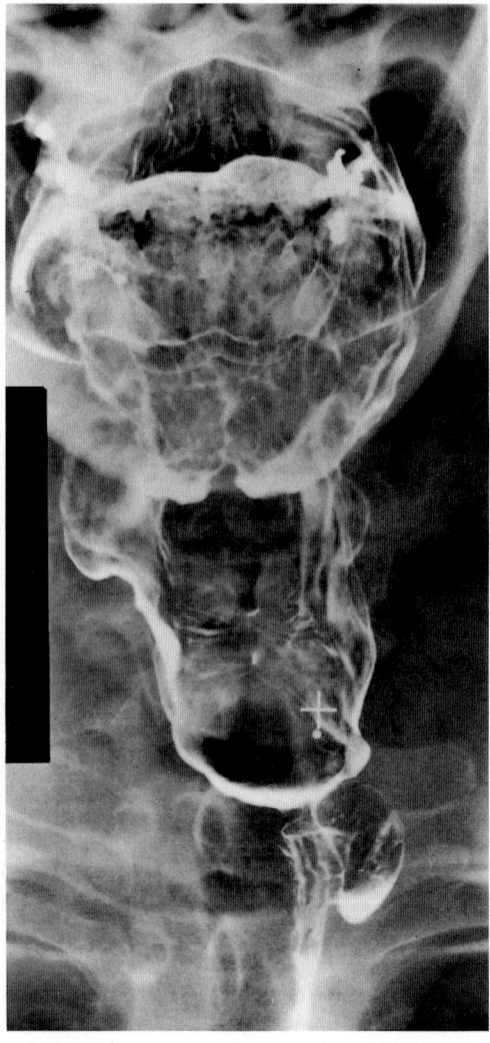

FIGURE 3.6. Value of insufflation. A frontal film (A) at rest and (B) during Valsalva maneuver. The Valsalva maneuver demonstrates normal bulging on the right side of the pharynx. Deformity and lack of distensibility on the left are due to scarring following resection of the left lobe of the thyroid. The frontal film at rest (A) is completely normal. There is also a lateral diverticulum at the pharyngoesophageal junction (arrow).

TABLE 3.7. Important technical factors.

> The patient's head must be straight (may be necessary to support during study).
> Careful collimation and centering.
> Do not "pan" too much or too fast.
> Videotape fluoroscopy for pharynx and esophagus.
> Cross-table fluoroscopy is useful in the debilitated or neurologically impaired patient.

sated swallow without aspiration may become one with severe aspiration in the horizontal position. Similarly, the right anterior oblique position (the common position for evaluating esophageal motility and single contrast evaluation of stricture) turns the head to the left, so if there is unilateral weakness on the right side of the pharynx, this position is contraindicated and the left anterior oblique position (which turns the head to the right) is preferable and safer.

4. It is more difficult to swallow with the **head in extension** because neck muscles are under tension in this position and the larynx has to rise further than in the neutral or flexed position. Also it has been shown that the lumen at the upper esophageal sphincter level is significantly narrower in the extended position than in the flexed position (18,19).

Extension may demonstrate abnormalities such as laryngeal penetration or retention not present in the neutral or flexed position. Conversely, head flexion (chin-tuck) during swallowing often improves swallowing; this is a common conscious or unconscious compensation in many patients with swallowing difficulty and is used extensively in swallowing therapy (see Chapter 14 for more head positioning used in therapy).

5. **Repetitive swallowing**: fatigue or signs of decompensation on rapid repetitive swallowing (such as retention or laryngeal penetration or aspiration) may be the only finding in early myasthenia gravis (20). "Fatigue," however, is not specific to myasthenia; many debilitated patients will tire over the course of a swallowing study.

Vary the Bolus Consistency or Characteristics

Solid Bolus

A solid bolus should be given if a subtle stricture, or solid-induced spasm, is suspected, or if a patient with symptoms of solid food dysphagia has a normal study with liquid barium. A solid bolus, however, should be given with caution to the patient with pharyngeal decompensation, especially if pharyngeal retention indicating pharyngeal weakness is seen with liquids. If laryngeal penetration or aspiration is seen with liquids, purée may be given first (sometimes with chin-tuck position), and depending on how the purée is handled, it may be possible to proceed with a small solid bolus.

Remember that patients with a neurological process involving the pharynx often cannot handle liquids without aspiration and actually may do better with thicker liquids and/or purée or solids (from the point of view of aspiration). However, if there is also pharyngeal paresis or decreased or absent tongue thrust the thicker boluses may result in increasing retention in the valleculae and piriform sinuses with the potential for overflow aspiration.

Examples of solid boluses include bread or bagel soaked in barium as advocated by Curtis et al. (21,22), barium paste on a cookie (graham cracker or Lorna Doone cookie), or Pill (12.5mm diameter, Bar-Test, Wolf Glenwood, Inc., New Jersey). The patient should be instructed not to chew the tablet but to swallow it "like an aspirin." Momentary holdup is to be expected at sites of normal anatomical narrowing such as cricopharyngeus, aortic arch, left main stem bronchus, left atrium, and gastroesophageal junction, but prolonged holdup through several swallows of water is abnormal (21,22). With prolonged holdup and no obvious narrowing previously noted, another swallow of thin barium should be given to see if there is *solid-induced spasm*.

Different Bolus Consistencies

Some patents have "bolus-specific dysphagia" and can safely swallow certain consistencies of bolus, whereas laryngeal penetration occurs with other consistencies (Figure 3.7). "Thin" barium, thick barium (high density), barium paste, barium paste mixed with applesauce to a purée, rice pudding, or graham crackers or Lorna Doone cookies are several possible consistencies.

Logemann advocates a technique known as the "modified barium swallow" in which very small volumes of liquid barium ($^1/_3$ teaspoon), barium paste (Esophatrast, $^1/_3$ teaspoon), and a cookie coated with Esophatrast ($^1/_4$ small cookie) are given to the patient (23). This approach, she feels, minimizes the risk of aspiration, but I prefer to stress the patient with larger volumes such as 5 and 10 mL and, presuming no aspiration with those boluses, with cup drinking and drinking through a straw. Otherwise the risk of aspiration during drinking and eating may be underestimated.

Sometimes we begin the examination with a small volume of Omnipaque and then move on to other bolus consistencies, beginning with what is felt to be the "safest" bolus (based on the clinical evaluation or swallowing history).

Recently several manufacturers have been working on test kits for swallowing evaluation. Food scientists are working on making puréed food more palatable and appealing to the eye as well as more varied in taste. The National Dysphagia Diet Project effort involves food scientists, speech-language pathologists, nutritionists, and dysphagia diet manufacturers, to name just a few (24).

Acidify the Barium Sulfate
(the Acid Barium Swallow)

To acidify $BaSO_4$, 0.5 mL of concentrated hydrochloric acid (37%) is added to 100 mL of single-contrast barium (such as Barosperse) in a glass beaker; this produces a pH of 1.6 to 1.7.

This test is a provocative one and is meant to reproduce what happens to the esophagus in the person whose esophagus has been regularly bathed with barium. The esophagus is then supposed to become acid sensitive and to respond with a motility abnormality.

Authorities, however, differ regarding the significance of a positive test. There is some correlation with gastroesophageal reflux and reflux esophagitis (25,26).

The test itself is as follows. Three swallows of the acidified barium are given to "sensitize" the esophagus; a fourth swallow is then observed fluoroscopically. The test is considered to be positive (an "acid-sensitive esophagus") if transient aperistalsis, spasm, or disorganized peristalsis is observed, or if the patient develops chest pain (25). An antacid such as Maalox is given to the patient after the acidified barium to counter its effect.

Chill the Barium

Esophageal motility may be normal with room temperature barium sulfate, whereas aperistalsis may occur with chilled barium. Ott, Gelfand, and their colleagues have advocated the use of chilled barium in double-contrast esophagography because it reduces primary peristalsis and improves distension of the lower esophagus and esophagogastric region (27), thus improving visualization of these areas.

In myotonic dystrophy, myotonia may develop in the pharynx only with chilled barium (28). We have seen two patients who complained of pain or dysphagia with cold liquids in whom esophageal spasm rather than aperistalsis was produced by chilled barium (personal observation).

Use of a Syringe or Spoon

The debilitated or neurologically impaired patient may be unable to drink through a straw or from a cup. A syringe attached to extension

FIGURE 3.7. Bolus-specific laryngeal penetration. (A) With thin liquid barium there is laryngeal penetration during swallowing (arrow). Contrast is seen entering the open, air-filled laryngeal vestibule (arrowheads) under the incompletely tilted epiglottis. Note also the squared-off valleculae (V), a sign of pharyngeal weakness. Posteriorly air is mixing with the barium bolus, producing a flow defect in the barium column. (B) With barium paste (Esophatrast), there is no laryngeal penetration because the bolus stays in a more condensed form. Note, however, that the laryngeal vestibule is still not closed, there being air in the laryngeal vestibule (arrows). Note also minimal nasal regurgitation (black arrow).

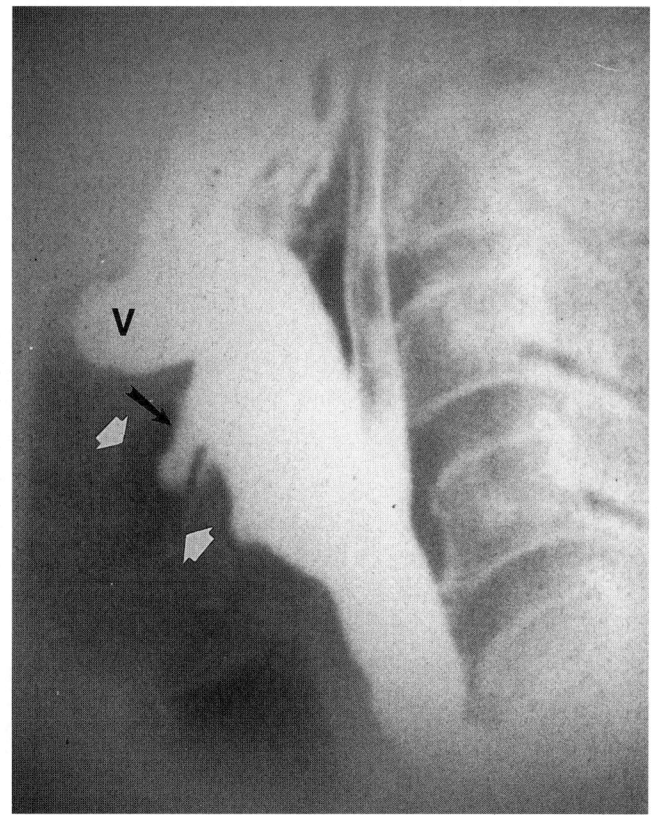

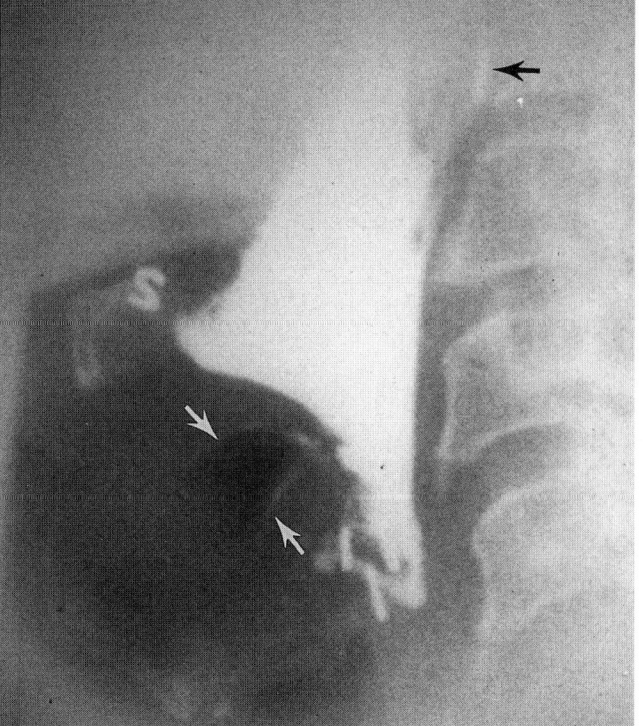

tubing can be used to insert small boluses (2–5 mL) directly into the mouth. Be sure to put the tip of the extension tubing into the front of the mouth; otherwise, the oral stage will be bypassed.

Conversely, of course, if the oral stage is compromised (by disease or surgery) it may be decided to try to bypass the oral stage by placing the tubing in the back of the mouth or by placing a glossectomy spoon in the back of the mouth.

These techniques should be used with caution: if tongue-palate competence is compromised, contrast will leak over the dorsum of the tongue into the pharynx prior to initiation of swallowing; this may then penetrate the unprotected larynx. Do not use water-soluble hypertonic agents, such as Gastrografin.

Spot Films of the Pharynx

Frontal and Lateral Views

Frontal and lateral double-contrast films are important to assess structure of the mouth and pharynx. Oblique films can give additional information under some circumstances, especially in the evaluation of the extent of a head and neck cancer.

Just as anywhere else in the gastrointestinal tract, it is important to take films at rest and during distension. In the frontal view this can be obtained during insufflation and in the lateral during phonation.

Insufflation (Valsalva)

The insufflated view will reveal asymmetry during distension, thus demonstrating areas with poor or absent distensibility (scarring, infiltration) or excessive distensibility (weakness) (Figure 3.6).

The Lateral View with Phonation

The lateral view at rest is really a partially collapsed view. Phonation distends the pharynx in an anteroposterior plane. This view is superior to one taken with the pharynx at rest in showing certain areas such as the tonsillar fossa, the base of the tongue, the aryepiglottic folds (12). During phonation (a prolonged "eee"), the soft palate elevates to appose Passavant's cushion, thus revealing the tonsillar fossa, which cannot be seen at rest or with bolus in the mouth, when the free edge of the soft palate rests against the dorsum of the tongue (Figures 3.4, 3.8–3.10). The undersurface of the elevated soft palate may also be seen better during phonation (Figure 3.8B). Phonation also causes the tongue to move forward, increasing the size of the valleculae and straightening the aryepiglottic folds (Figure 3.9). The maneuver also stretches the posterior wall of the pharynx and nodules in that area may become more obvious with prolonged phonation (Figure 3.10).

The Tube Esophagogram

The tube esophagogram is a relatively easy technique that is indicated in two different clinical situations: severe pharyngeal decompensation and question of tracheoesophageal fistula.

Severe Pharyngeal Compromise

In the presence of severe aspiration, the examination may be prematurely terminated because of the fear of further aspiration of contrast into the lungs. Furthermore, these patients cannot drink rapidly and repetitively enough to adequately distend the esophagus. The esophageal portion of the evaluation can then be performed by utilizing a tube esophagogram (29,30).

A small tube (red rubber catheter) is inserted into the esophagus and its tip positioned slightly above the aortic arch via mouth or nose, followed by injection of barium and/or air into the esophageal lumen. A peristaltic wave will be produced by esophageal distension (secondary peristalsis) and acceptable single and/or double-contrast views can be obtained by further injection of barium and air (Figure 3.11).

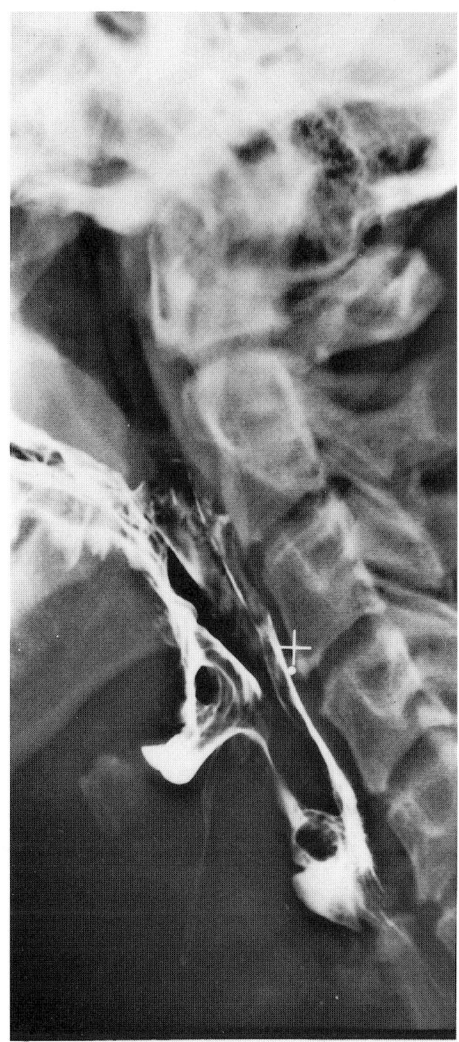 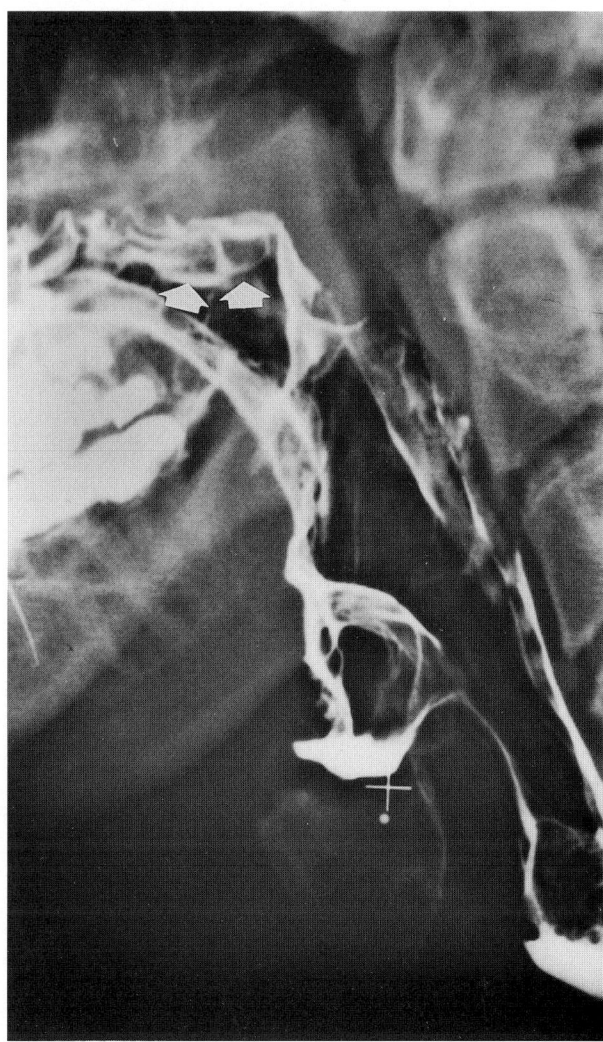

FIGURE 3.8. Value of phonation in diagnosis. (A) At rest, the soft palate abuts the tongue. No evidence of tumor can be seen. (B) During phonation, irregularity of the inferior surface of the elevated soft palate can be appreciated (arrows). Biopsy-proven Kaposi's sarcoma (KS).

Tracheoesophageal Fistula

The esophageal tube technique is also useful in cases of suspected tracheoesophageal fistula. Although this is an uncommon problem in the adult population, such a fistula is potentially fatal and may not be considered or may be misdiagnosed as aspiration. The tube should be positioned low in the distal esophagus and contrast (thin barium) injected as the tube is slowly withdrawn. Careful fluoroscopic monitoring is necessary to detect early filling of the tracheobronchial tree and so differentiate a fistula from overflow aspiration.

Radionuclide Scintigraphy

The technique of radionuclide scintigraphy, which can be used for the evaluation of pharyngeal and esophageal emptying as well as in the evaluation of aspiration, is outside the scope of this text.

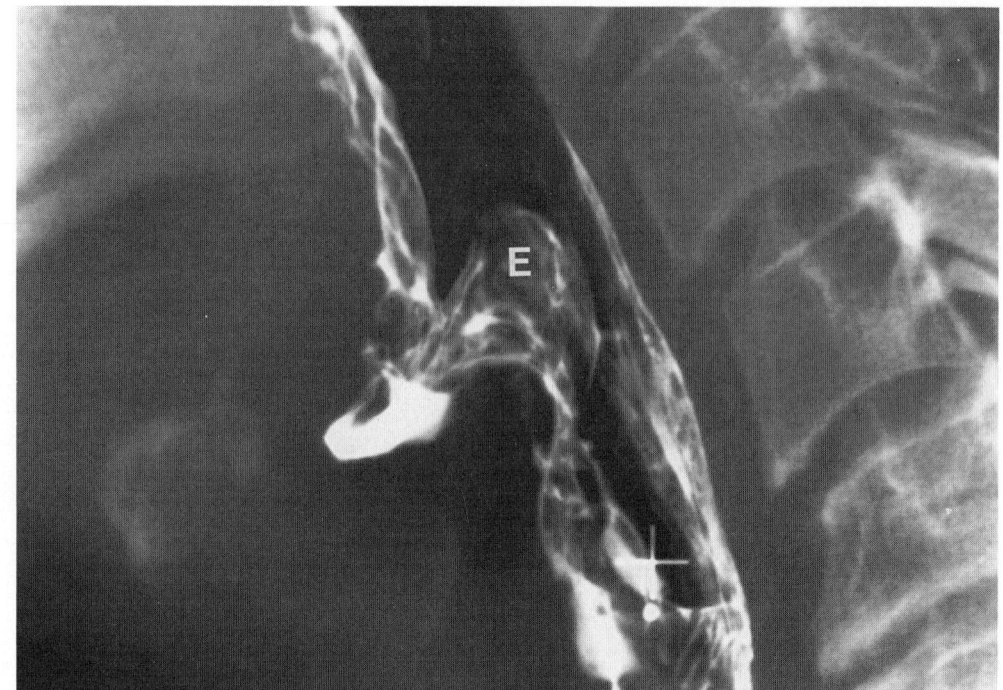

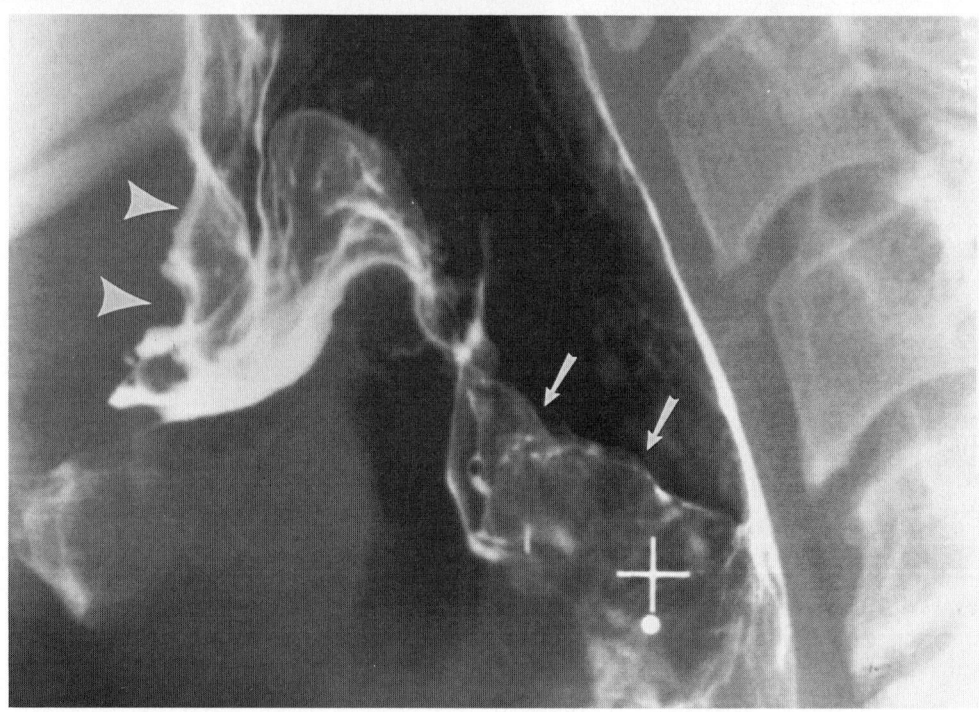

FIGURE 3.9. Another example of the value of phonation in diagnosis. (A) Lateral view of the pharynx coated with barium shows no real evidence of any tumor mass. There is thickening of the epiglottis (E) but no real evidence of any mass lesion. (B) When the patient phonates, there is obvious thickening of the epiglottis due to tumor invasion extending into one of the aryepiglottic folds seen as nodularity (arrows). There are also tumor nodules in the base of the tongue and the valleculae (arrowheads). (Reprinted with permission from Rubesin SE, Jones B, Donner MW. Contrast pharyngography: the value of phonation. *AJR Am J Roentgenol* 1987;148:269–272.)

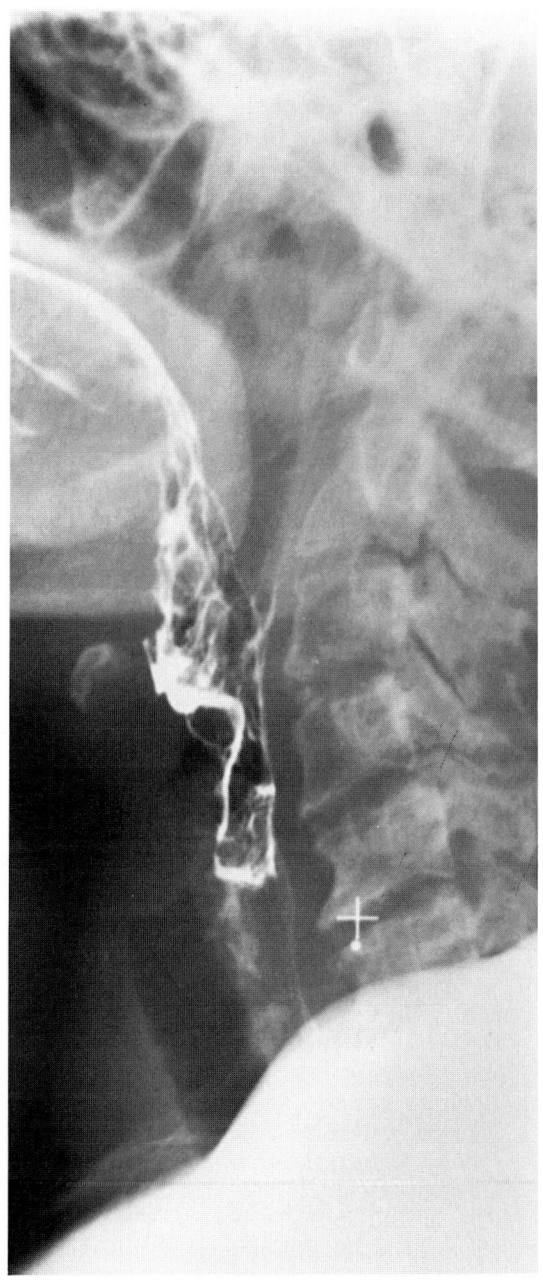 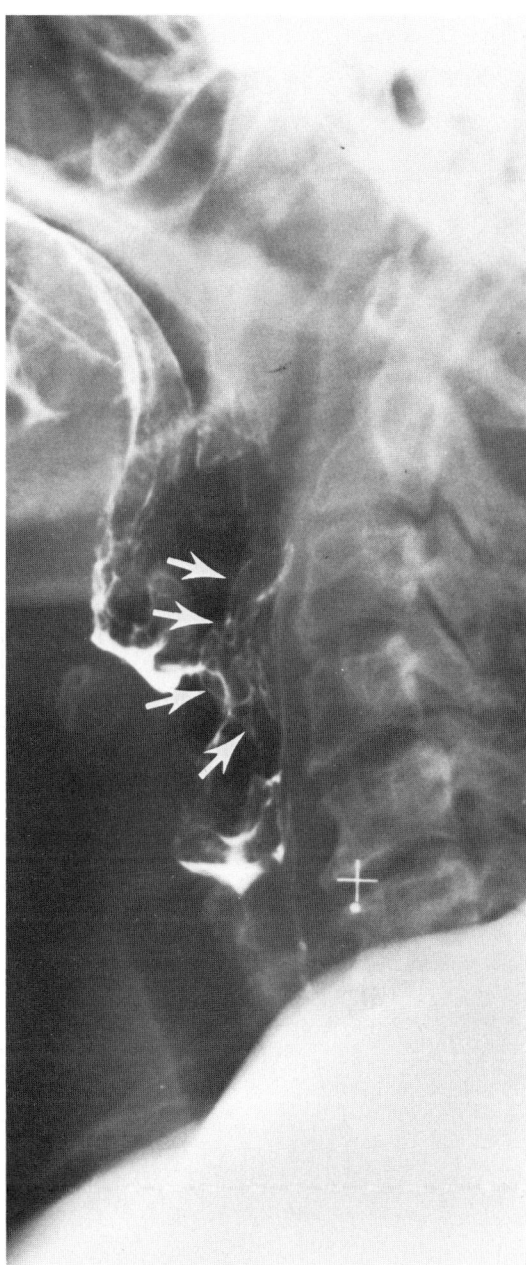

FIGURE 3.10. Further example of the value of phonation in diagnosis. (A) There is no suggestion of any mass lesion in the posterior wall of the pharynx on the view at rest. (B) With phonation, stretching and anterior movement of the pharynx, there is an obvious tumor nodule in the posterior wall (arrows). (Films courtesy of Dr. George P. Saba, Baltimore.)

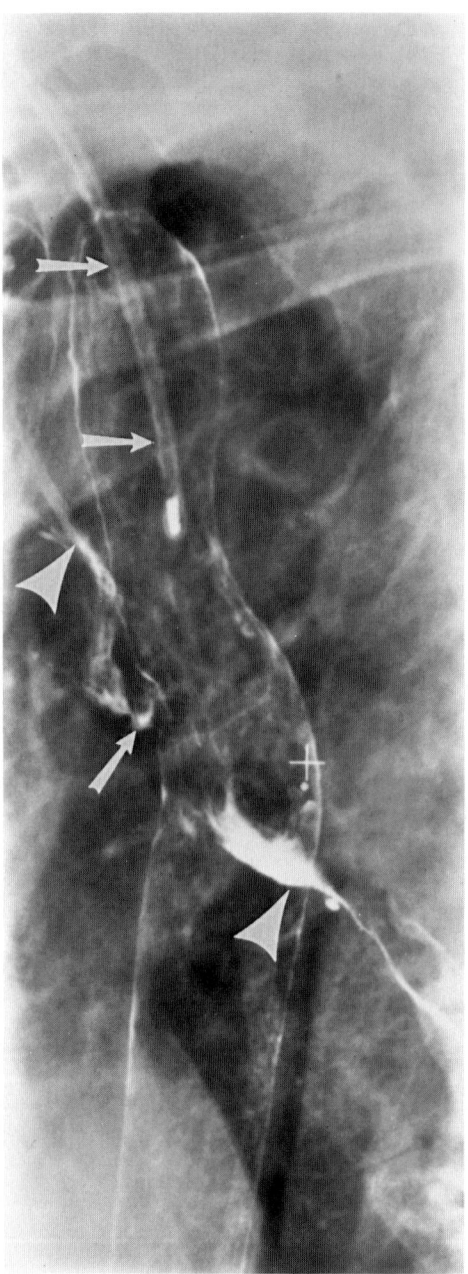

FIGURE 3.11. Tube esophagogram showing good coating and distension of the body of the esophagus following injection of high-density barium and air. The tube (horizontal arrows) is positioned high in the thoracic esophagus. There is also some contrast in bronchi (arrowheads) following aspiration (which prompted the tube study) and within a small diverticulum in the midesophagus (sloping arrow).

References

1. Jones B, Ravich WJ, Donner MW. Dysphagia in systemic disease. *Curr Imaging* 1991;3:158–171.
2. Kikendall JW, Friedman AC, Oyewole MA, et al. Pill-induced esophageal injury: case reports and review of the medical literature. *Dig Dis Sci* 1983;28:174–182.
3. Buchholz DW, Marsh BR. Multifactorial dysphagia—looking for a second, treatable cause. *Dysphagia* 1986;1(2): 88–90.
4. Jones B, Donner MW. Examination of the patient with dysphagia. *Radiology* 1988;167: 319–326.
5. Jones B, Kramer SS, Donner MW. Dynamic imaging of the pharynx. *Gastrointest Radiol* 1985;10:213–224.
6. Ekberg O, Nylander G. Double-contrast examination of the pharynx. *Gastrointest Radiol* 1985;10:263–271.
7. Edwards DAW. History and symptoms of esophageal disease. In: Vantrappen G, Hellemans J, eds. *Diseases of the Esophagus*. New York: Springer-Verlag; 1974.
8. Ott DJ, Gelfand DW, Wu WC, Castell DO. Esophagogastric region and its rings. *AJR Am J Roentgenol* 1984;142:281–287.
9. Chen YM, Ott DJ, Gelfand DW, Munitz HA. Multiphasic examination of the esophagogastric region for strictures, rings, and hiatal hernia: evaluation of the individual techniques. *Gastrointest Radiol* 1985;10:311–316.
10. Semenkovich JW, Balfe DM, Weyman PJ, Heiken JP, Lee JKT. Barium pharyngography: comparison of single and double contrast. *AJR Am J Roentgenol* 1985;144:715–720.
11. Apter AJ, Levine MS, Glick SN. Carcinomas of the base of the tongue: diagnosis using double-contrast radiography of the pharynx. *Radiology* 1984;151:123–126.
12. Rubesin SE, Jones B, Donner MW. Contrast pharyngography: the importance of phonation. *AJR Am J Roentgenol* 1987;148:269–272.
13. Cockerill EM, Miller RE, Chernish SM, McLaughlin GC III, Rodda BE. Optimal visualization of esophageal varices. *AJR Am J Roentgenol* 1976;126(3):512–523.
14. Linsman JF. Gastroesophageal reflux elicited while drinking water (water siphonage test): its clinical correlation with pyrosis. *AJR Am J Roentgenol* 1965;94:325–332.

15. Crummy AB. The water test in the evaluation of gastroesophageal reflux: its correlation with pyrosis. *Radiology* 1966;87:501–504.
16. Blumhagen JD, Christie DL. Gastroesophageal reflux in children: evaluation of the water siphon test. *Radiology* 1979;131:345–349.
17. Halpert RD, Spickler E, Feczko PJ. Dysphagia in patients with gastric cancer and a normal esophogram. *Radiology* 1985;154:589–591.
18. Ekberg O. Posture of the head and pharyngeal swallowing. *Acta Radiol Diagn* (*Stockh*) 1986;27(6):691–696.
19. Castell JA, Castell DO, Schultz AR, Georgeson S. Effect of head position on the dynamics of the upper esophageal sphincter and pharynx. *Dysphagia* 1993;8(1):1–6.
20. Silbiger ML, Pikheney R, Donner MW. Neuromuscular disorders affecting the pharynx: cineradiographic analysis. *Invest Radiol* 1967;2:442–448.
21. Curtis DJ, Cruess DF, Willgress ER. Normal solid bolus swallowing erect position. *Dysphagia* 1986;1:63–67.
22. Curtis DJ, Cruess DF, Willgress ER. Abnormal solid bolus swallowing in the erect position. *Dysphagia* 1987;2:46–49.
23. Logemann J. *Evaluation and Treatment of Swallowing Disorders*. Boston: College Hill Press; 1983:91.
24. Felt P. The National Dysphagia Diet Project: the science and practice. *Nutr Clini Pract* 1999;14(5):S60–S63.
25. Donner MW, Silbiger ML, Hookman R, Hendrix TR. Acid-barium swallows in the radiographic evaluation of clinical esophagitis. *Radiology* 1966;87:220–225.
26. McCall IW, Davieser ER, Delahunty JE. The acid-barium test as an index of intermittent gastro-oesophageal reflux. *Br J Radiol* 1973;46:578–584.
27. Ott DJ, Gelfand DW, Munitz HA, Chen YM. Cold barium suspensions in the clinical evaluation of the esophagus. *Gastrointest Radiol* 1984;9:193–196.
28. Bosma JF, Brodie DR. Cineradiographic demonstration of pharyngeal area myotonia in myotonic dystrophy patients. *Radiology* 1969;92:104–109.
29. Levine MS, Kressel HY, Laufer I, et al. The tube esophogram: a technique for obtaining a detailed double-contrast examination of the esophagus. *AJR Am J Roentgenol* 1974;142:711–714.
30. Halpert RD, Dubin L, Feczko PJ, Weitz J. Air contrast tube esophogram: technique and clinical examples. Technical note. *J Can Assoc Radiol* 1984;35:58–60.

4
Interpreting the Study

BRONWYN JONES

Radiographic Anatomy and Analysis of Function

The anatomy and physiology of swallowing were discussed in some depth in Chapter 2. However, it is important in this chapter to develop our knowledge of *radiographic* anatomy and the normal movements of individual structures that are analyzed in the radiographic study (such as tongue thrust, epiglottic tilt, hyoid elevation, etc.).

To understand the radiographic anatomy of the mouth and pharynx, it is essential to transpose what we know about the structure of the pharynx into the structures that are seen on a radiograph. Hence, sagittal and coronal anatomic line drawings are compared with corresponding radiographs (see Figures 4.1 and 4.2).

The functional aspects of the normal swallow can be seen in line drawings (Figure 4.3) and then in freeze-frame prints from a cinepharyngogram (Figure 4.4). The physiology of the normal swallow is presented in the accompanying legends as well as subsequently.

The interpretation will be approached from two aspects: functional or motion abnormalities, and anatomic or structural abnormalities. Functional abnormalities will be discussed first, followed by structural abnormalities in relation to specific anatomical areas.

Analysis of the Functional Aspects of Swallowing: The Videorecording

General Comments

In reviewing the examination, slow motion, backup, and stop-frame capability is essential. With these capabilities, the movement of individual structures may be observed, first in isolation, and then in combination with others. Individual structures that must be analyzed include tongue, palate, pharyngeal constrictor wave, epiglottis, hyoid and larynx, cricopharyngeus, and esophageal stripping wave. Each swallow may need to be analyzed several times to evaluate all the structures adequately in conjunction with the various radiographic signs (Table 4.1).

One must be familiar with the anatomy, the radiographic anatomy, and the physiology of the normal swallow (1–9), and one must be searching for signs of compensation and decompensation (see Chapter 5). In other words, sometimes it is necessary to look at the action of the structure; at other times it is what happens to the shape or position of the bolus that indicates abnormality. For example, does the bolus fragment? Does it pool in abnormal places such as floor of mouth or cheek? Is it misdirected, such as into the nasopharynx or larynx?

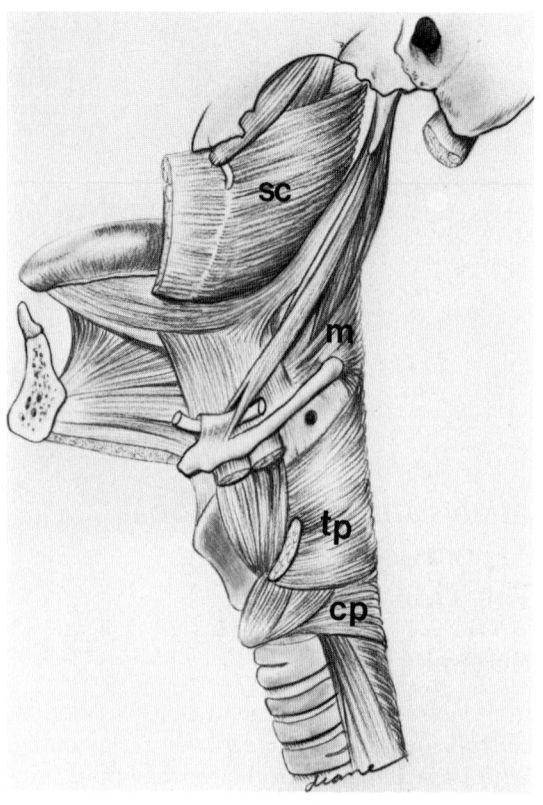
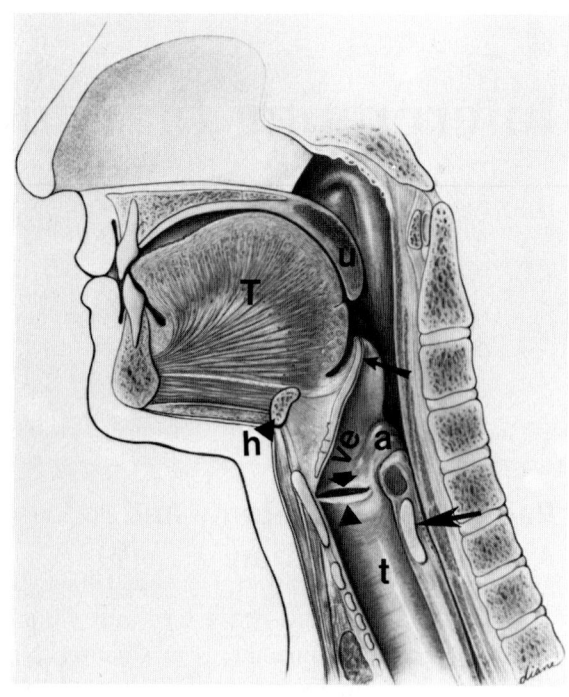

FIGURE 4.1. Lateral sagittal views of the pharynx comparing line drawings, plain films, and radiographs. (A) Line drawing indicates the constrictor and suspensory musculature of the pharynx viewed from the side. The constrictor muscles overlap, the inferior constrictor being the most external, the middle constrictor (m) in the middle layer, the superior (sc) the most internal. The inferior constrictor (ic) is continuous with the proximal circular muscle fibers of the esophagus and the fascicles of the cricopharyngeal (cp) portion of the inferior constrictor merge with the fascicles of the circular muscle of the esophagus (ce). (See also Figure 2.3, Chapter 2, for more in-depth labeling of anatomical structures.) (Reprinted with permission from Bosma JF, Donner MW, Tanaka E, Robertson D. Anatomy of the pharynx, pertinent to swallowing. *Dysphagia* 1986;1:23–33.) (B) Sagittal line drawing showing the structures in the sagittal plane including the tongue (T), soft palate (u), epiglottis (arrow), vestibule (ve), cords (false, arrow; true, arrowhead), arytenoid mass (a), cricoid cartilage (long arrow), and trachea (t). (Reprinted with permission from Donner MW, Bosma JF, Robertson DL. Anatomy and physiology of the pharynx. *Gastrointest Radiol* 1985;10:196–212.) (C) Lateral soft tissue view of the neck shows the corresponding structures, more clearly defines the valleculae (v) and the piriform sinus (p). Note the incomplete calcification of the thyroid cartilage (th), and the hyoid bone (h). (D) Lateral view of the pharynx, which has now been coated by high-density barium. One can now clearly see the soft palate (U), the dorsum of the tongue (T), the valleculae (v), the epiglottis (arrow), and the piriform sinus (p). There is minimal retention of contrast in the valleculae and piriform sinuses. (E) Lateral view during phonation, with the structures outlined by contrast. Note that the soft palate (U) has elevated to a right angle, revealing the tonsillar fossa (arrows), expanding the valleculae (V) and piriform sinus (P), and expanding the pharynx in the frontal plane.

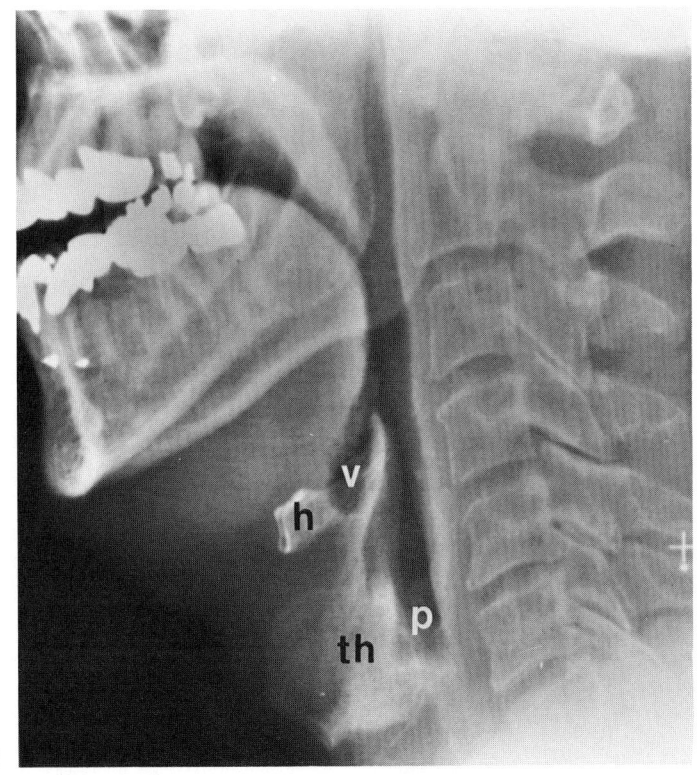

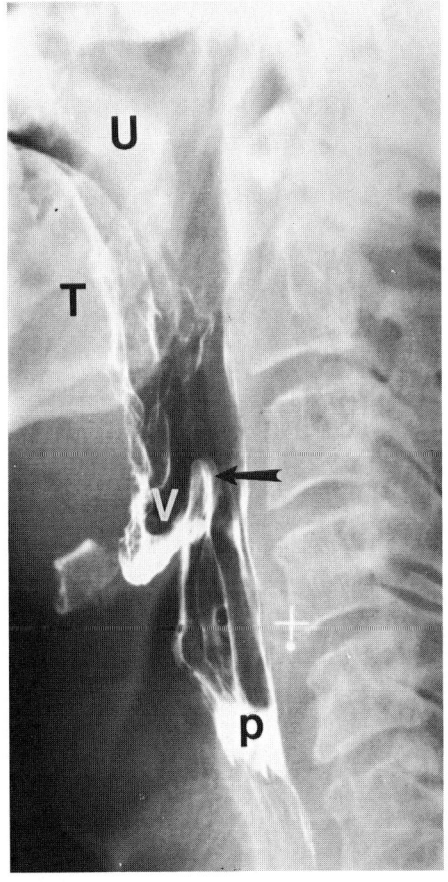

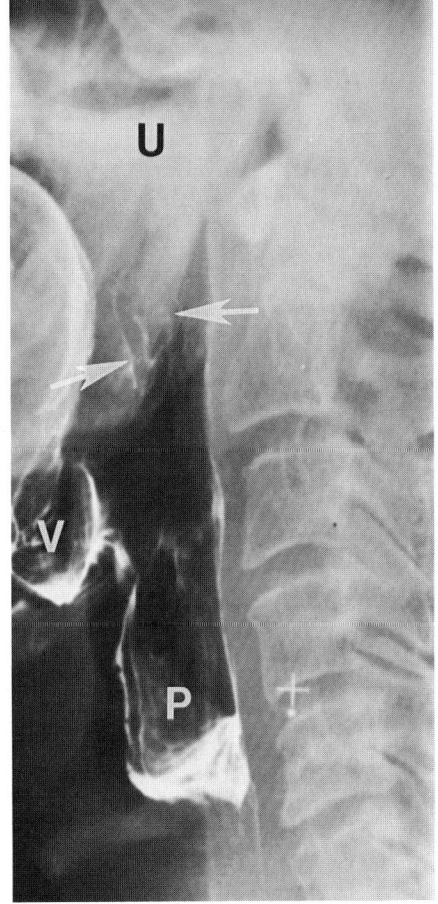

FIGURE 4.1. *Continued*

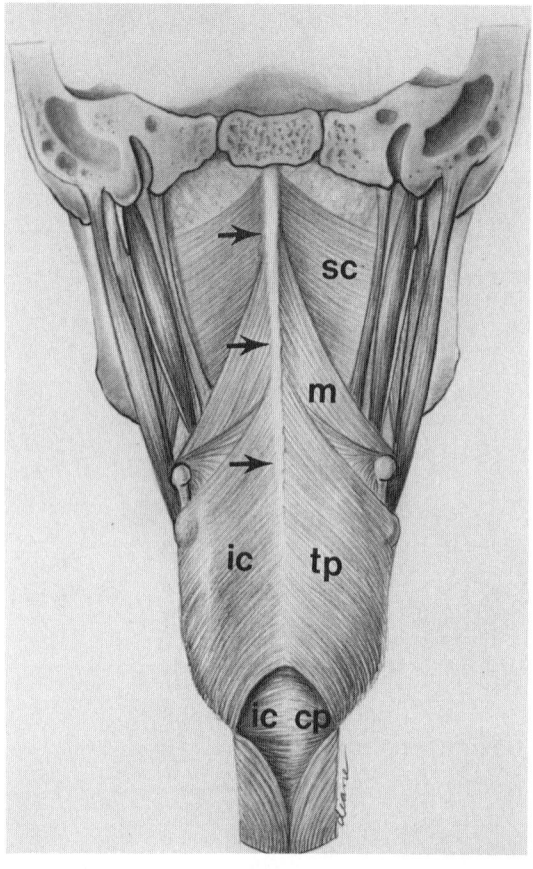 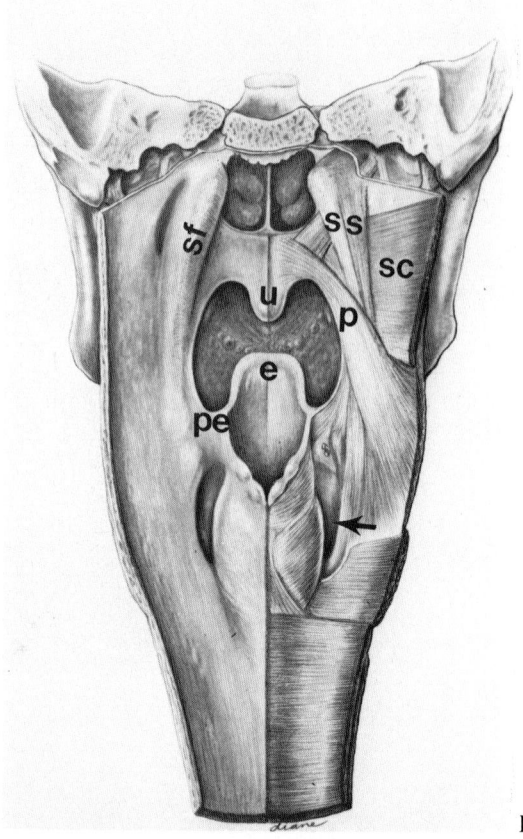

FIGURE 4.2. Comparisons can be made between line drawings and radiographs in the coronal (frontal) plane. (A) The constrictor and lateral suspensory muscles of the pharynx viewed from the posterior aspect: arrows, pharyngeal raphe; sc, superior constrictor; m, middle constrictor; ic, inferior constrictor; tp, thyropharyngeus; cp, cricopharyngeus. Note again that the constrictor muscles overlap, the inferior being the more external and the superior the more internal. Note, also, that the fibers of the cricopharyngeus or horizontal fibers of the inferior constrictor muscle merge with the fascicles of the proximal circular muscle of the esophagus. (B) The structures in the anterior wall of the pharynx as viewed from the posterior aspect: s, salpingopharyngeus; sf, salpingopharyngeal fold; sc, superior constrictor; p, palatopharyngeus; u, uvula; e, epiglottis; arrow, piriform sinus. The pharyngeal raphe and the posterior portion of the proximal cervical esophagus have been sectioned and each side drawn laterally to expose the structures. On the right side the mucosa has been stripped to demonstrate the underlying muscles, while on the left side, the mucosa remains intact. This drawing shows the contours of the valleculae and piriform sinuses and demonstrates the relationship of the valleculae to the base of the tongue and epiglottis. (Reproduced with permission from Donner MW, Bosma JF, Robertson DL. Anatomy and physiology of the pharynx. *Gastrointest Radiol* 1985;10:196–212.) (C) The pharynx has now been coated with high-density barium outlining the valleculae (v) and piriform sinuses (p). In this particular patient the epiglottis is not clearly visualized on this view at rest. (D) The patient demonstrates "blowing up a balloon," or a prolonged "oo" sound. The pharynx is now expanded especially in the region of the proximal portions of the piriform sinus. There is more symmetric distension proximally than distally because the superior portion lacks the support of the thyroid cartilage. (C and D, reproduced with permission from Jones B, Donner MW. Examination of the patient with dysphagia. *Radiology* 1988;167:319–326.)

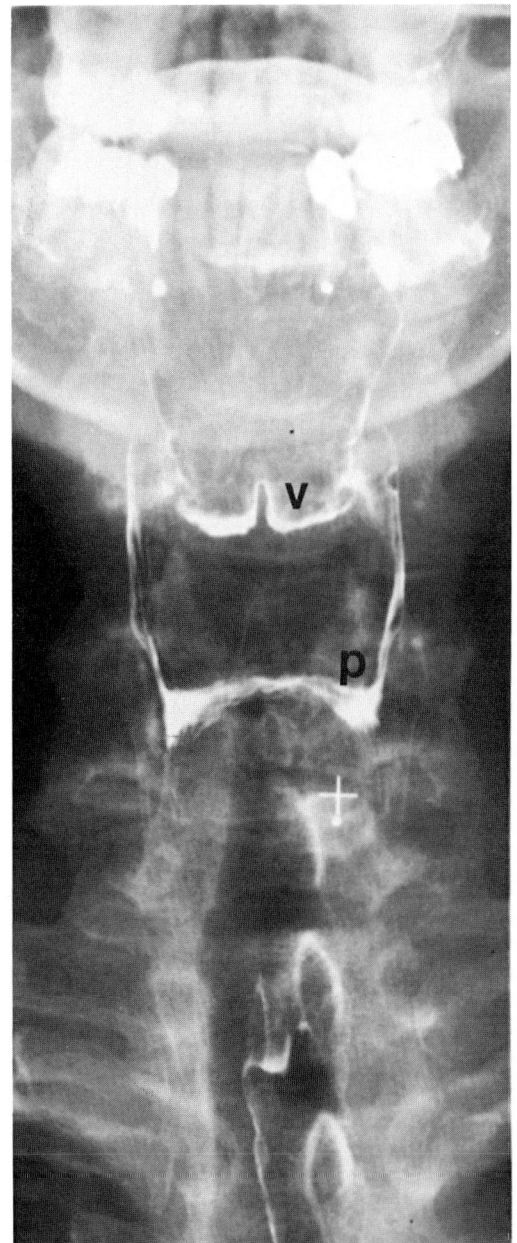
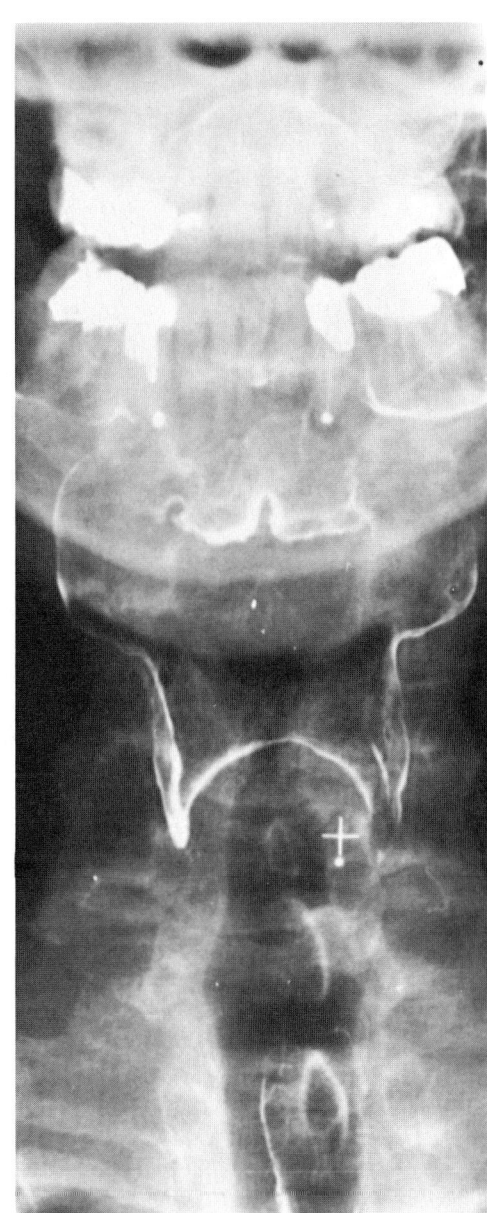

FIGURE 4.2. *Continued*

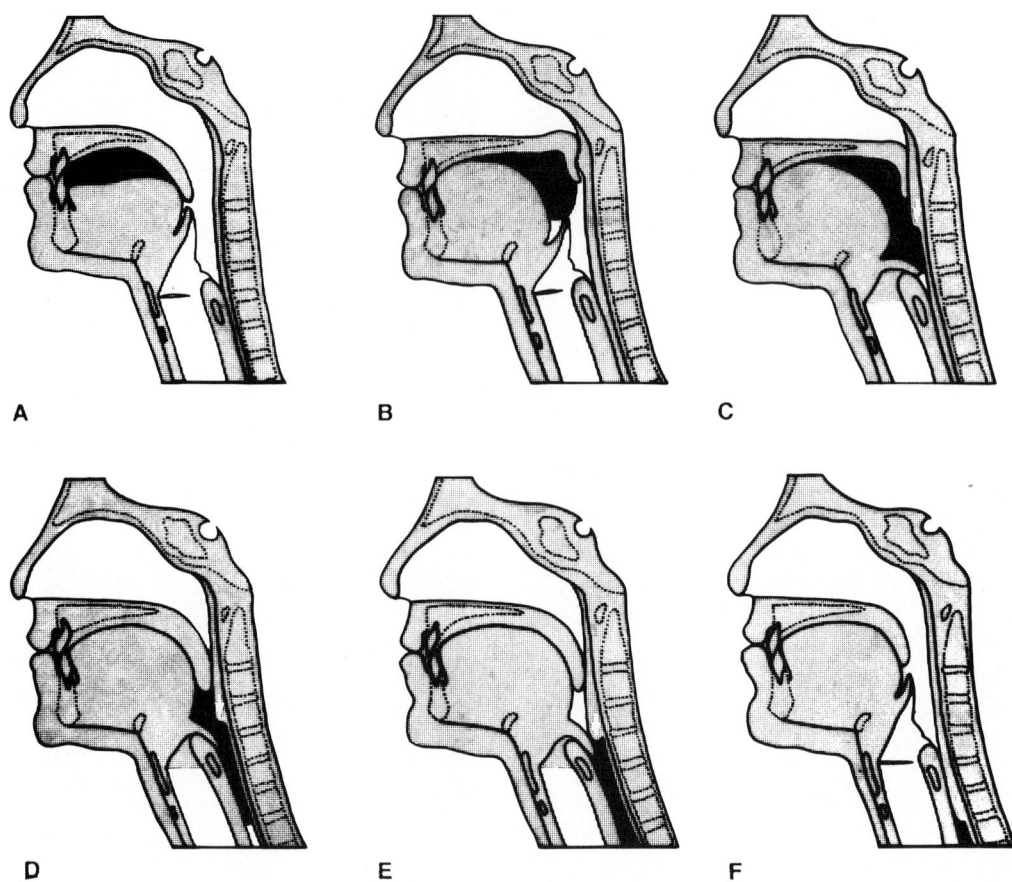

FIGURE 4.3. Line drawing of the normal swallow. (A) Bolus is held in the oral cavity by apposition of soft palate and tongue with the surrounding laryngeal structures and airway at rest. (B) Bolus is conveyed into the oropharynx by the tongue and the soft palate has elevated. The airway and surrounding larynx have elevated in preparation for swallow. (C) Bolus is descending into the hypopharynx on either side of the cricoid prominence. The larynx has reached its maximum elevation. (D) Bolus continues through the hypopharynx, through the open cricopharyngeal segment, and into the esophagus, with the peristaltic wave descending behind it. The nasopharynx begins to open and opening progresses in a descending sequence. (E) The wave of pharyngeal contraction has obliterated the oropharyngeal cavity and moved into the hypopharynx, with the bolus descending further through the open cricopharyngeal segment into the esophagus. The nasopharyngeal airway continues to open in a cephalocaudal fashion. (F) Bolus has disappeared into the esophagus. All structures have returned to the open position: the normal contours of the airway are again visible, although the larynx has not yet completed its descent to its original resting position. Barium is coating the valleculae and piriform sinuses. (Reproduced with permission from Donner MW, Bosma JF, Robertson DL. Anatomy and physiology of the pharynx. *Gastrointest Radiol* 1985;10:196–212.)

The Normal and Abnormal Swallow

Analysis of the swallow may be performed by breaking the swallow down into several phases:

1. the oral phase
2. tongue-palate seal
3. nasopharyngeal (soft palate–superior constrictor) seal
4. compression and propulsion of bolus
5. hyoid/larynx/epiglottic tilt (laryngeal complex)
6. cricopharyngeal opening
7. esophageal peristalsis.

These phases are discussed in turn.

The Oral Phase

Normal

The lips engulf the bolus, which is sized by the tongue and held at rest toward the front of the mouth. If mastication is necessary, the bolus is manipulated by the tongue and chewed by the teeth until it is judged "swallowable."

With increasing bolus size, the bolus is held further toward the back of the oral cavity (10).

Dodds et al. have characterized the normal oral transfer phase depending on where the bolus is positioned at the beginning of swallow. These authors identified the common "tipper swallow" (approximately 95% of people) and the uncommon "dipper swallow" (5%) (11). In the former, the bolus is held in a central groove in the tongue blade and is then transferred into the pharynx by a progressive upward and posterior movement of the tongue blade, moving the bolus posteriorly into the pharynx through the open fauces. The tongue motion completely obliterates the oral cavity behind the bolus, the tongue progressively abutting the hard palate.

In the "dipper swallow," the bolus is held under the tongue in the floor of the mouth and is transferred out of the floor of the mouth by a downward scooping movement of the tongue blade under the bolus, transferring it into the oral cavity, and from there it is transferred into the pharynx in the same way as a tipper swallow. Each individual's swallow is either a "tipper" or a "dipper" repetitively and does not switch back and forth between the two types.

Another way of handling the bolus in the mouth is the "chipmunk swallow"; that is, the bolus is partially held in the cheeks (often a large bolus) and the patient swallows several times to clear the oral cavity, each swallow decreasing the amount held in the cheeks. This behavior can usually be curtailed by instructing the patient to "put in your mouth only the amount you can swallow in one swallow" or "take in your mouth a volume that you would normally swallow." The average normal bolus size has been reported to be 23 mL by Ekberg et al. (12).

Abnormalities of the Oral Phase

Weakness of the lips results in drooling, and the side of the drooling may be helpful diagnostically, although it may also depend on the angle at which the bolus is presented to the mouth.

It is very important to observe both the bolus and the tongue movements to diagnose tongue weakness (Table 4.1). Malpositioning or fragmenting of the bolus, multiple tongue blade movements to propel the bolus posteriorly, tremor or myoclonus, undulations of tongue blade, failure to obliterate the oral cavity, atrophy of the tongue, and low hyoid position can all be signs of tongue weakness. In the frontal view, asymmetry of the tongue at rest or asymmetry of bolus position as well as preservation of air in the apex of the mouth during bolus transfer are all signs of weakness.

Also, be aware of the patient who has weakness of the tongue blade and cannot maintain the bolus in the central groove who may lose a portion of the bolus into the floor of the mouth (partially simulating a "dipper" position). In this situation the bolus has fragmented and probably will be left behind in the floor of the mouth after the swallow as retained bolus, an abnormal finding.

Weakness of the cheek can be appreciated also in the frontal position by ballooning during swallow or pooling or pocketing after swallow.

Tongue-Palate Seal

Normal

Normally the bolus remains in the mouth and does not leak out because there is competence of lip seal anteriorly and tongue-to-palate

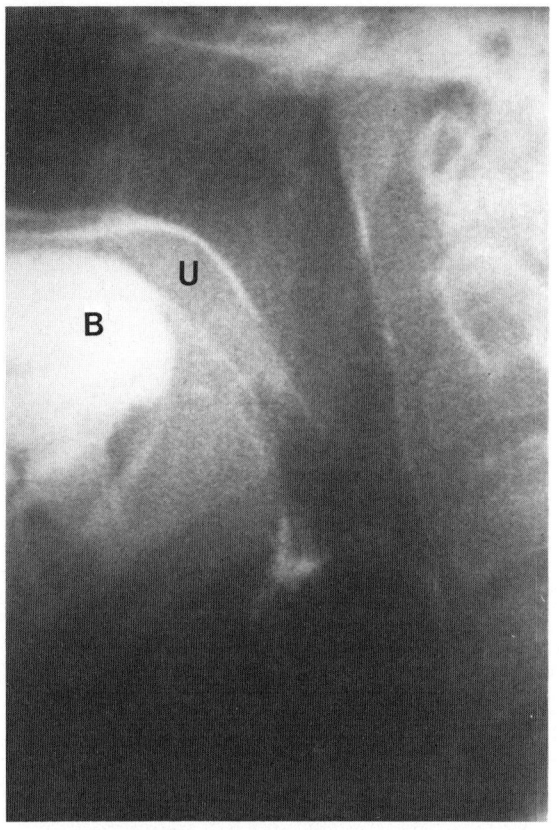 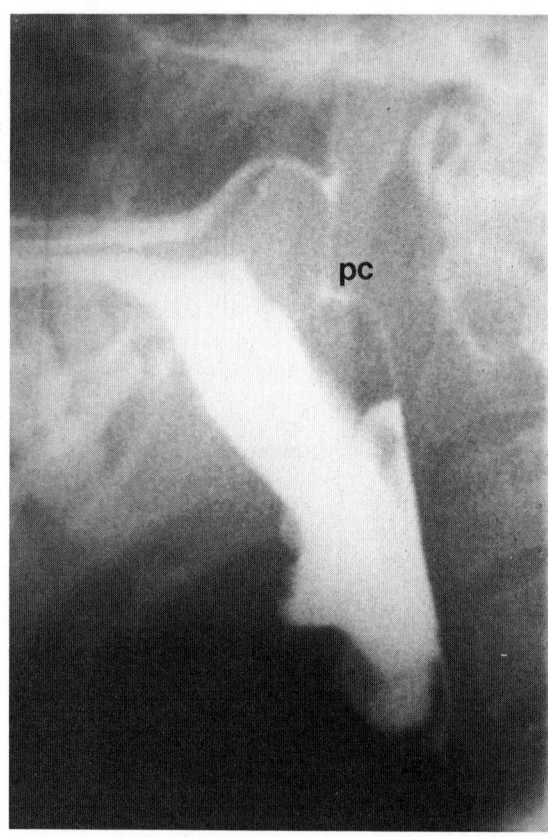

FIGURE 4.4. Selected stop-frame prints from a cine-pharyngogram demonstrate several stages of a normal swallow. (A) Bolus (B) is retained in the mouth by apposition of the posterior aspect of the tongue and the depressed soft palate (U). A small amount of contrast has been introduced through the nose and is coating the posterior nasopharyngeal wall and the superior portion of the soft palate. (B) As the bolus is propelled into the oropharynx, the soft palate elevates to a right angle and apposes to the converging posterior pharyngeal wall, Passavant's cushion (pc). (C) The soft palate (U), posterior pharyngeal wall, and dorsum of the tongue (T) remain closely in contact until bolus has cleared from the oropharynx. The proximal stripping wave (sw) has begun. (D) The posterior stripping wave (sw) has become more pronounced and is proceeding distally. The epiglottis has completely inverted and the vestibule is closed as the bolus passes through the hypopharynx. Note the closed larynx with the appearance of the conus (arrow) and the tracheal air column (T). The cricopharyngeus is completely open to allow easy passage of the bolus. There is a tiny amount of contrast in the entry to the vestibule, which is extruded as swallowing proceeds. (E) The stripping wave (sw) has proceeded further. There is a small amount of bolus (B) still trapped in the hypopharynx. The larynx is still closed. (F) The bolus has passed into the cervical esophagus. The laryngeal vestibule (L) has reopened and the epiglottis (arrow) is once more in an almost upright position. There is a small strand of contrast extending from the epiglottis to the posterior pharyngeal wall, presumably coating mucus. (A, B, C, D, and F reproduced with permission from Jones B, Kramer SS, Donner MW. Dynamic imaging of the pharynx. *Gastrointest Radiol* 1985;10:213–224.)

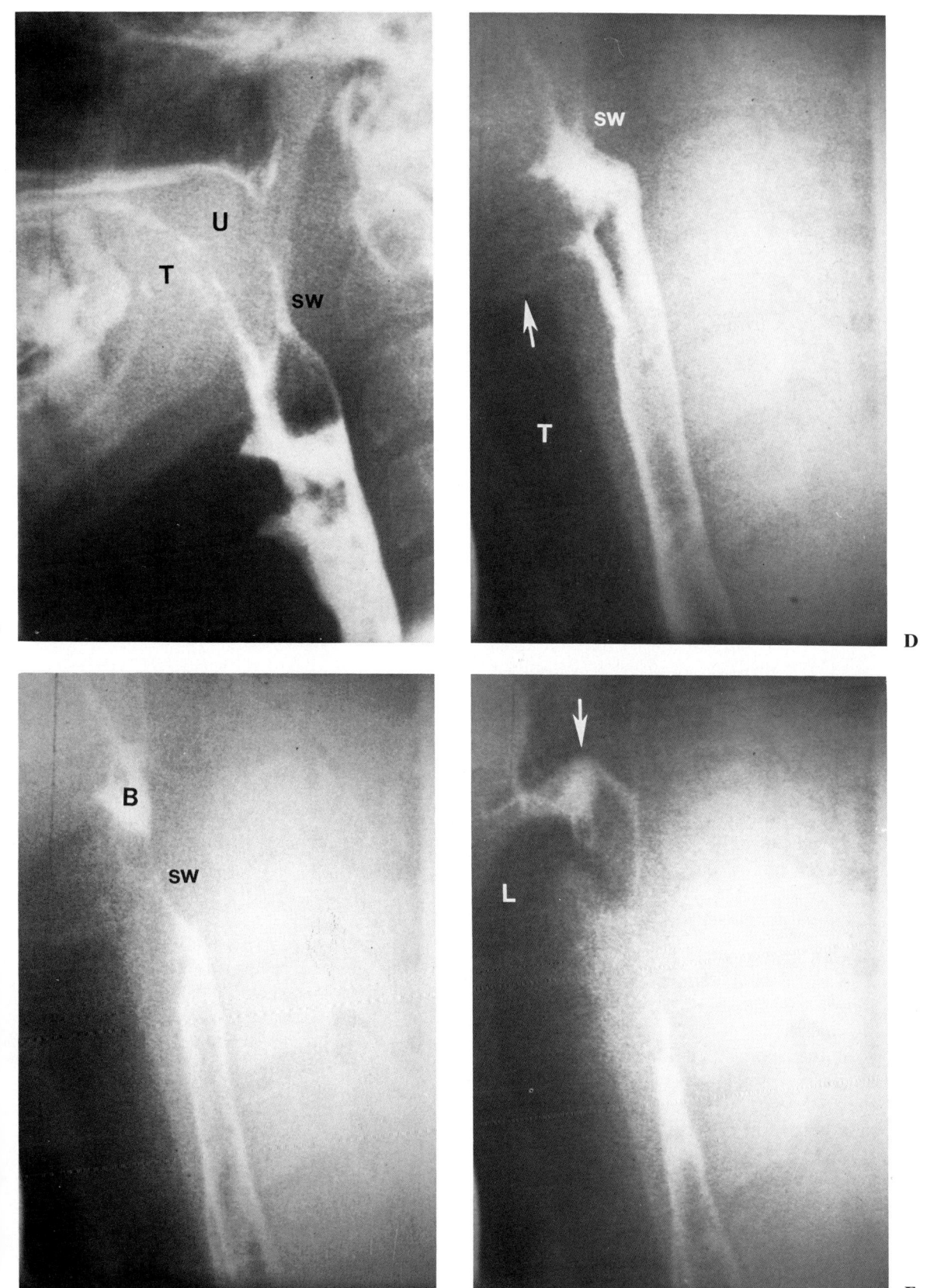

FIGURE 4.4. *Continued*

TABLE 4.1. Analysis of dynamic study.

Radiographic sign	Due to failure of	Associated radiographic findings
Abnormal oral phase	Tongue and/or lips	Drools, unable to propel bolus posteriorly, repetitive tongue movements with failure to propel bolus from front to back of mouth, pocketing in cheek or floor of mouth
Oral leakage	Tongue/palate competence; tongue atrophy or weakness	Unable to transfer bolus to back of mouth, low hyoid
	Palate weakness	Sluggish elevation of palate on speech and swallow
Nasal regurgitation	Palate/pharyngeal wall competence Palate	Sluggish elevation, failure to appose Passavant's cushion
	Posterior pharyngeal wall (superior constrictor)	Poor cushion (limited anterior movement of posterior pharyngeal wall)
Retention	Inadequate push (propulsion of bolus)	Poor or absent posterior stripping wave
		Poor or absent pharyngeal contraction
		Asymmetry of contraction or epiglottic tilt, overdistension on insufflation
	and/or distal obstruction (functional or structural)	Cricopharyngeal abnormality (opens late, incompletely, or closes early); web, stricture, tumor, etc.
Penetration	Laryngeal elevation	No or poor apposition of hyoid to mandible
	Laryngeal closure	Cord(s) remain(s) open during swallow, air in vestibule, no conus
	Epiglottic tilt	Epiglottis upright or not inverted during bolus passage
Aspiration	Retained bolus enters larynx after swallow	Retention postswallow, contrast in larynx and trachea, exclude pouch emptying postswallow, exclude tracheoesophageal fistula, mimicking penetration or aspiration

seal posteriorly. Normally the soft palate rests against the posterior tongue blade without any kinking when the patient is erect.

Abnormal Tongue-Palate Seal

A kink in the palate in the erect position is a sign of palatal *compensation* for a defective tongue (see Chapter 5) or a sign of soft palate weakness.

In the supine position, however, the palatoglossus muscle must contract to maintain the bolus within the oral cavity, producing a kink in the soft palate.

Incompetence of the seal between tongue and palate results in *premature leakage* from the mouth into the oropharynx before initiation of swallowing with the potential for aspiration into the open, unprotected larynx (Figure 4.5). In the frontal position, unilateral premature leakage versus central leakage points to the side of the weakness (Figure 4.5B).

Soft Palate–Passavant's Cushion Seal-Normal

As the bolus is propelled into the oropharynx by an upward, backward movement of the blade of tongue, the soft palate elevates to a right angle, apposing Passavant's cushion, a focally converging segment of the superior pharyngeal wall, produced by focal contraction of the upper fibers of the superior pharyngeal constrictor muscle. This apposition prevents *nasopharyngeal regurgitation* (Figure 4.6).

Bolus Compression and Propulsion

Progressive contraction of the superior, middle, and inferior constrictors and the retraction

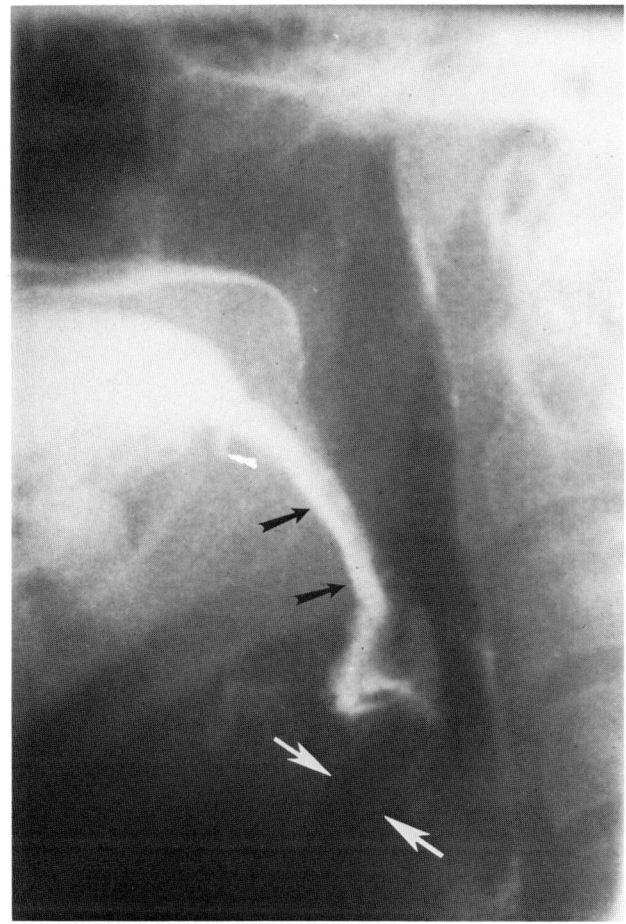 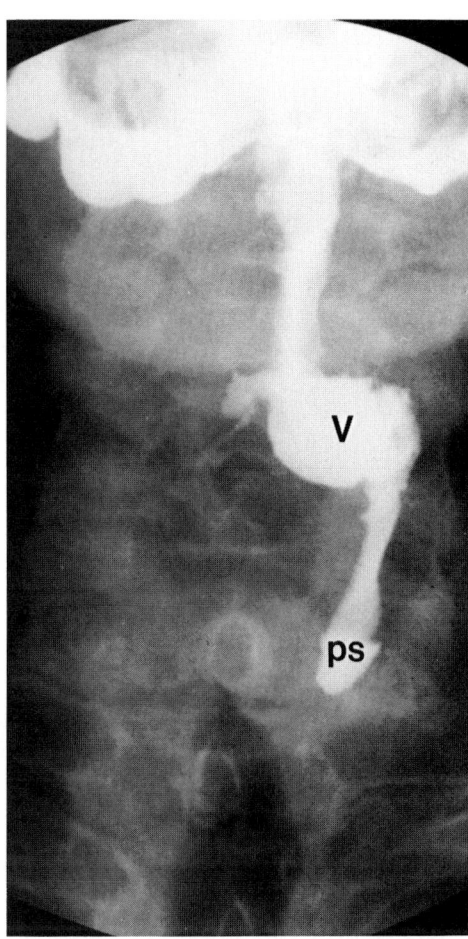

FIGURE 4.5. Premature leakage. Films from two separate patients reveal the appearance of premature leakage from the mouth. (A) This still frame from a cinepharyngogram in the lateral projection demonstrates contrast leaking over the dorsum of the tongue into the valleculae (arrows). Note that no swallow has occurred and that the soft palate (u) is incompletely apposed to the posterior portion of the tongue. There is thus the potential for overflow aspiration into the open vestibule of the larynx (white arrows). (B) In the AP projection there is unilateral leakage over the back of the left side of the tongue into the left vallecula (V) with overflow into the left piriform sinus (ps). Lateralization of leakage is an important piece of information for the therapist because exercises can be directed at that side. Injections to increase bulk or a prosthesis may be indicated.

of the base of the tongue propel the bolus through the pharynx. The constrictor stripping wave can be observed on lateral views as a progressive forward movement of the posterior pharyngeal wall. On frontal views, the wave can be appreciated as the motion of the lateral walls of the pharynx to the midline, obliterating the pharyngeal cavity behind the bolus.

Pharyngeal Paresis/Paralysis

Failure of the lateral pharyngeal walls to come to the midline indicates pharyngeal paresis. No movement or bulging during swallow indicates paralysis.

Unilateral weakness results in asymmetry in the frontal view and can actually cause a confusing appearance, which can be solved with careful

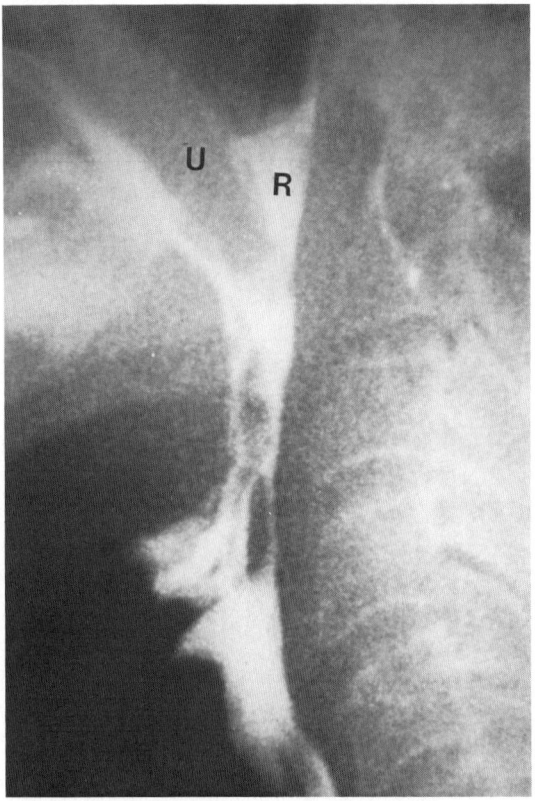 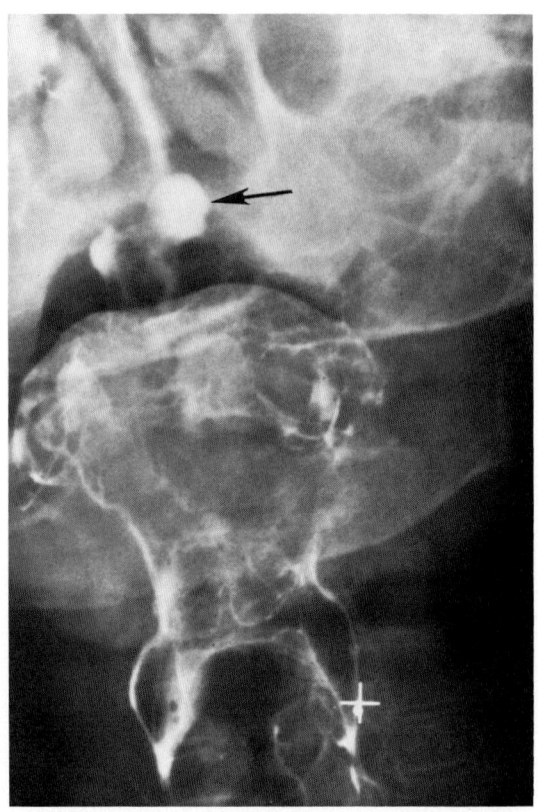

FIGURE 4.6. Nasal regurgitation. (A) A still frame from a cinepharyngoesophagogram demonstrates lack of elevation of the soft palate (U) and no evidence of Passavant's cushion, with resultant nasopharyngeal regurgitation (R). The epiglottis is upright even though the bolus is passing behind the larynx. (B) The appearance of nasal regurgitation (arrow) in the frontal plane.

analysis of the dynamic images. The contracting normal side can divert the bolus across to the atonic side, causing it to pass down the paralyzed side. Under some circumstances the contracting normal side may be misinterpreted as a mass, whereas the abnormality is actually on the non-contracting, bulging side (Figure 4.7).

Effect of Head Position

Turning the head to one side results in the bolus passing down the opposite "food channel." This can be a useful therapeutic maneuver in patients with unilateral paresis. Turning the head toward the paretic side results in the bolus passing down the normal side, which may improve clearance and/or laryngeal penetration (see Chapter 14).

Pharyngeal peristalsis proceeds much faster than esophageal peristalsis (12–25 cm/s vs 1–4 cm/s). This is why dynamic imaging is essential to detect subtle alterations in pharyngeal function. Constrictor action may be affected by intrinsic disease of the pharyngeal muscles or neuromuscular diseases, or by local factors such as fibrosis (e.g., following head and neck surgery, radiation, or cervical spine diseases such as degenerative disease, ankylosing spondylitis, or surgical fusion). Such local scarring may compound difficulties in swallowing by also restricting laryngeal elevation (13). Cervical osteophytes may also hinder or even prevent downward tilt of the epiglottis if they are located in a strategic position (Figure 4.8).

Hyoid Elevation, Laryngeal Closure and Epiglottic Tilt

Hyoid and Laryngeal Action During Swallow

As the bolus enters the oropharynx, the larynx begins to elevate, moving upward and forward.

Laryngeal movement can be appreciated by observing the upward and forward movement of the hyoid bone during swallowing. The reader is referred to an excellent review of laryngeal dynamics by Curtis (14).

Dodds et al. have shown that there is a direct correlation between maximal excursion of the hyoid bone and the volume of swallowed bolus (mean 13.0 and 13.5 mm movements in women and men, respectively, with a 2 mL bolus, increasing to 14.8 and 16.7 mm with a 10 mL bolus) (15).

The hyoid bone, according to Ekberg, may elevate in a one-step fashion (in 20%) or a two-step fashion (in 80%); in the latter case, the first smaller movement is backward and superiorly, followed by a superior and anterior movement (16). Laryngeal elevation occurred simultaneously with hyoid elevation but continued for a short period after the hyoid had reached its peak elevation, so-called laryngeal shortening. Descent of the hyoid to its resting position occurred in a one-step fashion, this movement occurring simultaneously with upward tilting of the epiglottis to its resting position. Mandibulohyoid distance at rest in this series was 4 to 27 mm (mean 15 mm). During swallowing, the hyoid apposes the angle of the mandible.

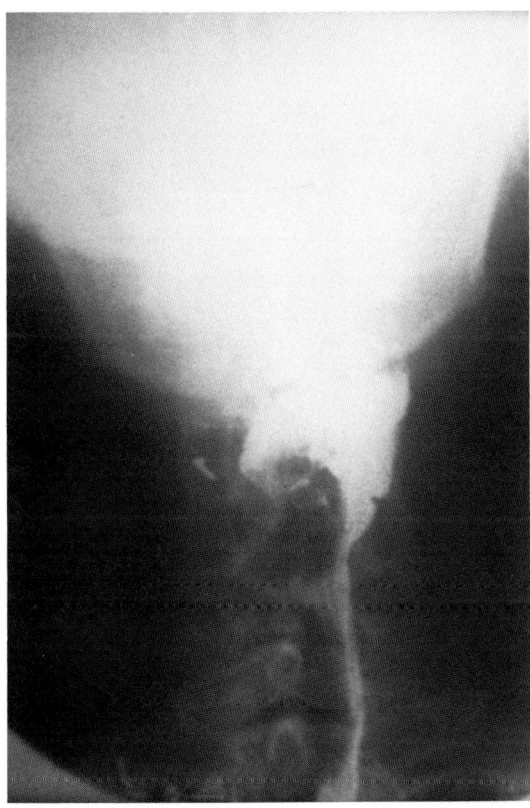 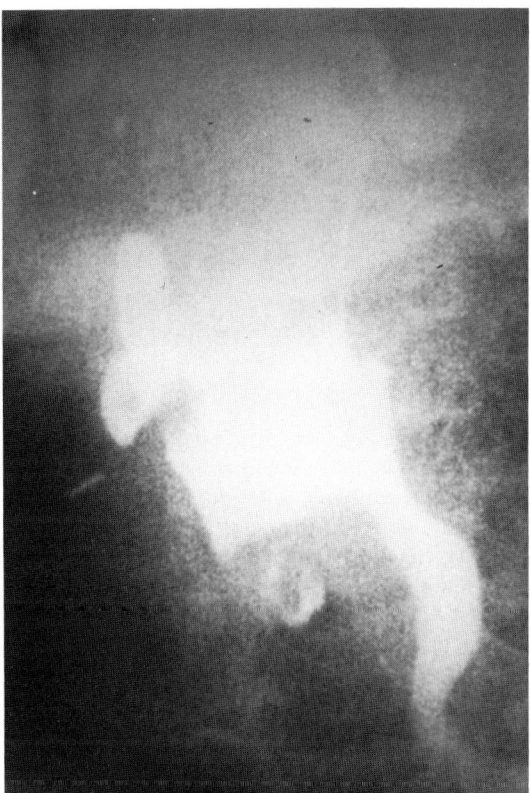

FIGURE 4.7. (A) and (B). Unilateral pharyngeal paresis in films from two patients. In both patients there is failure of contraction on the left side. Contraction of muscles on the normal right side have caused the barium to pass down the atonic left side. The apparent filling defect on the right side could easily be mistaken for a pharyngeal mass on static spot films. The asymmetry of unilateral pharyngeal paresis should not be confused with an intrinsic tumor or with pressure from an extrinsic mass. (B reprinted with permission from Jones B, Donner MW. In: *Radiology: Diagnosis Imaging Intervention*, Taveras JM, Ferrucci JF, eds. The Pharynx in Radiology/Diagnosis—Imaging—Intervention. Philadelphia: JB Lippincott; 1990.)

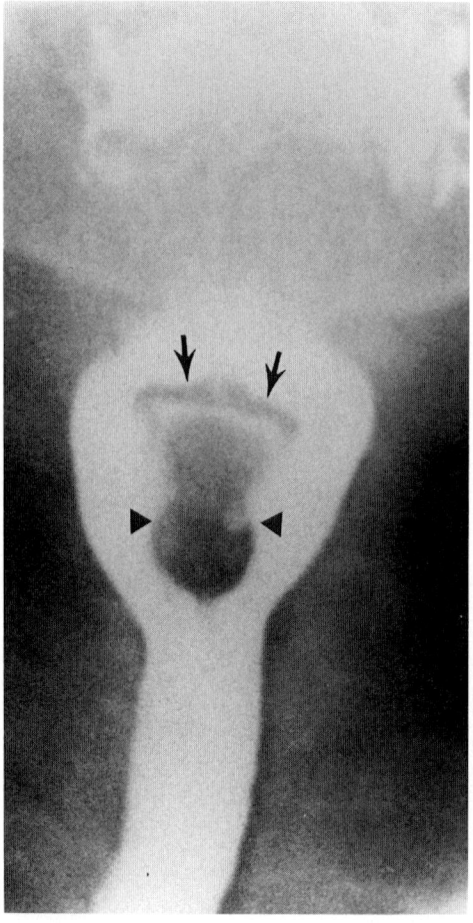 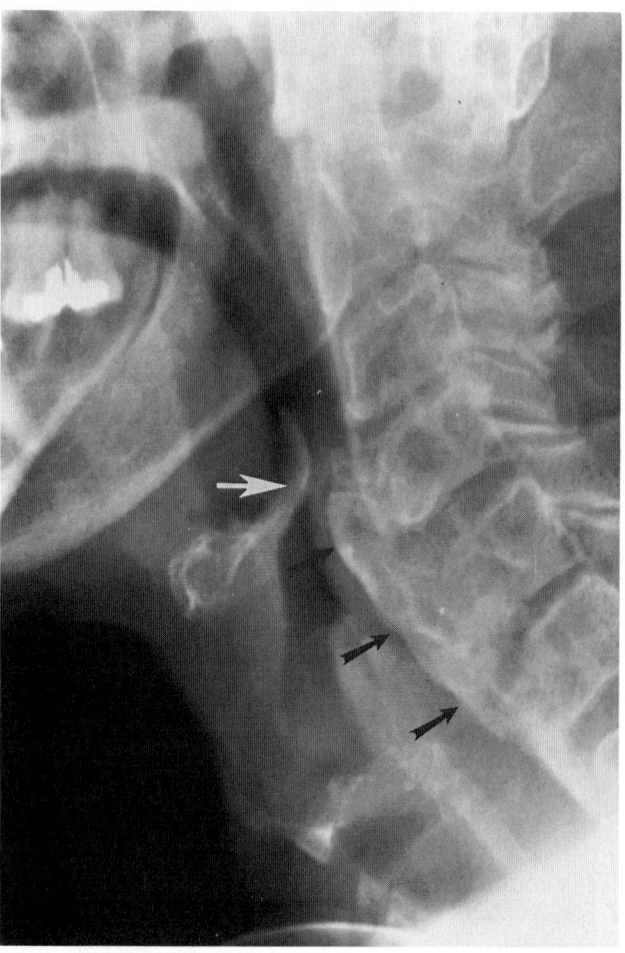

FIGURE 4.8. Epiglottic tilt. (A) Pseudomass created by tilt of the epiglottis. The epiglottis itself can be seen as a "seagull" or inverted flat "V" (arrows). The tilted epiglottis has deflected the bolus into the lateral food channels, creating a filling defect (arrowheads). (B) Inadequate tilt (plain film). A lateral plain film of the neck shows evidence of Forestier's arthritis with flowing osteophytes and a large bony ledge extending down the anterior cervical spine from C3 down (black arrows). Note that even in this view at rest, the epiglottis (white arrow) almost abuts the bony ridge. (C) Inadequate tilt (contrast study). In another patient with focal Forestier's arthritis, the epiglottis is unable to invert, remaining at an oblique or semiupright position, and there is immediate laryngeal penetration (arrow). Note also retention in the valleculae (V).

Epiglottic Tilt

Epiglottic tilt appears to occur as a two-step procedure in most individuals. The first movement (to the horizontal position) is probably a passive one, induced by hyoid elevation and tongue thrust. The second movement (to the inverted position) is thought to be an active one and is probably brought about by contraction of the thyroepiglottic muscle (17). A minority of individuals fail to completely invert the epiglottis, tilting only to the horizontal or oblique position. In the frontal view, the completely inverted epiglottis may be seen as a "sea gull-shaped" filling defect (Figure 4.8A). Deflection of bolus into the lateral food channels may produce a flow defect, which should not be misinterpreted as a mass (Figure 4.8B).

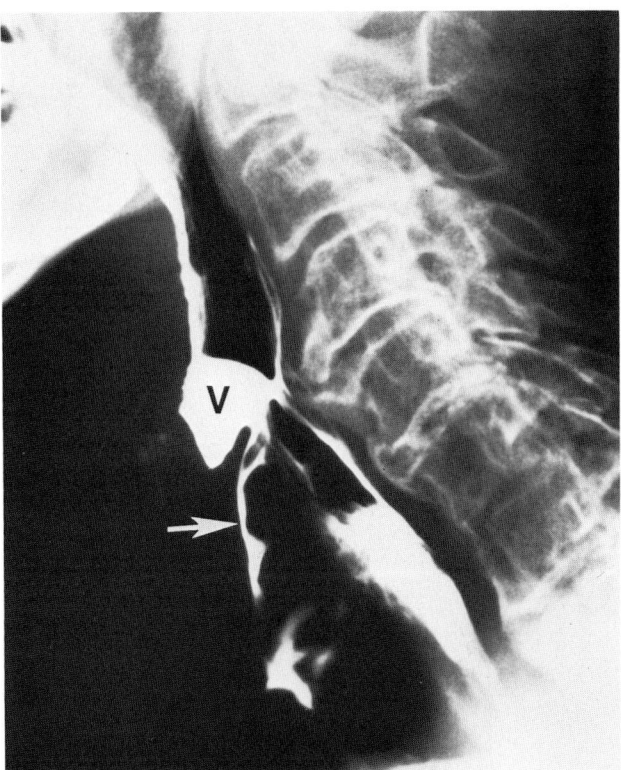

C

FIGURE 4.8. Continued

What Prevents Aspiration?

Laryngeal protective mechanisms are complex. Vital components include good laryngeal elevation and competent laryngeal closure as well as epiglottic tilt.

These three functions should be examined carefully if laryngeal penetration or aspiration is seen during the study. When the aspiration occurs is also important. Laryngeal penetration or aspiration through the vocal folds into the trachea may occur *during* swallow (Figure 4.9A), *prior* to swallow (Figure 4.9B), or *after* swallow (Figure 4.9C). Aspiration prior to swallow often is due to premature leakage of bolus from the mouth. Aspiration after swallow can result from many causes (e.g., failure to clear the pharynx or mouth of retained bolus with overflow aspiration) or from regurgitated (e.g., achalasia) or refluxed bolus (GER) (see Table 4.2).

The *timing* of the aspiration has important therapeutic implications. Various *therapeutic modifications* of head position (chin-tuck, head turn, or tilt) laryngeal elevation, bolus size, and swallow/respiration/cough sequencing (the supraglottic and supersupraglottic swallow) can be tried based on analysis of *why* and *when* aspiration is occurring (see Chapter 14).

It is also important to observe whether the aspiration produces a reflexive cough or is

TABLE 4.2. Aspiration.

Timing	Cause
Prior to swallowing	Failure of the glossopalatal seal with premature leakage from the mouth and entry into the open larynx
During swallowing	Poor laryngeal elevation Poor laryngeal closure Incomplete epiglottic tilt
After swallowing	Overflow of retained bolus Late emptying of a pouch or diverticulum Regurgitation from the esophagus Gastroesophageal reflux

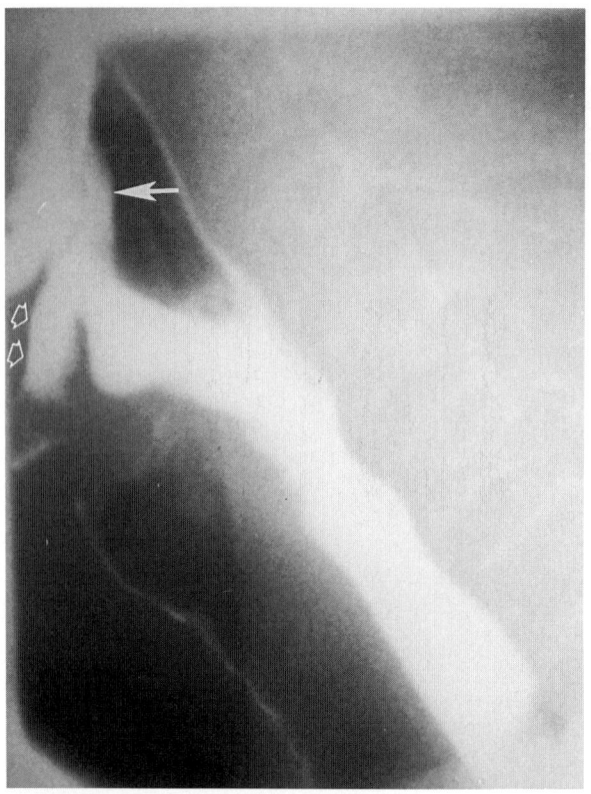
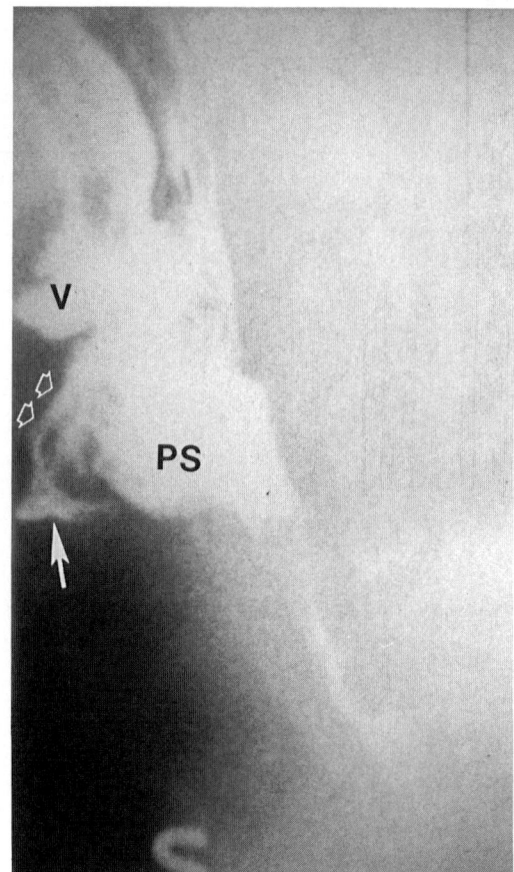
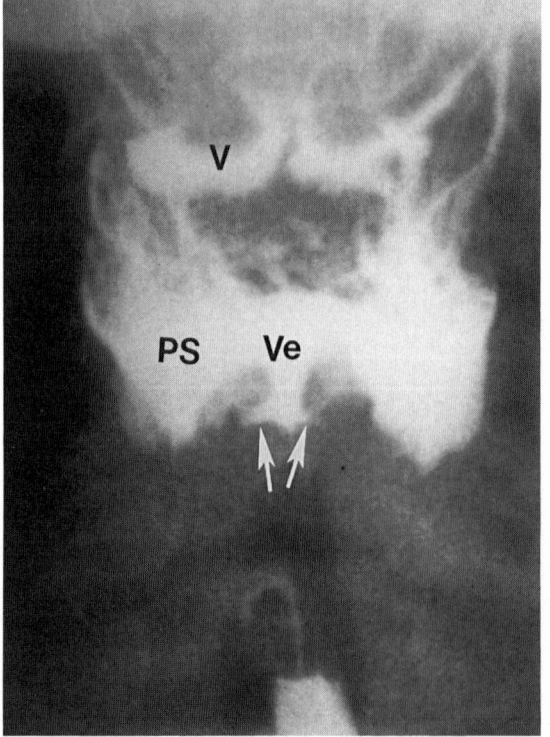

FIGURE 4.9. Aspiration. (A) Aspiration during a swallow. There is entry of bolus (arrowheads) into the vestibule down to the level of the closed true vocal cords. The epiglottis is still upright (arrow). There has been previous aspiration with barium coating the anterior wall of the trachea and inferior surface of the cords. Lateral (B) and frontal (C) views of the pharynx demonstrate aspiration of retained bolus. Note that there is retention of contrast in the valleculae (V) and piriform sinuses (PS). No swallow is taking place, yet there is entry of contrast into the laryngeal vestibule [arrowheads, (B)], Ve, (C) and between the vocal cords in the ventricle (arrows).

"silent." Many patients with chronic aspiration are *silent* aspirators (presumably due to loss of sensation, i.e., the afferent input for the cough reflex). In this group of patients especially, bedside evaluation will underestimate the extent of aspiration. Even with the most intensive physical examination and multiple predictors, clinical evaluations predict the presence of aspiration correctly in less than 50% of cases (18,19).

The Cricopharyngeal Area

The cricopharyngeus muscle is actually a portion of the inferior constrictor muscle (the horizontal portion arising from the cricoid cartilage). There is a zone of sparse musculature above (Killian's triangle) and below (area of Laimer) the cricopharyngeus where there is the potential for herniation and diverticular formation.

The upper esophageal sphincter (UES) consists of a zone of high pressure consisting of some fibers of the inferior constrictor muscle, the cricopharyngeal muscle, and some circular fibers of the proximal cervical esophagus. The cricopharyngeus is closed between swallows, presumably to prevent overdistension of the esophagus during respiration. This area must relax and open completely to allow unimpeded passage of bolus from the pharynx into the cervical esophagus.

The cricopharyngeus may open late, incompletely, or it may close early, sometimes trapping fluid in the "sphincter segment."

What Opens the Lumen at the Cricopharyngeal Level?

Several factors contribute to the opening of the pharyngoesophageal segment: cricopharyngeal relaxation, superior and anterior elevation of the hyoid and larynx, the "push" from contraction of the pharyngeal constrictors (and probably tongue base), and the thrust from the bolus itself. Thus, in pharyngeal paresis, prominence of the cricopharyngeus is common. However, it is the pharyngeal milieu that is abnormal (i.e., lack of "push") rather than the cricopharyngeus itself. One can be taught to relax and open the cricopharyngeal sphincter area voluntarily (e.g., to produce esophageal speech following laryngectomy). In this technique there is a controlled release of swallowed air from the thoracic esophagus into the pharynx. A study by Gatenby et al. documented failure of achievement of esophageal speech postlaryngectomy with abnormal motion of the cricopharyngeal area (20). An extreme example of voluntary relaxation of cricopharyngeus is seen in beer guzzlers and sword swallowers (see later: Figure 5.1).

Radiographically, a posterior indentation at the pharyngoesophageal junction during bolus passage indicates the level of the cricopharyngeus (Figure 4.10). There are conflicting opinions in the literature about the significance of such an indentation (i.e., cricopharyngeal prominence) (21–30). Some authorities believe mild indentation is within the range of normality, since this finding can be seen in an asymptomatic population, especially with increasing age. Significant luminal narrowing (>50%), however, can definitely produce symptoms of dysphagia (Figure 4.10).

Experimental and postmortem data correlating radiographic findings of cricopharyngeal prominence of "pharyngeal bars" with those from dissection specimens of patients do not demonstrate conclusively whether this radiographic appearance represents muscular hypertrophy or spasm (21).

In rare instances, there may be what appears to be a second sphincteric mechanism (an "accessory sphincter") about 1 to 1.5 cm below the cricopharyngeus (31). Donner observed that the esophagus between the two "sphincters" appears to be atonic in such cases, and bolus may be trapped (Donner, unpublished personal communication).

Radiographic Observations and Manometric Measurements

We have already seen that cricopharyngeal relaxation (as measured by manometry) is only one of the factors involved in the opening of

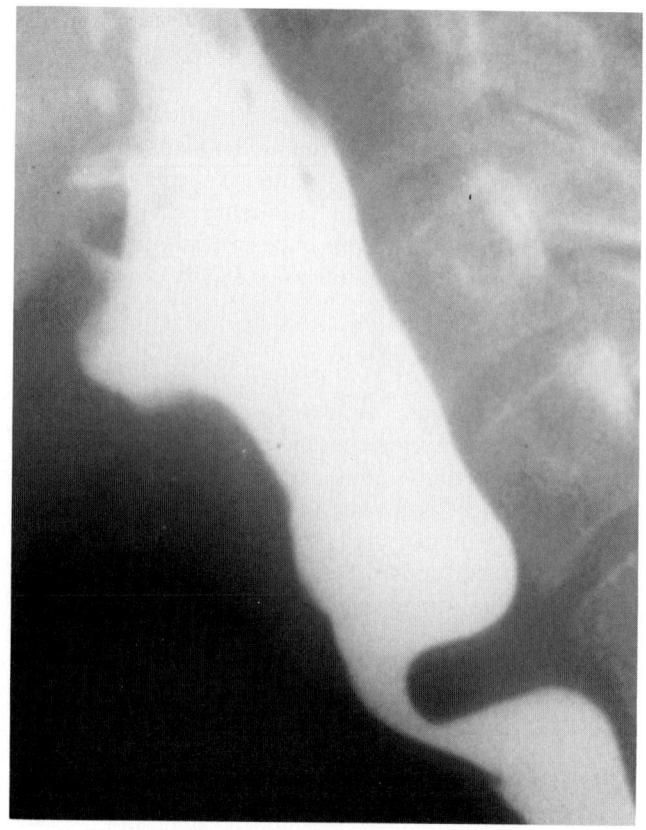

FIGURE 4.10. Cricopharyngeal prominence. A lateral still-frame print from a cinepharyngoesophagram demonstrates marked cricopharyngeal prominence during passage of a large bolus, with luminal compromise of about 80%. Despite this, the patient's dysphagia responded to dilatation. Note that giving such a patient a solid bolus is unnecessary and may be potentially dangerous!

the pharyngoesophageal segment; laryngeal movement, pharyngeal contraction, and the bolus itself all have a role. Thus there often is a discrepancy between radiographic observation, which demonstrates luminal size, and manometry. Manometric measurements are well discussed in a review by Dodds et al. (32).

Bolus size also plays a role. In 1988 Kahrilas et al. demonstrated that larger boluses produced both an increased anteroposterior diameter and prolongation of the time the sphincter was relaxed. As the interval of relaxation increased, the period for laryngeal elevation was prolonged, the UES relaxed earlier and contracted later, and the interval between the onset of elevation of the larynx and pharyngeal contraction increased. The amount of superior movement of the cricopharyngeus was also directly related to bolus volume (33).

Does "Cricopharyngeal Achalasia" Exist?

The cricopharyngeus may fail to relax completely, may open late, or may close early and thus trap a portion of the bolus above it. (Careful frame-by-frame analysis of the recorded dynamic imaging will determine the timing of the abnormality.)

True "cricopharyngeal achalasia," defined manometrically as "complete failure of the cricopharyngeus to relax," is very rare. Much more common is prominence due to aging, in combination with pharyngeal paresis, or in association with an esophageal disease such as gastroesophageal reflux or spasm (see Chapter 6, Tables 6.1 and 6.2). In the extreme case of complete incoordination or failure of the swallow reflex to trigger (absence or a swallow), the sphincter does not receive the normal signal to relax and will therefore appear prominent or even fail to open at all. Simultaneous videofluorography and manometry may be useful in the evaluation of patients with cricopharyngeal bars (34,35).

Oral Decompensations and Pharyngeal Decompensations: Relative Importance and Frequency

How common are tongue weakness and oral decompensation compared with pharyngeal decompensation? Several fairly recent studies have focused on and highlighted the potential dangers of oral phase abnormalities.

Oral decompensation may be more important in choking and aspiration than has been recognized. For example, in a survey of 75 patients who survived a near-fatal choking episode, Feinberg and Ekberg found abnormalities in 58 (36). Interesting, oral stage dysfunction was the predominant problem occurring in 32 patients, with pharyngeal abnormalities in 19, pharyngoesophageal segment abnormalities in 28, and esophageal abnormalities in 23. Alcohol had been ingested prior to the choking episode in 11 of the patients and may have played a role.

Similarly, the same authors studied a group of 50 elderly aspirators (mean age, 87 years) and found oral stage dysfunction to be the cause of the aspiration in 23 (37). Pharyngeal stage dysfunction, such as defective laryngeal closure or incomplete bolus transport, was the cause in one fifth of the patients, and combined oral and pharyngeal function was the cause in 17 cases. The authors concluded that "oral stage dysfunction is at least as important as pharyngeal dysfunction in causing aspiration in the elderly."

Chen et al. (38) studied the frequency of oral findings in 46 patients with dysphagia following cerebrovascular accidents. These authors found combined oral and pharyngeal findings in 39 patients, with oral stage abnormalities alone in 2 and pharyngeal findings alone in 9.

Oral findings may be the only sign of a neuromuscular condition, especially in the radiographic diagnosis of Parkinson's disease. For example, Leopold and Kagel studied 72 patients with Parkinson's disease and found "pre-pharyngeal dysphagia" in over 60% (39). Findings included tremor, impulsive feeding, impaired volume regulation, and abnormal lingual transfer movements.

Similarly, Nilsson et al. examined 75 patients with the same disease and reported oral or pharyngeal findings in almost all (40). Interestingly, the Hoehn and Yahr score of the Parkinson's disease did not correlate with the swallowing impairment.

Oral findings may also offer clues to the diagnosis of "psychogenic dysphagia" or dysphagic symptoms in a patient with an otherwise negative videofluorographic swallowing study (VFSS) and a strong psychological overlay to his or her symptoms. We have reported 26 patients thought to have psychogenic dysphagia and found abnormal oral movements to be a strong indicator of this condition (41). Abnormal oral behavior suggestive of psychogenic overlay includes rocking the bolus, swirling the bolus around the mouth, a pharyngeal swallow without oral transfer, and multiple tongue movements without oral transfer. Fear of swallowing (phagophobia) is often an integral part of psychogenic dysphagia (42).

To test whether we could accurately differentiate patients with psychogenic dysphagia from the those with true neurological disease, we compared 10 patients with neurological disease with 12 patients who had a diagnosis of "psychogenic dysphagia" (43). A radiologist (BJ), blinded to the diagnoses, evaluated the VFSS findings and classified these patients into two groups based on the oral and pharyngeal findings alone. In the psychogenic group there were oral findings alone with a normal pharyngeal phase. In the remainder (except for one patient with an oral tremor thought to represent Parkinson's disease), there were a combination of oral and pharyngeal findings. Oral findings thought to represent neurological disease included drooling, inability to transfer bolus, tongue atrophy or decreased tongue thrust, multiple tongue movements, premature leakage, piecemeal swallow, and lingual tremor.

We subsequently studied this group via a follow-up telephone questionnaire. Twenty-

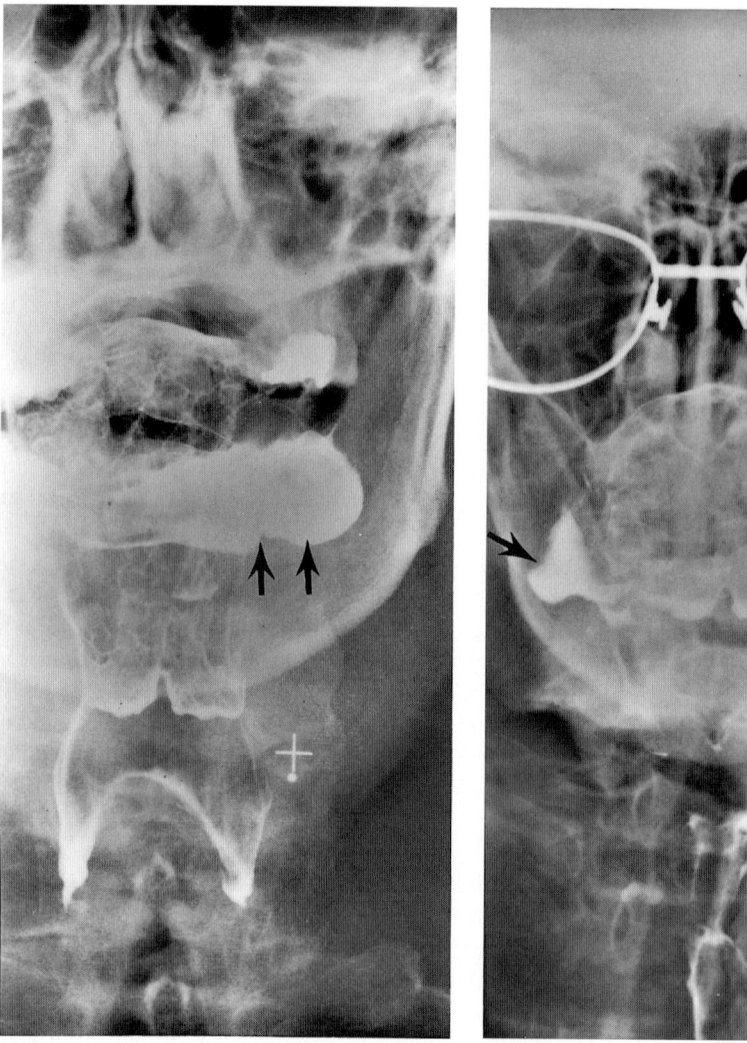

FIGURE 4.11. Oral decompensations with abnormal retained bolus. Two patients demonstrate pooling in the floor of the mouth (A) (arrows) and in the cheek (B) (arrow).

one patients were contacted and 19 were willing to participate in the study. Of these, *none* had developed further problems and none had developed a neurological condition (43) other than glossopharyngeal neuralgia, a condition associated with throat pain but not with dysphagia (44).

Thus, it is extremely important to be able to recognise oral decompensations and to differentiate between abnormal oral behavior and oral decompensations that indicate a neurological process (Figure 4.11).

On the other hand, is a negative VFSS adequate to exclude functional abnormalities of the pharynx? In 1995 Olsson et al. (45) reported the manometric findings in 19 patients with a negative VFSS and found manometric abnormalities in 14. Abnormalities included 5 patients with high UES resting pressures, 5 patients with high residual UES pressures, 3 with weak pharyngeal contractions, 3 with pharyngeal "spasms," 7 with prolonged contraction/relaxation times, 5 with reduced UES compliance, and 7 with UES/P incoordination.

The authors advise caution in equating a negative VFSS with normality. Further studies are indicated to clarify the role of manometry in the presence of a negative VFSS.

4. Interpreting the Study

Analysis of Esophageal Peristalsis

Pharyngeal constrictor activity merges with the peristaltic wave in the cervical esophagus, which in turn merges with the wave in the thoracic esophagus (although esophageal peristalsis is much slower). The bolus is then propelled into the stomach.

Peristalsis is evaluated by observing a single swallow and following it from mouth to stomach. "Double" swallowing inhibits the stripping wave; some patients fail to understand the instructions and continue to swallow; in such cases the wave of the final swallow can be observed. The stripping wave may be lost if the patient is nauseated or by pathological processes such as achalasia, scleroderma, diabetes, alcohol, disturbances of the central nervous system, vagotomy (e.g., pseudoachalasia following heart-lung transplantation), and some medications.

The Role of Saliva

For many years it was believed that the only important function of saliva was to assist in moistening and preparing the bolus, especially the dry, textured, or solid kind. Other functions, however, include a barrier against injury, prevention of desiccation, and control of oral microbial flora by acting as a buffer, resisting a change in pH protective against caries (46,47). Prevention of dryness is certainly an important function of saliva, and patients with decreased saliva production (such as Sjögren's syndrome) may complain of dysphagia, especially in the oral or initiation phase of swallowing.

In the esophagus, saliva has been regarded merely as a vehicle of lubrication to assist passage of the bolus. Recent evidence, however, suggests a potentially very important function in esophageal clearance of acid. Deficient saliva production may thus compound the harmful effects of refluxed gastric acid. Esophageal clearance proceeds as a two-step process; esophageal emptying, followed by acid neutralization (48). Peristaltic activity empties most of the refluxed acid from the esophagus, and the remainder is neutralized by swallowed saliva. Therefore, patients with low salivary flow rates may be more at risk for the development of reflux esophagitis. Indeed, xerostomia following radiotherapy has been reported to be associated with impaired esophageal acid clearance and resultant esophageal inflammation (48).

Analysis of Structure

Tongue and Mouth Abnormalities

The tongue may be affected by neuromuscular disorders that may produce fasciculation, weakness or atrophy (e.g., amyotrophic lateral sclerosis), and difficulty in *initiating* swallowing (pseudobulbar palsy), by chorea (rapid repetitive movements interfering with initiation of swallowing), or by dystonia (the hypertonic tongue being situated in a high position in the posterior aspect of the mouth: the so-called fisted tongue) (Figure 4.12A).

The tongue may be enlarged in an infiltrative disease such as *amyloidosis*, and the sheer bulk of it may compromise both initiation and propulsion (Figure 4.12B), causing painful bullae or ulcers, as well.

Both the tongue blade and the base of the tongue may be involved with carcinoma (Figure 4.12C). Following resection (Figure 4.12D), especially if the resection includes the base of the tongue, there may be either difficulty with leakage prior to swallowing or difficulty with propulsion. It is being increasingly recognized that the tongue base plays a major role in propulsion of the bolus, a function that until fairly recently was thought to be the responsibility primarily of the pharyngeal constrictor muscles.

Soft Palate Abnormalities

The interested reader is referred to two excellent articles by Rubesin et al. (49,50) for a review of the radiological anatomy of the soft palate.

The upper surface of the soft palate can be coated by nasal instillation of heavy-density barium (patient sniffs to help in coating). Smooth asymmetry is best appreciated on the lateral view as a double white line. The *site* of the double white line is different depending on whether the levator veli palatini (superior

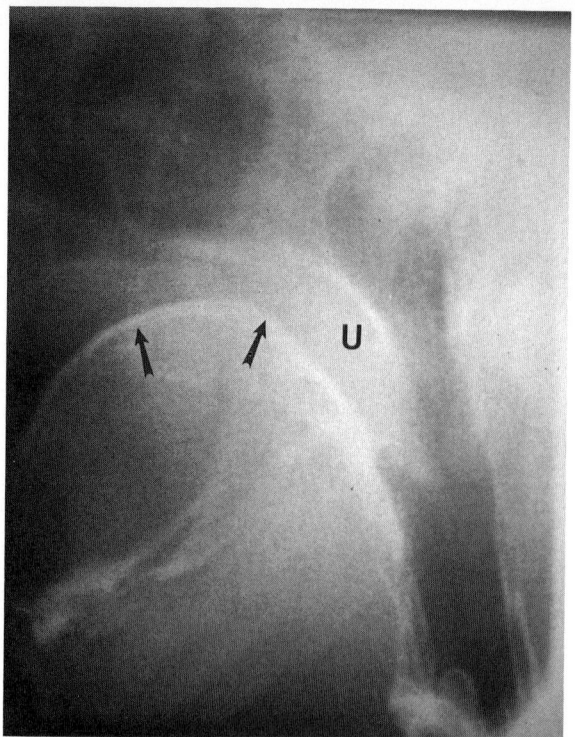
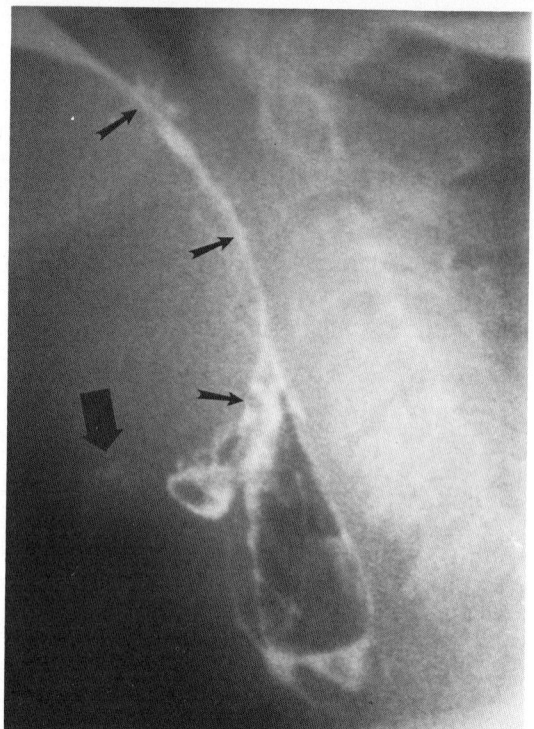
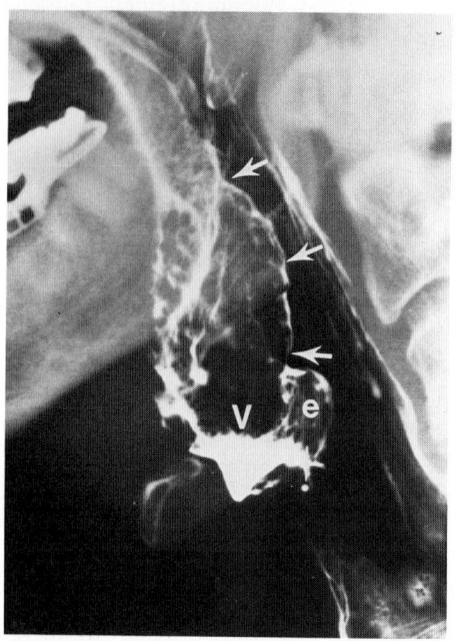
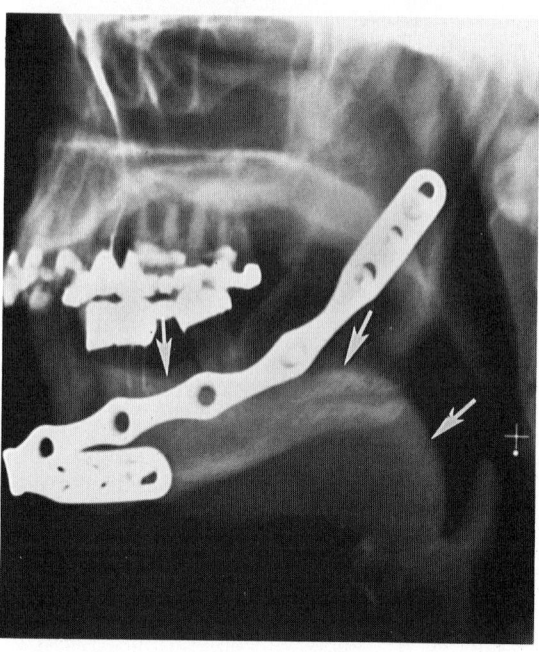

FIGURE 4.12. Tongue abnormalities. (A) Myotonic dystrophy. In this patient with dystonia, the firm tongue (arrows) is situated posteriorly in the mouth as a result of muscle bunching. This is the "fisted tongue." The superior surface of the uvula (u) has been coated with contrast by nasal instillation of barium. Arrows indicate the surface of the tongue blade. (B) Amyloidosis. The tongue blade and dorsum are markedly enlarged, severely compromising the pharyngeal airway (arrows) and displacing the epiglottis. The hyoid bone is displaced inferiorly by the bulk of the tongue (large arrow). Note also that there is retention in the valleculae and piriform sinuses due to pharyngeal paresis and failure to clear the pharynx. (Reprinted with permission from Jones B, Gayler BW, Donner MW. Pharynx and cervical esophagus. In: Levine MS, ed. *Radiology of the Esophagus*. Philadelphia: WB Saunders; 1989.) (C) Carcinoma of the tongue base. There is a large, bulky soft tissue mass (arrows) involving the base of the tongue, widening the vallecula (V) and displacing the epiglottis (e) downward from its normally upright position. (D) Resection. The patient has had a partial glossectomy, radical neck dissection and hemimandibulectomy for carcinoma of the floor of the mouth. Note the diminished tongue bulk (arrows). There is a metal prosthesis in one of the mandibles.

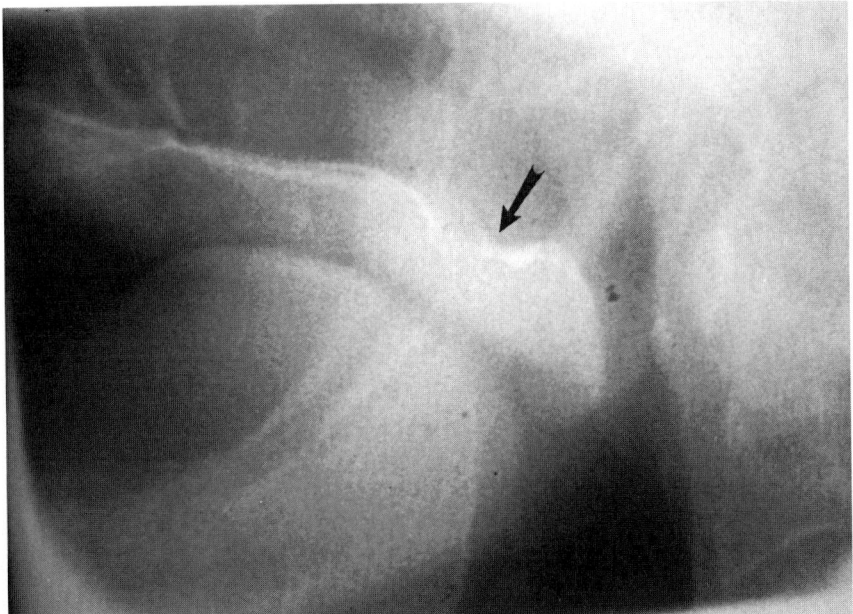

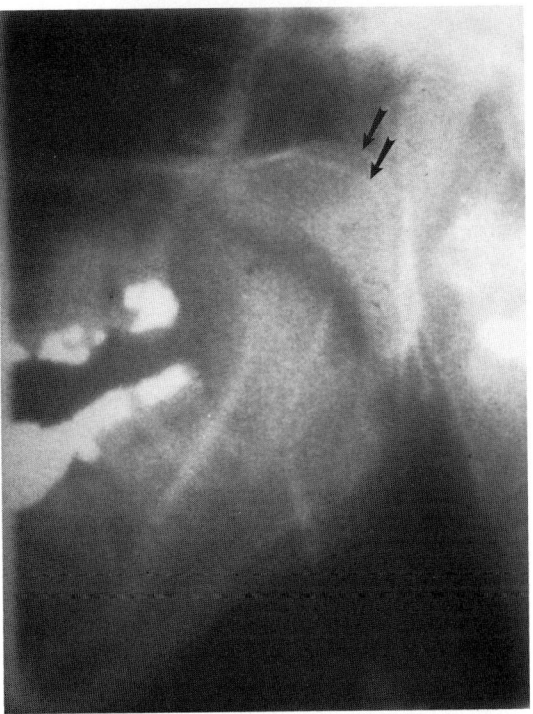

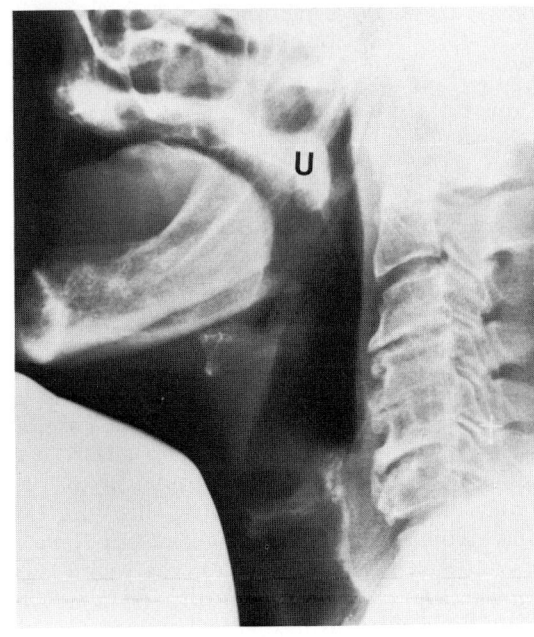

FIGURE 4.13. Soft palate abnormalities. (A) Kinking of the soft palate as a sign of compensation. Note that the superior surface of the soft palate has been coated by barium instillation through the nose. There is a kink partway down the uvula (arrow), which in the erect position is a sign of compensation. (B) Asymmetry of the soft palate. The posterior surface of the soft palate has been coated by nasal instillation of barium. There are two coated surfaces on the superior portion (arrows) indicating asymmetric weakness of one side of the soft palate. (C) Rigid soft palate following lye ingestion. The soft palate (U) is in an unusual position, neither apposed to the back of the tongue nor apposed to Passavant's cushion. The patient is not swallowing, yet the soft palate is elevated; it also is shorter than normal owing to contracture. During swallowing there was both leakage of contrast over the back of the tongue and nasopharyngeal regurgitation. Note also that the patient is edentulous as a result of damage to the mouth and gums from lye ingestion.

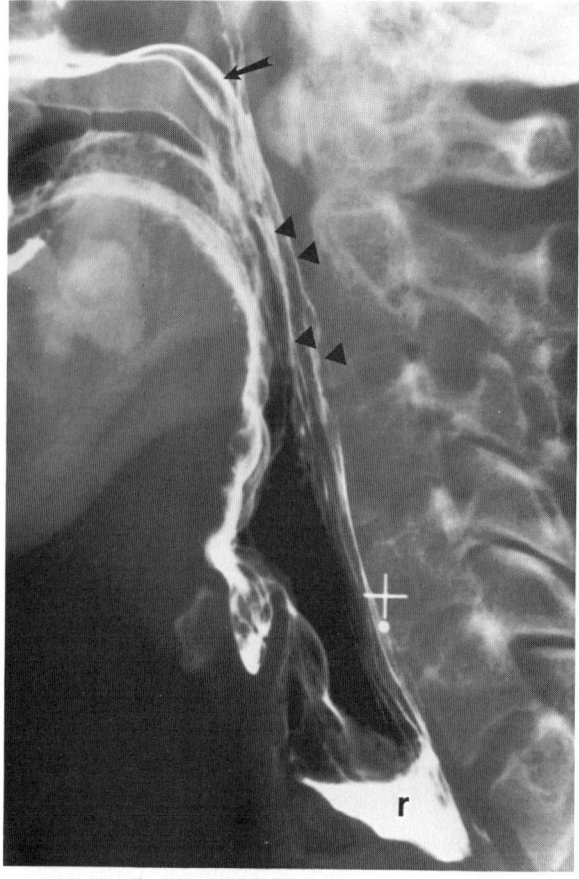 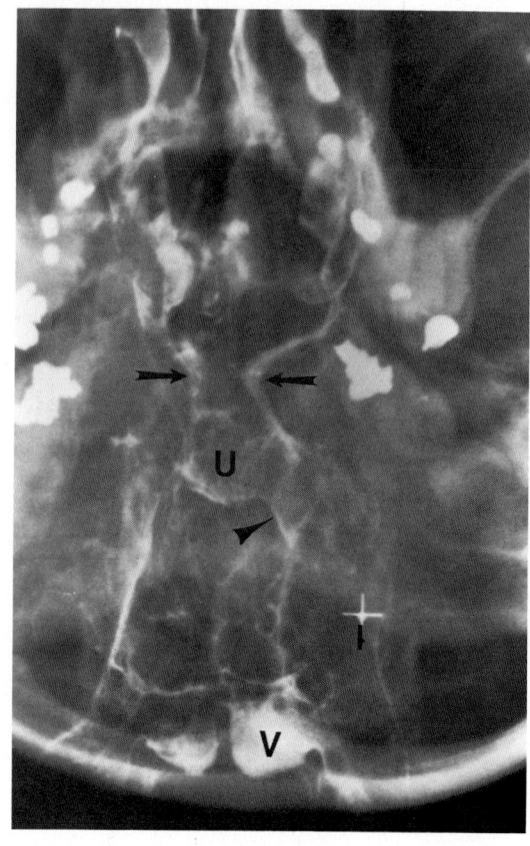

FIGURE 4.14. The sphinx view. This patient, with a history of poliomyelitis at the age of 5, presented with dysphagia secondary to right-sided pharyngeal paresis. (A) At rest, a lateral view of the pharynx shows a "double soft palate" due to asymmetric elevation of the soft palate (arrow) primarily due to asymmetric action of the palatopharyngeal muscle. There is mild nasopharyngeal regurgitation. There is also asymmetry of the posterior pharyngeal wall (arrowheads) and moderate retention (r) in the piriform sinuses due to pharyngeal paresis. (B) The "sphinx view" taken during phonation shows midline movement of the lateral pharyngeal walls, the movement being somewhat asymmetric (arrows). The palatopharyngeal fold moves toward the midline on the left (arrowhead) but shows no sign of movement on the right. The uvula (U) and valleculae (V) can also be seen with some retention in the valleculae. (Reproduced with permission from Rubesin SE, Jones B, Donner MW. Radiology of the soft palate. *Dysphagia* 1987;2:8–17.)

surface) or the palatopharyngeus (descending portion) is involved (Figures 4.13 and 4.14).

The "sphinx view" (a basal view with the patient positioned as an Egyptian sphinx) has been used to evaluate velopharyngeal portal closure in patients with cleft palate or nasal speech (51). In this view, the patient lies prone on the fluoroscopic table with arms outstretched, the head is positioned until the velopharyngeal portal can be seen as a barium-outlined oval (Figure 4.14). Anteriorly, the oval is bordered by the soft palate and uvula, laterally by the lateral pharyngeal walls, and posteriorly by the posterior pharyngeal wall.

The Pharynx Itself

Definition of the three anatomical compartments of the pharynx is important in discussing the location of lesion in, for example, the naso- (epi), oro- (meso-), and hypopharynx.

Nasopharynx

The nasopharynx extends from the base of the skull to the superior surface of the soft palate and is not a part of the alimentary tract.

Oropharynx

The oropharynx extends from the pharyngeal aspect of the palate above to the base of the tongue and the hyoid bone below; hence, the valleculae are part of the oropharynx. The dorsum of the tongue forms the anterior border, and the middle and part of the inferior constrictor muscles form the lateral and posterior walls.

Hypopharynx

The hypopharynx extends from the valleculae at the base of the tongue to the pharyngo-

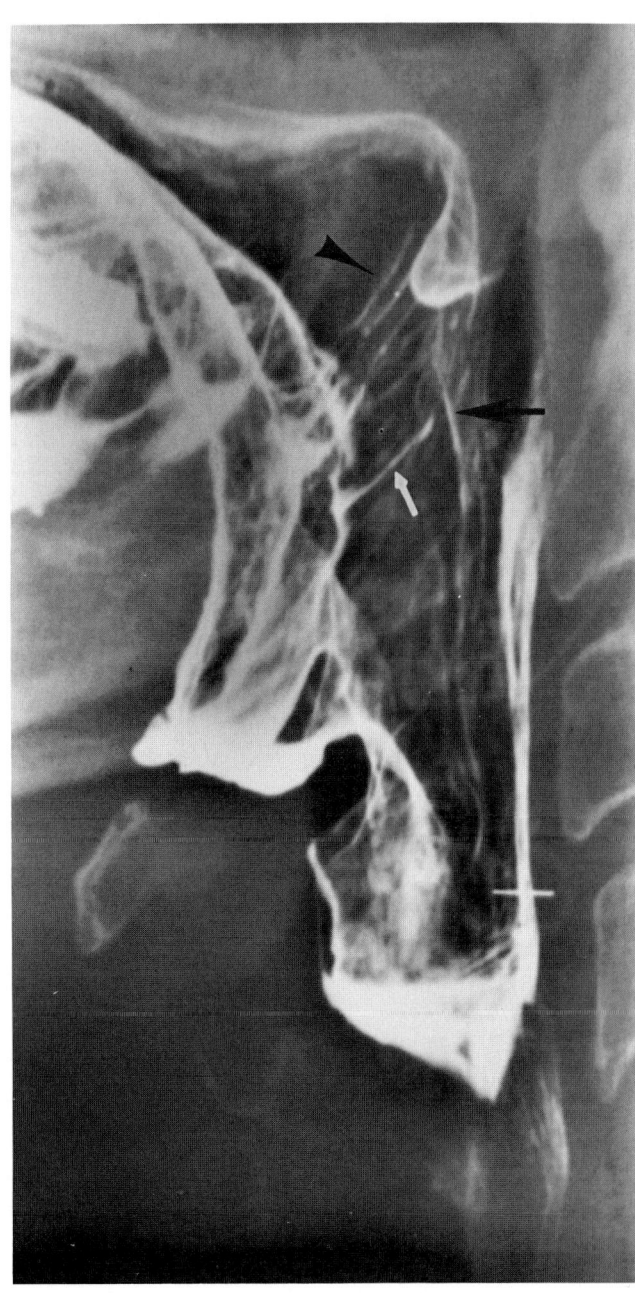

FIGURE 4.15. Lines of the pharynx. Double-contrast lateral view of the pharynx filmed while the patient phonates "eee" demonstrates paired palatoglossal folds (arrow) covering the palatoglossus muscle. The palatopharyngeal fold (curved arrow) covers part of the palatopharyngeus and salpingopharyngeus muscles. The pharyngoepiglottic fold (white arrow) is superficial to the internal fibers of the stylopharyngeus muscle. (Reproduced with permission from Rubesin SE, Jessurun J, Robertson D, Jones B, Bosma JF, Donner MW. Lines of the pharynx. *RadioGraphics* 1987;7(2):217–237.)

esophageal segment ending at the lower border of the cricopharyngeal muscle.

Valleculae and Piriform Sinuses

Spaces are created by loose mucosa covering the cartilaginous framework of the larynx. The piriform sinuses are created by the larynx protruding into the hypopharynx, and the contour is molded somewhat by the overlying thyroid cartilage and thyrohyoid ligament. The medial border of the piriform sinus consists of the aryepiglottic fold.

The medially situated glossoepiglottic fold divides the area at the base of the tongue anterior and lateral to the epiglottis into the paired symmetric valleculae. The lateral glossoepiglottic folds form the lateral wall of the valleculae, whereas the pharyngoepiglottic fold forms the posterior aspect of the valleculae.

Lines of the Pharynx

Rubesin et al. coined the phrase "lines of the pharynx" in a study correlating line drawings, anatomy, and radiographic anatomy (52). The phraseology arose from the fact that the mucosa of the pharynx is thrown into linear or nodular folds by underlying structures such as muscles, cartilage, or lymphoid tissue (Figure 4.15).

The *longitudinal muscle layer* consists of three muscles: the salpingopharyngeus (not seen on barium swallow because it lies superior and posterior to the soft palate), the palatopharyngeus, and the stylopharyngeus. The latter two muscles together elevate the mucosa to form the palatopharyngeal fold (Figure 4.15). The mucosa over the palatoglossus muscle produces the palatoglossal fold. Transverse folds overlie the arytenoid and cricoid cartilage.

References

1. Donner MW, Bosma JF, Robertson DL. Anatomy and physiology of the pharynx. *Gastrointest Radiol* 1985;10:196–212.
2. Bosma JF, Donner MW, Tanaka E, Robertson D. Anatomy of the pharynx, pertinent to swallowing. *Dysphagia* 1986;1:23–33.
3. Curtis DJ. Radiographic anatomy of the pharynx. *Dysphagia* 1986;1:51–62.
4. Rubesin SE, Jessurun J, Robertson D, Jones B, Bosma JF, Donner MW. Lines of the pharynx. *RadioGraphics* 1987;7:217–237.
5. Bosma JF. Deglutition: pharyngeal stage. *Physiol Rev* 1957;37:275–300.
6. Miller AJ. Deglutition. *Physiol Rev* 1982;62:129–184.
7. Miller AJ. Neurophysiological basis of swallowing. *Dysphagia* 1986;1:91–100.
8. Miller AJ. Swallowing: neurophysiologic control of the esophageal phase. *Dysphagia* 1987;2:72–82.
9. Dodds WJ, Stewart ET, Logemann JA. Physiology and radiology of the normal oral and pharyngeal phases of swallowing. *AJR Am J Roentgenol* 1990;154:953–963.
10. Dantas RO, Kern MK, Massey BT, Dodds WJ, Kahrilas PJ, Brasseur JG, Cook IJ, Lang IM. Effect of swallowed bolus variables on oral and pharyngeal phases of swallowing. *Am J Physiol* 1990;258(5 pt 1):G675–G681.
11. Dodds WJ, Taylor AJ, Stewart ET, Kern MK, Logemann JA, Cook IJ. Tipper and dipper types of oral swallows. *AJR Am J Roentgenol* 1989;153:1197–1199.
12. Nilsson H, Ekberg O, Olsson R, Hindfelt B. Quantitative assessment of swallowing in healthy adults. *Dysphagia* 1996;11(2):110–116.
13. Zerhouni EA, Bosma JF, Donner MW. Relationship of cervical spine disorders to dysphagia. *Dysphagia* 1987;1:129–144.
14. Curtis DJ. Laryngeal dynamics. *CRC Crit Rev Diagn Imaging* 1982;19:29–80.
15. Dodds WJ, Man KM, Cook IJ, Kahrilas PJ, Stewart ET, Kern MK. Influence of bolus volume on swallow-induced hyoid movement in normal subjects. *AJR Am J Roentgenol* 1988;150:1307–1309.
16. Ekberg O. The normal movements of the hyoid bone during swallow. *Invest Radiol* 1986;5:408–410.
17. Ekberg O, Sigurjonsson S. Movements of the epiglottis during deglutition: a cineradiographic study. *Gastrointest Radiol* 1982;7:101–107.
18. Linden P, Siebens AA. Dysphagia: predicting laryngeal penetration. *Arch Phys Med Rehabil* 1983;64(6):281–284.
19. Linden P, Kuhlemeier KV, Patterson C. The probability of correctly predicting subglottic penetration from clinical observations. *Dysphagia* 1993;8(3):170–179.

20. Gatenby RA, Rosenblum JS, Leonard CM, Moldofsky PJ, Broder GJ. Esophageal speech: double-contrast evaluation of the pharyngoesophageal segment. *Radiology* 1985;157:127–131.
21. Torres WE, Clements JL, Austin GE, Knight K. Cricopharyngeal muscle hypertrophy: radiologic anatomic correlation. *AJR Am J Roentgenol* 1984; 141:927–930.
22. Seaman WB. Functional disorders of the pharyngoesophageal junction: achalasia and chalasia. *Radiol Clin North Am* 1969;7:113–119.
23. Sokol EM, Heitman P, Wolfe BS, Cohen BR. Simultaneous cineradiographic and manometric study of the pharynx, hypopharynx, and cervical esophagus. *Gastroenterology* 1966;51:960–974.
24. Templeton RE, Kredel RA. Cricopharyngeal sphincter: roentgenologic study. *Laryngoscope* 1943;53:1–12.
25. Crichlow TVL. Cricopharyngeus in radiography and cineradiography. *Br J Radiol* 1956;29: 546–556.
26. Seaman WB. Cineroentgenographic observations of the cricopharyngeus. *AJR Am J Roentgenol* 1966;96:922–931.
27. Palmer ED. Disorders of the cricopharyngeus muscle: a review. *Gastroenterology* 1976;71: 510–517.
28. Roed-Peterson K. The pharyngo-esophageal sphincter: a review of the literature. *Dan Med Bull* 1979;26:275–281.
29. Ekberg O, Nylander B. Dysfunction of the cricopharyngeal muscle. *Radiology* 1982;143: 481–486.
30. Curtis DJ, Cruess DF, Berg T. The cricopharyngeal muscle: a videorecording review. *AJR Am J Roentgenol* 1984;142:497–500.
31. Ekberg O, Borgstrom P, Lindgren S. Is there an accessary sphincter of the cervical oesophagus? *Br J Radiol* 1988;61:341–343.
32. Dodds WJ, Kahrilas PJ, Dent J, Hogan WJ. Considerations about pharyngeal manometry. *Dysphagia* 1987;1:209–214.
33. Kahrilas PJ, Dodds WJ, Dent J, Logemann JA, Shaker R. Upper esophageal sphincter function during deglutition. *Gastroenterology* 1988;95: 52–62.
34. Ekberg O. Cricopharyngeal bar: myth and reality. *Abdom Imaging* 1995;20(2):179–180.
35. Olsson R, Ekberg O. Videomanometry of the pharynx in dysphagic patients with a posterior cricopharyngeal indentation. *Acad Radiol* 1995; 2(7):597–601.
36. Feinberg MJ, Ekberg O. Deglutition after near-fatal choking episode: radiologic evaluation. *Radiology* 1990;176(3):637–640.
37. Feinberg MJ, Ekberg O. Videofluoroscopy in elderly patients with aspiration: importance of evaluating both oral and pharyngeal stages of deglutition. *AJR Am J Roentgenol* 1991; 156(2):293–296.
38. Chen MY, Ott DJ, Peele VN, Gelfand DW. Oropharynx in patients with cerebrovascular disease: evaluation with videofluoroscopy. *Radiology* 1990;176(3):641–643.
39. Leopold NA, Kagel MC. Prepharyngeal dysphagia in Parkinson's disease. *Dysphagia* 1996;11(1): 14–22.
40. Nilsson H, Ekberg O, Olsson R, Hindfelt B. Quantitative assessment of oral and pharyngeal function in Parkinson's disease. *Dysphagia* 1996;11(2):144–150.
41. Buchholz D, Barofsky I, Edwin D, Jones B, Ravich W. Psychogenic oropharyngeal dysphagia: report of 26 cases. *Dysphagia* 1994;9: 267–270.
42. Shapiro J, Franko DL, Gagne A. Phagophobia: a form of psychogenic dysphagia. A new entity. *Ann Otol Rhinol Laryngol* 1997;106(4):286–290.
43. Barofsky I, Ravich W, Buchholz D, Jones B. Oral findings on videoswallowing study in neurogenic and psychogenic dysphagia. Paper presented at: 25th Annual Meeting of the Society of Gastrointestinal Radiologists; 1996; Bermuda.
44. Neumann S, Buchholz D, Ravich W, Jones B. Psychogenic dysphagia: a long-term follow-up study. *Dysphagia* 1999;14(2):128.
45. Olsson R, Castell JA, Castell DO, Ekberg O. Solid-state computerized manometry improves diagnostic yield in pharyngeal dysphagia: simultaneous videoradiography and manometry in dysphagia patients with normal barium swallows. *Abdom Imaging* 1995;20(3):230–235.
46. Herrera JL, Lyons MF II, Johnson LF. Saliva: its role in health and disease. *J Clin Gastroenterol* 1988;10:569–578.
47. Helm JF. Role of saliva in esophageal function and disease. *Dysphagia* 1989;4:76–84.
48. Helm JF, Dodds WJ, Pelc LR, Palmer DW, Hogan WJ, Teeter BC. Effect of esophageal emptying and saliva on clearance of acid from the esophagus. *N Engl J Med* 1984;310: 284–288.
49. Rubesin SE, Jones B, Donner MW. Radiology of the adult soft palate. *Dysphagia* 1987;2:8–17.

50. Rubesin SE, Rabischong P, Bilaniuk LT, Laufer I, Levine MS. Contrast examination of the soft palate with cross-sectional correlation. *RadioGraphics* 1988;4:641–665.
51. Skolnick ML. Videofluoroscopic examination of the velopharyngeal portal during phonation in lateral and base projections—a new technique for studying the mechanisms of closure. *Cleft Palate J* 1970;7:803–816.
52. Rubesin SE, Jessurun J, Robertson D, Jones B, Bosma JF, Donner MW. Lines of the pharynx. *RadioGraphics* 1987;7:217–237.

5
Adaptation, Compensation, and Decompensation

BRONWYN JONES

The 26th edition of *Stedman's Medical Dictionary* offers the following definitions:

Adaptation: an advantageous change in function or constitution of an organ or tissue to meet new conditions (p. 23).
Compensation: term used to describe a process in which a tendency for a change in a given direction is counteracted by another change so that the original change is not evident (p. 372).
Decompensation: a failure of compensation (in heart disease) (p. 445).

When these words are used to describe a swallow, they indicate certain changes implied in the foregoing definitions (1).

Adaptation

The process of adjustment of the *normal* swallow to different stimuli is called **adaptation**. The pharynx must adapt to its various functions, namely, respiration, speech, and swallowing. Changes in head, neck, and body position may alter the anatomical relationships of the area. The effect of gravity is also important. Think about how much additional muscular strength must be generated in the pharyngeal constrictor muscles to swallow in the supine or prone position or even standing on one's head (2). Similarly, it takes more tongue thrust to swallow in the prone position than in the supine position.

The pharynx must also adjust to the bolus, since individual boluses may vary in size, temperature, consistency, weight, viscosity, and elasticity. The effect of different boluses can be seen during videofluoroscopy by observing the difference between distension of the lumen with a swallow of thin liquid barium and one of the same volume of barium paste: the "weight" of the paste bolus results in the lumen size becoming wider, usually.

Over a lifetime the pharynx ages with the rest of the body and swallowing is altered by the anatomical and physiological changes that occur with the aging process (see Chapter 12). At the other end of the spectrum, a baby feeds by suckling, and the shape of the oral cavity and pharynx and the relationship of the pharynx and larynx to the base of the skull are quite different in the neonate and in the adult (see Chapter 11).

One form of adaptation occurs in persons who can voluntarily open the cricopharyngeus such as sword swallowers (Figure 5.1) and beer guzzlers. Others allow controlled release of esophageal air such as in esophageal speech.

Compensation

A very important concept to understand is that a **compensated** swallow indicates *already impaired swallowing*. Compensation for impaired swallowing may be conscious and voluntary, or subconscious and involuntary. Conscious effects of compensation include a change in the speed and style of eating, or in the types of food eaten. Some patients will limit

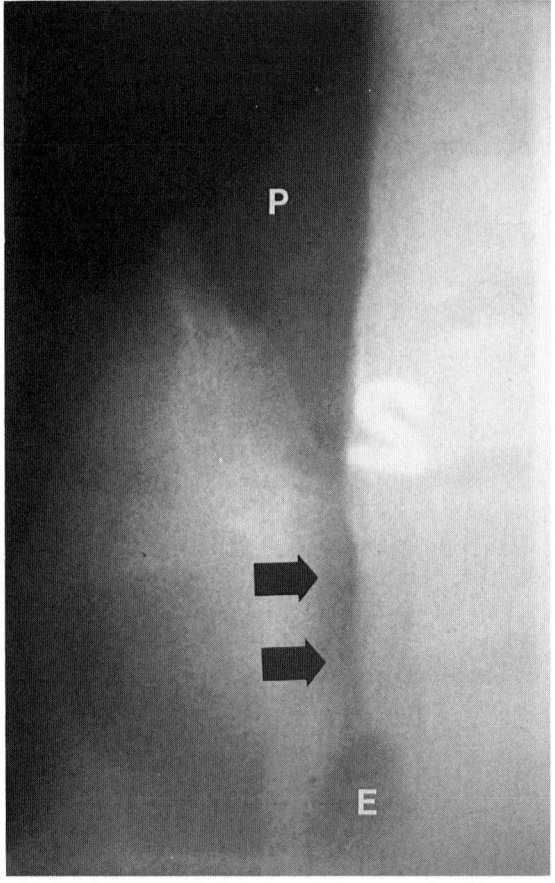 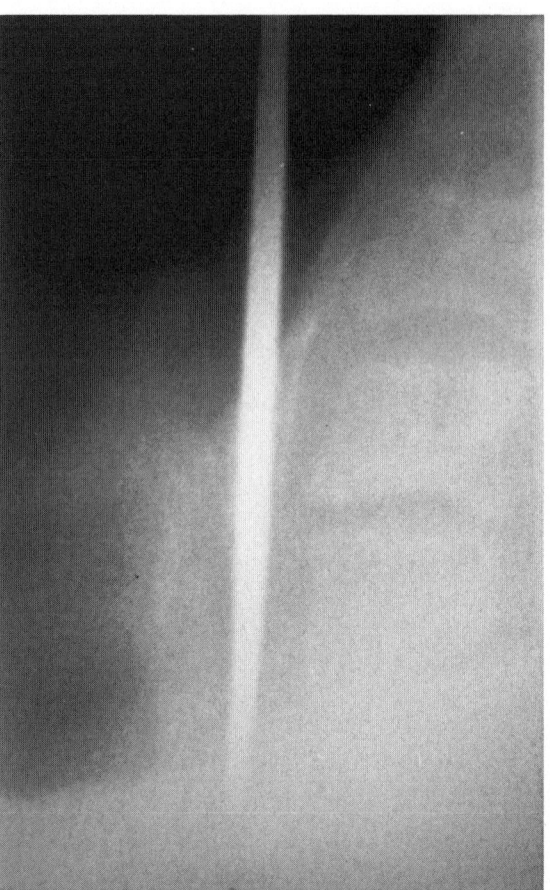

FIGURE 5.1. Voluntary opening of the cricopharyngeal segment. This individual, a sword swallower, is able to open the cricopharyngeus muscle at will. (A) Air can be seen in the pharynx (P) above the cricopharyngeus and in the esophagus (E) below the cricopharyngeus with air in the sphincter zone (arrowhead) in a slightly more narrowed lumen (arrows). While the cricopharyngeus remains open, a sword can be passed through the area. (B) A sword is extending from the pharynx down through the cricopharyngeus. It was subsequently passed down to about the level of the tracheal bifurcation.

what they eat, omitting solid foods and substituting purées, or even restricting their diet to liquids only. Some patients will eat very slowly or wash the solid food down with liquids.

When swallowing is impaired but compensated, careful history taking may provide important clues. A patient may report that feeding has become more arduous and time-consuming. Food may have to be specially prepared, either by vigorous chewing or mechanical blending, and certain foods may be avoided entirely. Frequent small meals make feeding easier, and individual bolus size may be voluntarily reduced. Double swallowing may help to clear retained material from the pharynx. The patient may have found through experimenting that certain postures help. Momentary flexing of the chin down during swallow is a common early sign of compensation. This maneuver, interestingly, is a minor variation on the "chin-tuck" commonly used in swallowing therapy. A patient with unilateral weakness may have discovered independently, again by experimentation, that the swallow is improved by turning or tilting the chin toward the weak side (see Chapter 14 for these and other techniques used in swallowing therapy).

5. Adaptation, Compensation, and Decompensation

Sometimes, postural support muscles of the head and neck can be recruited to aid in swallowing, and in such a case the recumbent or semirecumbent position, with the head resting on a pillow, may improve the swallow by allowing the postural muscles to be used for swallowing. Even the basic method of feeding may be altered, as when suckle feeding (sipping liquids repetitively, through a straw or artificial nipple) may be useful (3).

When swallowing is impaired, it is possible for one structure to **compensate** for a deficiency in an adjacent structure, with the result that swallowing may still be effective and safe without overt signs of dysfunction. *These compensatory signs are visible on the dynamic imaging study* (Figures 5.2–5.6, 5.7A, E, F). Remember, the presence of these findings indicates an impaired swallow.

Compensation occurs slowly and implies that the impairment has been a gradual process. Compensation occurs in some patients with an impaired swallow and not in others. It is not known why some patients with impaired swallowing develop compensatory changes and others do not, although neural plasticity has been implicated in this process (4,5). Compensation also tends to occur when one of the organs is weak and the other strong (e.g., weak soft palate, strong tongue, or vice versa).

If the insult to the swallow is a sudden one (e.g., a massive cerebrovascular accident), there is usually no time for compensation, whereas with a slowly progressive process there is time for compensation to develop.

It cannot be stressed too much that these signs of compensation indicate that swallowing is already compromised; further deterioration may overwhelm the compensatory process and overt signs of abnormal swallowing may appear, such as nasopharyngeal regurgitation or aspiration with cough-choke episodes. The swallow has now *decompensated* (Figures 5.2–5.6, 5.7B, C, D).

The swallow can be broken down into five distinct stages, each of which has a characteristic pattern of compensation and decompensation (Table 5.1; Figures 5.2–5.6) (1). The five stages are as follows:

1. Control of the junction of mouth and pharynx (to prevent premature leakage)
2. Closure of the palatopharyngeal isthmus (to prevent nasopharyngeal regurgitation)
3. Compression and propulsion of the bolus (by the pharyngeal constrictors and back of tongue)
4. Closure of the larynx
5. Opening of the pharyngoesophageal (P-E) segment

At the first step, for example, deficiency of the tongue (atrophy, weakness, surgery) may be compensated by downward displacement or kinking of the soft palate; conversely, upward backward displacement of the tongue may compensate if the soft palate is weak. Decompensation of this stage results in premature leakage prior to swallow with the risk of aspiration prior to swallow. (Figures 5.2–5.6 and Table 5.1 illustrate and explain steps 1–5. Some radiographic examples of compensation and decompensation are demonstrated in Figure 5.7.)

Compensatory changes can also occur under different circumstances. If, for example, there is an obstructing lesion in the pharynx or cervical esophagus, the constrictor wave may become deeper and presumably stronger as a compensatory phenomenon to overcome the distal obstruction. Such a prominent wave is not uncommon if there is prominence of the cricopharyngeus or a cervical esophageal web (Figure 5.7).

If signs of compensation are seen, one may need to perform additional maneuvers to stress the swallow in order to show that the swallow may decompensate in certain circumstances. If, for example, kinking of the soft palate is seen in the erect position, tongue abnormalities may be brought out by having the patient swallow against gravity in the prone position. Similarly, eliminating the effects of gravity by examining the patient in the supine position with a cross-table tube or in the lateral supine position may demonstrate nasal regurgitation not evident before (see also Chapter 3). Stressing the tongue-palate seal in the supine position may also reveal premature leakage.

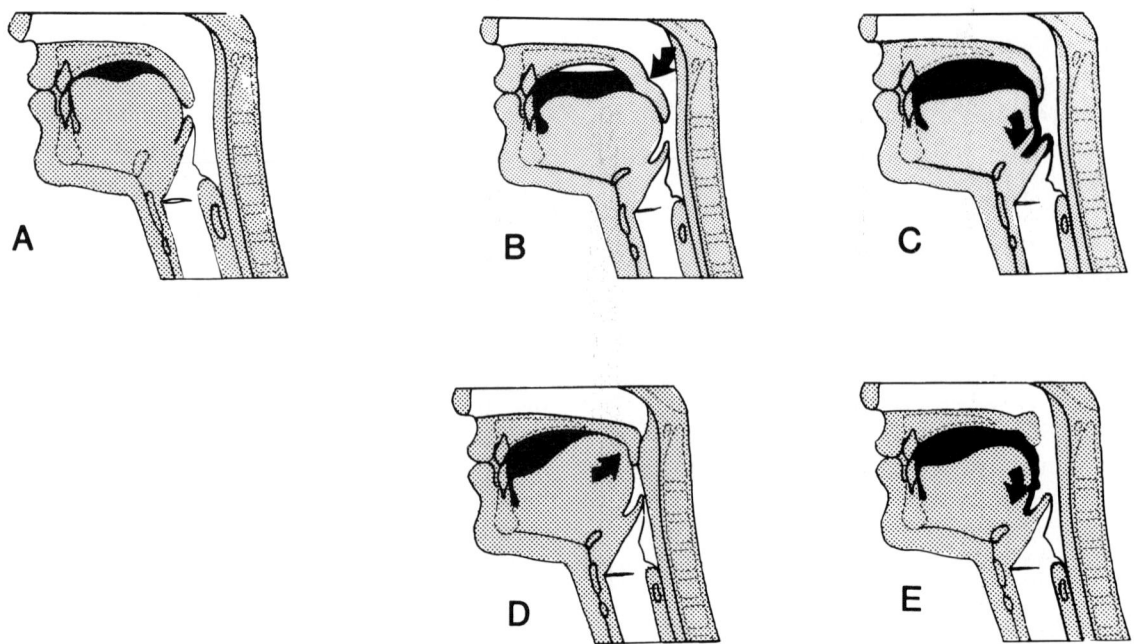

FIGURE 5.2. Control of junction of mouth and pharynx. (A) In the normal situation, the soft palate abuts the posterior portion of the tongue, preventing premature leakage from the back of the mouth. (B) Deficiency of the tongue due to atrophy, weakness, incoordination, or postsurgical defect may be compensated for by downward displacement of the palate, which "kinks" to appose the tongue. Conversely, palatal deficiency is compensated by upward posterior displacement of the tongue (D). Note that the bolus is held further forward in the mouth under these circumstances. (C, E) Decompensation, with premature leakage of oral contents into the pharynx with the potential for aspiration. (Figures 5.2, 5.3, 5.4, 5.5, and 5.6 reprinted with permission from Buchholz DW, Bosma JF, Donner MW. Adaptation, compensation and decompensation of the pharyngeal swallow. *Gastrointest Radiol* 1985;10:235–240.)

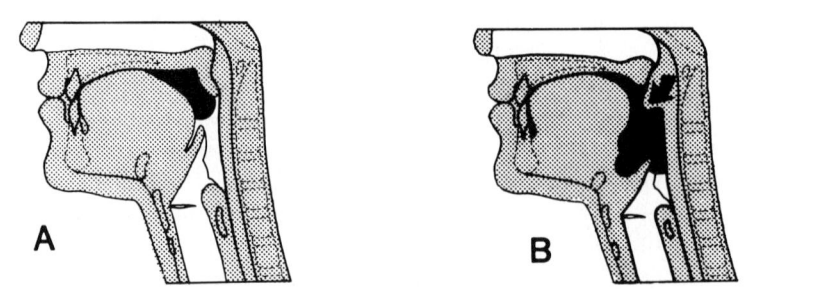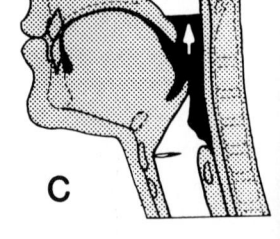

FIGURE 5.3. Closure of palatopharyngeal isthmus during swallowing. (A) In normal closure, the soft palate is elevated to a right angle to abut Passavant's cushion and thus prevent nasopharyngeal regurgitation. (B) Deficiency of the palate may be compensated for by increasing convergence of the superior pharyngeal constrictor muscles, resulting in a very prominent Passavant's cushion. (C) Decompensation will result in nasopharyngeal regurgitation through the palatopharyngeal isthmus.

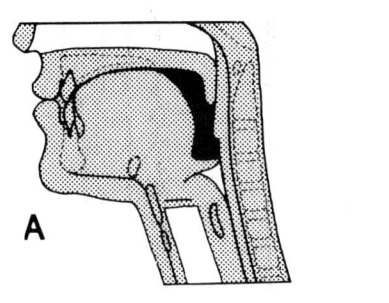
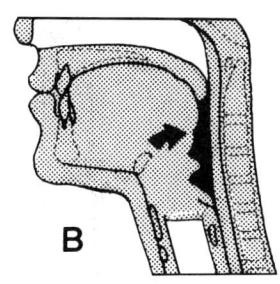
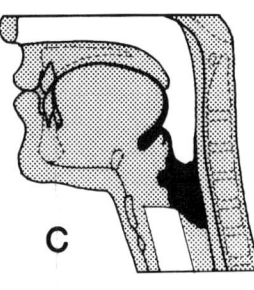
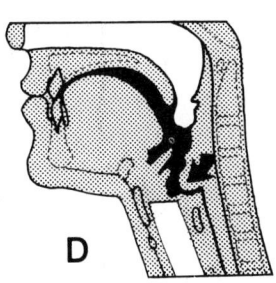
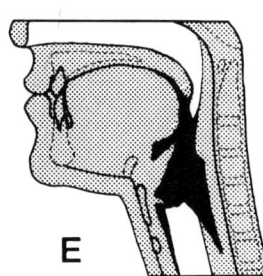

FIGURE 5.4. Compression of the bolus. (A) Normal compression. (B) Deficiency of the constrictor muscles may be compensated for by increased upward and posterior displacement of the tongue and larynx. Deficiency of the tongue in bolus compression may be followed by increased anterior movement of the constrictor muscles (D), resulting in a very prominent pharyngeal stripping wave. Decompensation due to inadequate bolus compression will result in bolus retention in the valleculae and piriform sinuses after swallowing (C) with the potential for overflow aspiration (E).

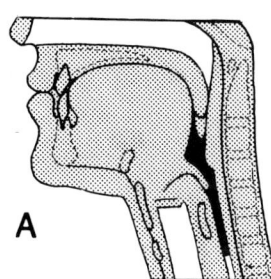
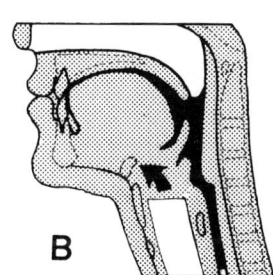
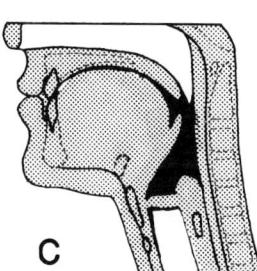

FIGURE 5.5. Closure of the larynx. (A) In normal closure and elevation of the larynx, there is the appearance of the "conus," with the epiglottis completely tilted and inverted to cover the entrance to the laryngeal aditus. (B) With poor epiglottic tilting or glottic closure, there may be increased upward and anterior displacement of the larynx. Occasionally under these circumstances there will also be increased size of the arytenoid masses as a sign of compensation (not illustrated). (C) Decompensation produces laryngeal penetration or aspiration (with or without reflexive cough).

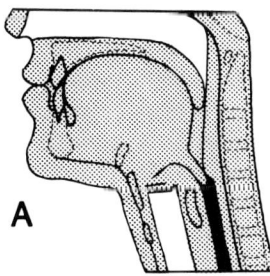
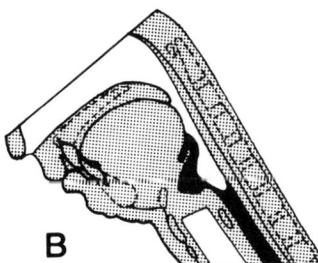
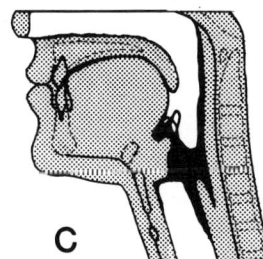

FIGURE 5.6. Opening of the pharyngoesophageal segment. (A) Normal opening of the P-E segment. (B) Diminished superior and anterior laryngeal movement (which contributes to opening of the P-E segment) may result in head and neck flexion and/or forward thrusting of the jaw during swallowing. (C) Decompensation will result in poor pharyngoesophageal segment opening, with retention in the piriform sinuses and the risk of overflow aspiration.

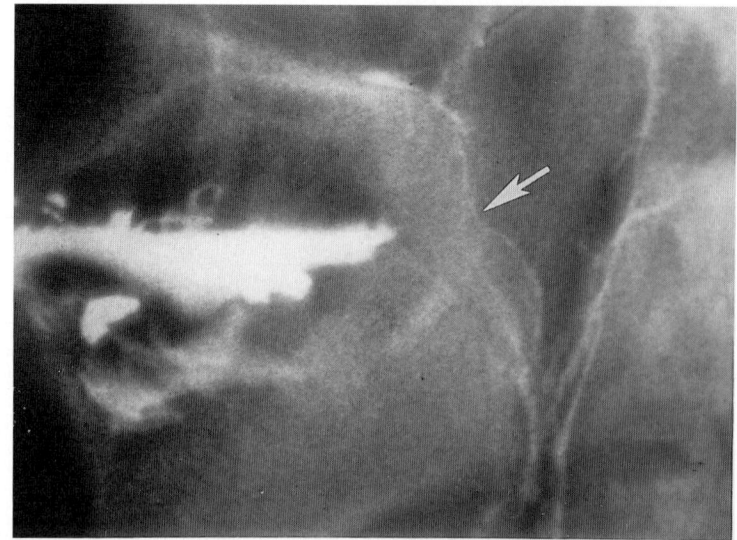

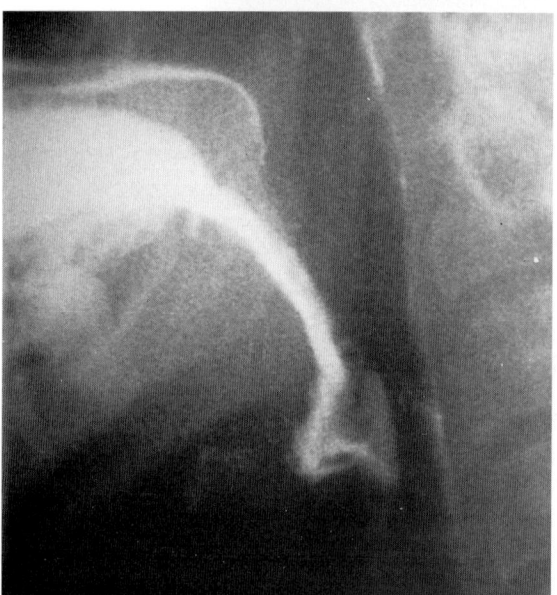
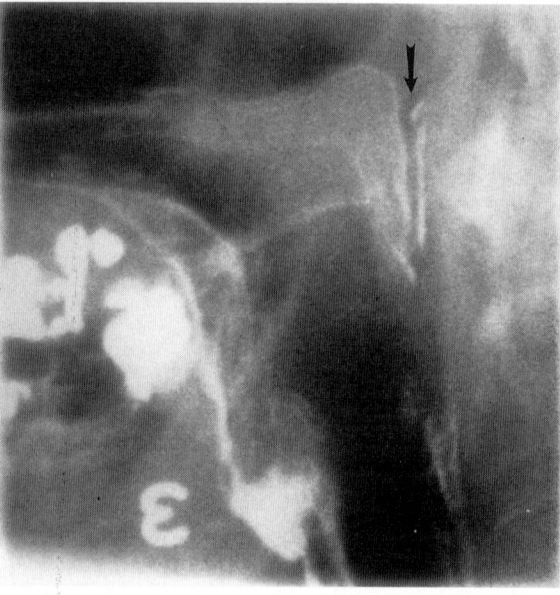

FIGURE 5.7. Some signs of oropharyngeal compensation and decompensation. (A) The palate kinks (arrow) in an effort to appose the tongue to maintain the bolus within the mouth. This is an abnormal finding in the erect position (note the air-fluid level in the mouth, indicating the patient is erect). (B) If further decompensation occurs, bolus may leak over the back of the tongue into the valleculae prior to swallowing, creating the potential for aspiration. (C) Incomplete elevation of the soft palate during enunciation of the word "candy" indicates that there is incomplete posterior movement of the soft palate with incomplete obliteration of the nasopharyngeal isthmus (arrow). There has also been some nasopharyngeal regurgitation on a previous swallow, and there is retention in the valleculae. (D) Examination in the supine position with a cross-table tube demonstrates nasopharyngeal regurgitation (arrows). Note the air-fluid level in the posterior aspect of the oral cavity. Note also that the contrast is layered along the posterior wall of the pharynx in this position. (The letters OO indicate zero degrees, i.e., the horizontal position.) (E) There is a very prominent stripping wave superiorly (arrows), raising the question of whether this is a compensatory phenomenon. The reason for the prominent wave is twofold: a cricopharyngeal bar (arrowheads) and a web on the anterior wall of the cervical esophagus (short arrow). (Reproduced with permission from Jones B, Donner MW. The pharynx. In: Taveras JM, Ferrucci JT, eds. *Radiology: Diagnosis Imaging Intervention.* Philadelphia: JB Lippincott, 1990.) (F) There is excessive posterior movement of the base of the tongue (T) in this patient with pharyngeal paralysis (in an attempt to clear the pharynx of bolus).

5. Adaptation, Compensation, and Decompensation

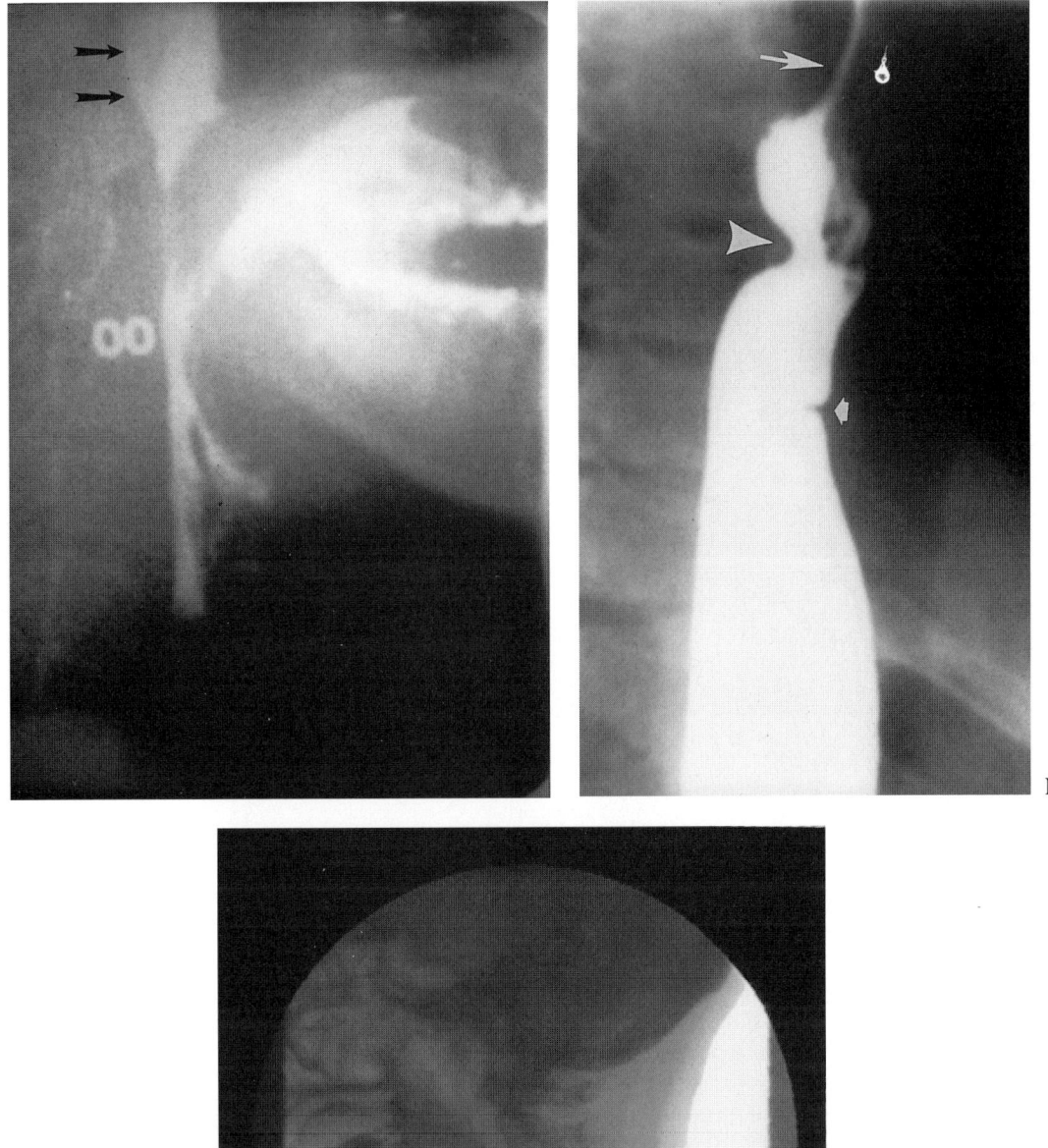

FIGURE 5.7. Continued

TABLE 5.1. The five stages of swallowing.

Step	Site	Area of deficiency	Signs of Compensation	Decompensation
1	Control of junction of mouth and pharynx pharynx (tongue/palate competence)	Tongue	Palate kinks to appose tongue (this is *normal* in the supine position but not in the erect position)	Leakage into pharynx prior to swallow
		Palate	Posterior aspect of tongue upward	Leakage into pharynx prior to swallow
2	Closure of palatopharyngeal isthmus (palate/constrictor competence)	Palate	Greater convergence of constrictor wall (prominent Passavant's cushion)	Nasopharyngeal regurgitation
3	Compression of bolus	Constrictor muscles	Tongue and larynx displaced posteriorly	Retention in valleculae and piriform sinuses after swallow
		Tongue base	Greater convergence of constrictor wall (prominent stripping wave)	Retention in valleculae and piriform sinuses after swallow
4	Closure of larynx	Intrinsic laryngeal muscles	Further displacement of larynx upward and forward	Laryngeal penetration or aspiration
5	Opening of P-E segment	P-E segment opening	Head flexion	Retention and/or overflow aspiration of retained bolus

It is important to report any radiographic findings of compensation to the referring physician. The patient needs to know that the swallow, although symptomatically not necessarily a problem, is impaired. Advice should include additional care when eating or drinking quickly or under conditions of decreased concentration such as in a social situation. Medications such as sedatives, antidepressants, and painkillers, or alcohol may also depress the function of the oral and pharyngeal musculature and may change an impaired but compensated swallow into a decompensated swallow.

References

1. Buchholz DW, Bosma JF, Donner MW. Adaptation, compensation, and decompensation of the pharyngeal swallow. *Gastrointest Radiol* 1985;10: 235–239.
2. Bruhlmann W. *Die roentgenkinematographische Untersuchung von Störungen des Schluckaktes.* [habilitationsschrift]. Zurich; 1982.
3. Ramsey WO. Suckle facilitation of feeding in selected adult dysphagic patients. *Dysphagia* 1986; 1:7–12.
4. Seitz RJ, Huang Y, Knorr U, Tellmann L, Herzog H, Freund HJ. Large-scale plasticity of the human motor cortex. *Neuroreport* 1995;6(5):742–744.
5. Atwood HL, Wojtowicz JM. Silent synapses in neural plasticity: current evidence. *Learn Mem* 1999;6(6):542–571.

6
Pharyngoesophageal Interrelationships and Reflexes Involved in Airway Protection

BRONWYN JONES

Do the mouth, pharynx, and larynx operate independently, or are there feedback mechanisms between the pharynx and esophagus?

Are there any reflexes that cause the cricopharyngeus muscle to contract, raise the upper esophageal sphincter (UES) pressure, or cause hypertrophy of the cricopharyngeus? What is the effect of gastroesophageal reflux on the UES, pharynx, or larynx? What effect does sensory input from the pharynx or larynx have on the esophagus?

Does esophagopharyngeal regurgitation of gastric acid harm the pharynx, and can this result in dysphagia?

This chapter hopes to answer some of these questions and to present the latest research on the subject of pharyngoesophageal interrelationships.

Oropharyngeal Dysphagia: The Potential Role of The Esophagus

Symptoms

It is a widely held misconception that the level of an obstructing esophageal lesion can be accurately pinpointed by the patient. Edwards, however, in a study of 383 patients with obstructive symptoms and known structural lesions of the esophagus, found that approximately one-third of those with distal esophageal obstruction had symptoms referred to the neck (1). Distal localization of a proximal lesion is much less common. Edwards concluded: "The site at which obstruction is localized by the subject is so frequently incorrect that no importance can be attached to it." Figure 6.1 summarizes Edwards's results, incorporating modifications by Jones et al. (2).

Experimental Studies

Intraluminal Foreign Bodies and Balloon Distension

Intraluminal foreign bodies lodged in the hypopharynx or upper esophagus may produce cricopharyngeal spasm (3). In cats, it has been shown that stimulation of afferent receptors in the hypopharynx or upper cervical esophagus evokes reflex contraction and spasm in the cricopharyngeal muscle with an increase in intraluminal pressure in the sphincter segment. Similarly, esophageal distention by liquids or an intraluminal balloon in humans results in elevated pressure in the sphincter segment (4–7).

Gastroesophageal Reflux and the Cricopharyngeus: Manometric Data

Reports in the manometry literature vary with respect to whether acid bathing the esophagus produces a rise in pressure in the sphincter segment. Early work in the 1970s (in human volunteers), which featured the use of perfused catheters to infuse the esophagus with saline or acid solution, reported elevated pressures in the sphincter segment (8,9). The closer the infusion was to the cricopharyngeal sphincter, the greater was the increase in pressure.

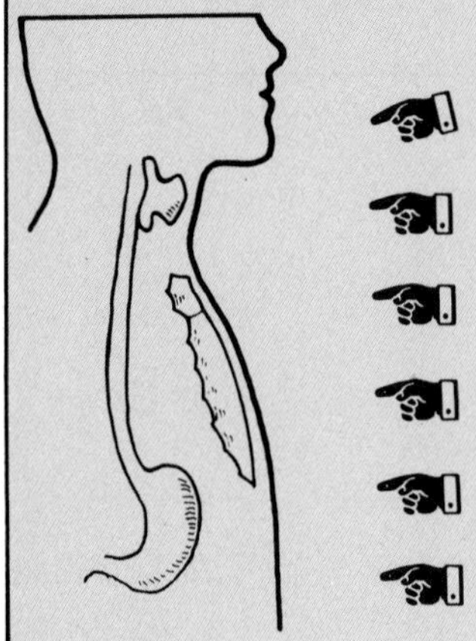

Site at which subject localizes block	Actual site of upper level of lesion				
	ACHALASIA	LOWER ESOPH. STRICT.	FUNDAL CANCER	MID ESOPH. STRICT.	UPPER ESOPH. STRICT.
	0	5	0	2	0
	28	6	1	3	6
	27	23	4	8	10
	42	25	5	11	2
	69	50	19	18	2
	7	10	3	2	0

FIGURE 6.1. Approximately one third of 383 patients with obstructive symptoms and distal esophageal abnormalities, such as achalasia and lower esophageal stricture, localize their symptoms at or above the suprasternal notch. [Modified from Edwards (1) and reproduced from Jones et al. (2), with permission.]

More recent work, using a modified sleeve sensor, compared UES pressures in 17 volunteers and 16 patients with esophagitis (10) and reported absence of an upper esophageal sphincter response to acid reflux. Neither group showed any change in the resting pressure in the UES with acid perfusion, although the patients with esophagitis developed severe heartburn.

More recent manometric studies, in general using solid-state catheters, have produced a wealth of data about the complex interactions of the lower esophageal sphincter (LES), gastroesophageal reflux (GER), intraesophageal pressure changes, and changes in pressure in the upper esophageal sphincter. Several new reflexes have been described.

UES Contractile Response to GER

Shaker et al. compared UES pressure changes in normal controls and patients with reflux esophagitis during 35 spontaneous reflux events (11). Most of the controls and patients showed a significant abrupt increase in UES pressures (UESP) as well as in intraesophageal pressure (IPI) in response to episodes of GER (11).

Pharyngo-UES Contractile Response

Mechanical stimulation of the pharynx in cats (12) and water stimulation in humans (13) produces an increase in the UES resting tone. As little as 0.1 mL of water resulted in this reflex. A higher volume of water infusion in humans results in what has been named a "pharyngeal swallow" (this may be produced in animals also by mechanical stimulation). This swallow (also called a secondary swallow) is similar to the pharyngeal phase of a normal swallow but excludes the oral phase of lingual propulsion and bolus transport. It is thought that these swallows both activate glottal closure as a protective reflex and clear the pharynx of any refluxed material or prematurely leaked fluid from the mouth. Much larger volumes of fluid need to be infused in elderly patients than in younger people to invoke this reflex, another sign of diminished sensation with aging (14). Much larger volumes were needed also in a study of patients with posterior laryngitis (thought to be reflux induced) perhaps because of diminished sensation due to acid damage to the pharyngeal mucosa (15).

There are also reflexes between the esophagus and pharynx and the glottis.

Esophagoglottal Closure Reflex

Esophageal distension during GER could potentially overwhelm the UES with the potential for overflow aspiration. In the early 1990s a reflex was described in both humans (16) and cats (17) in which esophageal distension results in reflex adduction of the glottis. This distension may be produced focally (e.g., by a balloon), by diffuse distension (e.g., by air insufflation), or by a GER episode.

This reflex is postulated as one of the airway protective mechanisms against retrograde esophageal transit such as during belching (18), regurgitation, GER (19), and possibly vomiting.

Pharyngoglottal Adduction Reflex

Injection of minute amounts of water into the pharynx results in brief closure of the vocal cords. This is thought to be a protective maneuver to prevent aspiration (20). Significantly higher volumes of fluid are necessary to evoke this reflux in the elderly than in young people (14).

Gastroesophageal Reflux and the Cricopharyngeus: Pathological Data

Chronic inflammatory changes have been found in the cricopharyngeus in myotomy specimens from patients with cricopharyngeal dysphagia and documented gastroesophageal reflux (21).

Two studies commented on the histopathology of cricopharyngeus muscle in patients with Zenker's diverticulum, a process often accompanied by esophageal diseases such as GER. Atrophy and degeneration of muscle fibers were found in both studies (22,23).

Gastroesophageal Reflux and the Lungs

Direct Damage to the Lungs

Acute aspiration pneumonia, due either to aspiration prior to or during swallowing or to overflow aspiration of retained, regurgitated, or refluxed material, is well recognized clinically (24). Less well appreciated are other long-term effects of chronic aspiration such as interstitial fibrosis or progressive deterioration in pulmonary function (25).

Indirect Effects

Even less known is coughing or asthma caused by gastroesophageal reflux. Acid bathing the distal esophagus is associated with a reflex constriction of the bronchioli. Hence, it is not surprising that GER has been documented as a causative factor in late-onset adult asthma (26,27) and in young children with chalasia (28–30). Response to antireflux therapy in patients with asthma and documented reflux can be dramatic. In such patients, symptoms of reflux may be subtle or even absent.

The Larynx

Other respiratory lesions have been reported in association with gastroesophageal reflux; these include inflammation of the arytenoids, laryngeal granuloma, posterior laryngitis, and contact ulcers of the larynx (31–33). The lesions may respond to antireflux therapy. These findings explain the presenting symptoms of hoarseness and sore throat of which some patients with reflux complain.

Reflux has also been indicated as an etiological factor in the development of laryngeal cancer (34,35).

Similarly, a more recent study at the Johns Hopkins Medical Institutions of patients with large hypopharyngeal cancer requiring laryngopharyngoesophagectomy found esophageal disease in just over half (36). Secondary esophageal squamous cell carcinomas were found in about 25% of the specimens, many of which were small and not suspected clinically prior to surgery. In 33% of the 24 patients, there was pathological evidence of gastroesophageal reflux as evidenced by either Barrett's esophagus or esophagitis.

Gastroesophageal Reflux and Other Reflexes

There are also numerous reports of other reflux-induced changes in the cardiorespiratory cycles including tachycardia, bradycardia,

TABLE 6.1. The many facets of gastroesophageal reflux.

Pharynx
Pain and/or lump or foreign body sensation ("globus")
Prominent cricopharyngeus
Asymmetry of contraction
Lateral pharyngeal pouches
Zenker's diverticulum
Larynx
Chronic cough
Pain and hoarseness
Laryngitis
Contact granuloma
Laryngeal ulcer
Laryngospasm
Laryngeal cancer
Lung
Aspiration pneumonia
Chronic lung disease
Asthma
Sleep apnea
Heart
Tachycardia
Bradycardia
Arrhythmias
Syncope

syncope, laryngospasm, and apnea. The reader is referred to a review of normal and abnormal reflexes between swallowing and other symptoms (37). Table 6.1 suggests the multifaceted nature of this condition.

Clinical Studies

Pharyngeal symptomatology in GER was first stressed in the radiology literature by Cherry et al. (38). In our experience at the Johns Hopkins Swallowing Center (admittedly a biased population), pharyngeal symptomatology is a common presentation in patients with gastroesophageal reflux. For example, over a 2-year period, one third of the patients seen at the Johns Hopkins Swallowing Center had GER as their underlying condition, and of these, approximately one third presented with pharyngeal symptoms such as globus sensation, cough-choke episodes, sore throat, pain on swallowing, or hoarseness (Jones, personal observation). Many of these patients had been evaluated at other institutions, where, in many cases, diagnostic evaluations had been restricted to the symptomatic area, hence explaining the lack of a diagnosis.

Swallowing Center Studies

To demonstrate the importance of evaluating both pharynx and esophagus in all patients with dysphagia, the following observations are presented.

Cricopharyngeal Prominence on Cineradiography

The esophageal findings in 24 consecutive patients with prominence of the cricopharynges on dynamic imaging were analyzed (2). All but two had findings in the esophagus, including a positive acid-barium test, hiatal hernia or Schatzki's ring, and spasm. In seven patients, gastroesophageal reflux was observed (Table 6.2). Asymmetry of pharyngeal contraction was

TABLE 6.2. Esophageal and pharyngeal findings in patients with cricopharyngeal prominence.[a]

Findings	Number of patients
Esophageal	
Segmental spasm	12
Acid sensitivity	10
Hiatus hernia	10
Reflux (in many cases up to cricopharyngeal segment)	7
Schatzki's ring	3
Severe esophagitis with long stricture	2
Multiple webs, cervical esophagus	2
Absent peristalsis	2
Normal esophagus	1
Pharyngeal	
Asymmetry with retention	7
Lateral pharyngeal pouch	6

[a] Findings in 24 consecutive patients with cricopharyngeal prominence shown on cineradiography; multiple findings in each patient.
Source: Reprinted with permission from Jones B, Ravich WJ, Donner MW, Kramer SS, Hendrix TR. Pharyngoesophageal interrelationships: observations and working concepts. *Gastrointest Radiol* 1985;10:225–233.

present in seven patients; lateral pharyngeal pouches were found in six patients, with cervical esophageal webs being present in two.

Recently a new radiographic sign of GER was reported, namely, premature closure of the cricopharyngeus (CP) (39).

Unexplained Pharyngeal Dysphagia

Forty patients with dysphagia localized at or above the suprasternal notch, in whom outside evaluations had been negative, were reviewed (26). In 14 of the 40 patients (35%), the pharynx was normal but there was an esophageal abnormality, either a structural lesion or a motility disorder. The lesions were not inconsequential and included compression from a mediastinal mass and a midesophageal stricture.

Of additional interest in this study was the frequency of simultaneous abnormalities in pharynx and esophagus (Figure 6.2). Eleven of the 40 patients (27.5%) had combined disorders, each of which was capable of causing dysphagia.

While these observations may have been coincidental, the possibility that a disorder in one region may be causally related to dysfunction in the other must be considered.

Zenker's Diverticulum

In 1991, twenty-seven patients with Zenker's diverticulum (Figure 6.3) were entered in the Swallowing Center database, and of these 23 had either Schatzki's ring, hiatal hernia, GER, or spasm. An additional two had achalasia.

An unpublished more recent review of the database revealed 67 patients with Zenker's diverticulum evaluated by the multidisciplinary team at the Johns Hopkins Swallowing Center. Of the 67 patients, 63 were found to have esophageal pathology of some kind, such as hiatal hernia, GER, or esophageal spasm (T. Karaho, unpublished observations).

The pivotal structure central to these observations is the UES (or CP). Studies from Cook et al. have shown a high intrabolus pressure in these patients (41,42), which can be abolished by CP myotomy (43). Prior studies had failed to show incoordination between CP relaxation and pharyngeal contraction (44,45).

Achalasia

The videofluorographic studies of 21 consecutive patients with achalasia were reviewed; 11 had pharyngeal findings (46). Of this group, 4 had been previously dilated either by bougie or pneumostatic technique. The most common radiographic finding was lateral pharyngeal pouches (9 patients); these were bilateral in 8 patients, and 5 emptied postswallow into the valleculae or piriform sinuses. Abnormalities of the pharyngoesophageal segment were found in 8 patients, the cricopharyngeus being prominent in 7 (Figure 6.4) and having an unusual spiral appearance in the eighth. This patient had had a Heller myotomy in the past, followed by gastroesophageal reflux disease complicated by a Barrett's esophagus.

Asymmetry of pharyngeal contraction was seen in 7 patients, asymmetry of epiglottic tilt in 2 and a Zenker's diverticulum in 2. A third patient had had resection of a Zenker's diverticulum approximately 10 years earlier. In 2 patients there was laryngeal penetration during swallowing.

Two manometric studies have validated the theory that there are changes in the CP segment in patients with achalasia. Dudnick et al. (47) demonstrated abnormal UES function in 19 patients with achalasia who showed increased residual pressure in the UES, decreased duration of UES relaxation, and more rapid onset of pharyngeal contraction. Not long afterward, Zhang and Diamant (48) reported on 216 motility studies in 156 achalasia patients. One hundred five patients in 125 studies had repetitive upper esophageal contractions and/or repetitive contractions of the UES. The study concluded that this was a potential mechanism for proximal symptomatology and for the development of a CP bar in these patients.

Psychogenic Dysphagia and Globus Hystericus

Over an 18-month period, there were 23 patients referred to the Johns Hopkins

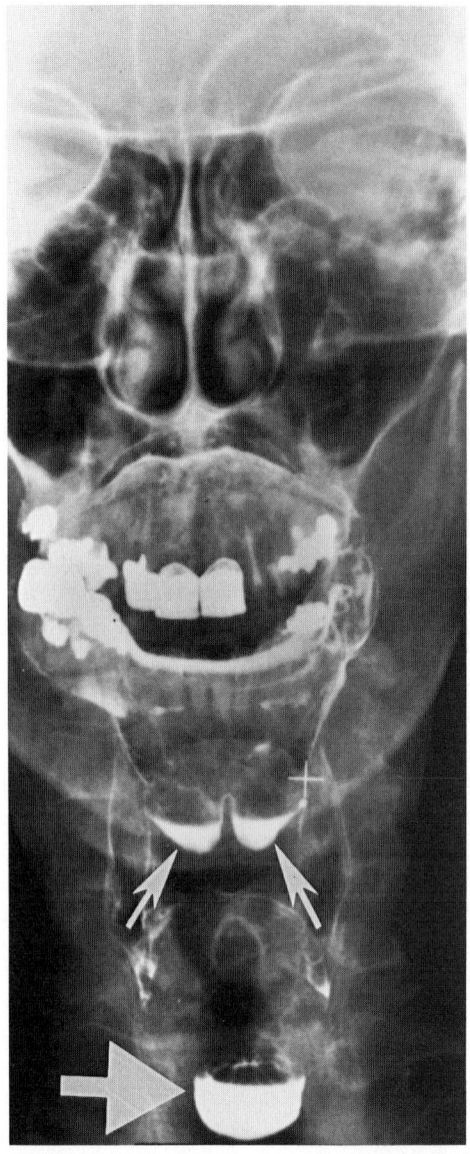 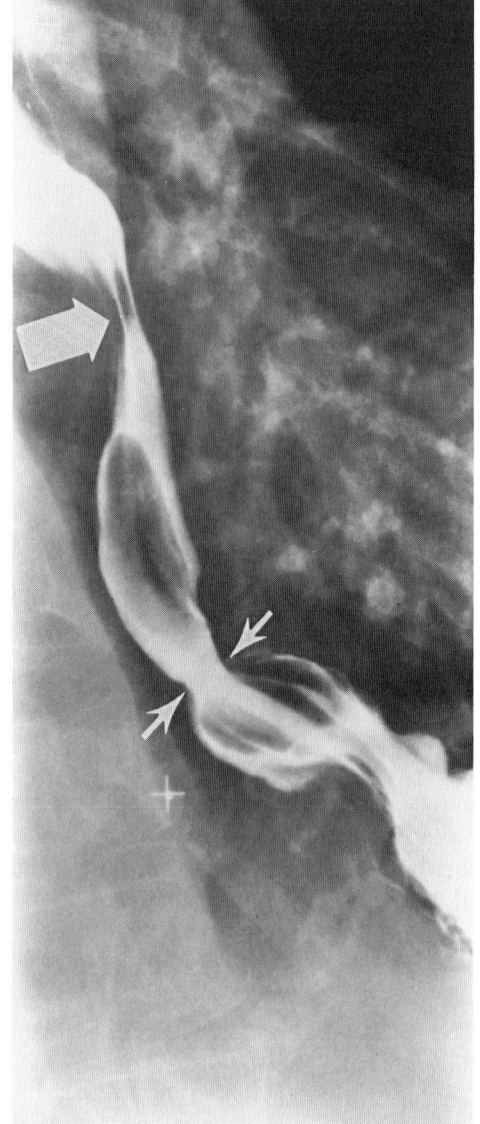

FIGURE 6.2. Esophageal findings in a patient with Zenker's diverticulum. (A) A 2 cm Zenker's diverticulum (large arrow) has remained filled following passage of bolus. Note, also, the retention in the valleculae and piriform sinuses (small arrows). (B) There is a small, sliding hiatal hernia with subtle narrowing of the gastroesophageal junction due to a peptic structure (arrows). There is a prominent impression on the midesophagus from tortuosity of the aorta (large arrow).

Swallowing Center who satisfied the criteria of either "psychogenic dysphagia" (15 patients) or "globus hystericus" (8 patients) (49). Evaluation at other institutions had been negative. In 15 of the group of 23 patients, a cause was found for the dysphagia. Findings included pharyngeal dysfunction in 4 (due to amyotrophic lateral sclerosis and tongue chorea in 1 each), structural obstruction in 5 (periesophageal mass in 2, pharyngeal cancer, aberrant subclavian artery, peptic stricture 1 each) and esophageal dysmotility in 6, with gastroesophageal reflux in 5 of the 6. No abnormality could be demonstrated in 8 of the 23 patients.

This again underscores the fact that esophageal disorders commonly present with pharyngeal symptoms. It also indicates that the diagnoses of "psychogenic dysphagia" and "globus hystericus" should be made only after thorough evaluation. It is especially important to reevaluate such patients if there is any change or progression of symptoms. As mentioned previously, esophageal pathology is common in patients with globus sensation, and the term "globus hystericus" should be used with caution.

On the other hand, a manometric study of 22 patients with globus pharyngeus in 1994 by Chen et al. (50) demonstrated abnormal results in the pH probe test in the pharynx in only 2 patients and in the esophagus in only 4 patients. The researchers concluded that most patients with globus pharyngeus had normal results on pH monitoring. Similarly, most of the videofluoroscopy studies showed no evidence of pharyngeal pathology.

Subsequently we have evaluated the videofluoroscopic studies of 11 patients with "psychogenic dysphagia" and compared them with results from a group of 12 patients with neurogenic dysphagia (51). Findings in the psychogenic group included very small boluses, multiple tongue movements, complex oral motions such as rocking, swirling, bouncing, and pumping, or a pharyngeal swallow without oral propulsion of bolus. This was in contrast to the neurogenic group, who had abnormal find-

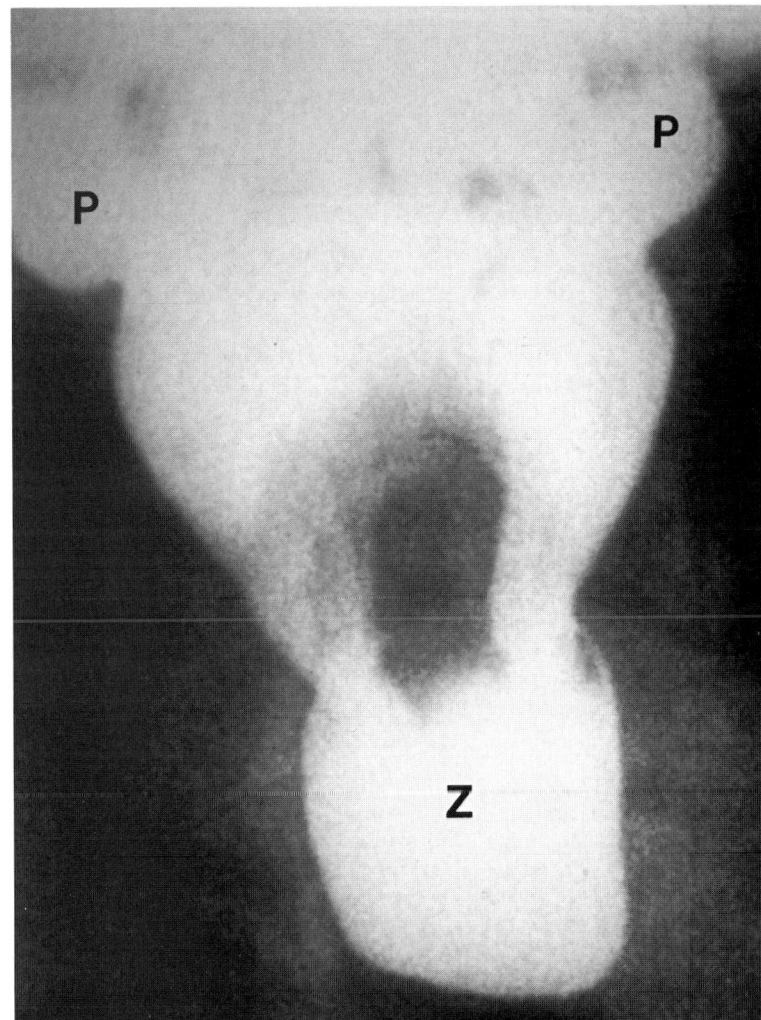

FIGURE 6.3. Achalasia with lateral pharyngeal pouches and Zenker's diverticulum. During swallowing, there are large bilateral pharyngeal pouches (P) and a large Zenker's diverticulum (Z). (Reproduced with permission from Jones B, Donner MW, Rubesin SE, Ravich WJ, Hendrix TR. Pharyngeal findings in 21 patients with achalasia. *Dysphagia* 1987;2(2):87–92.)

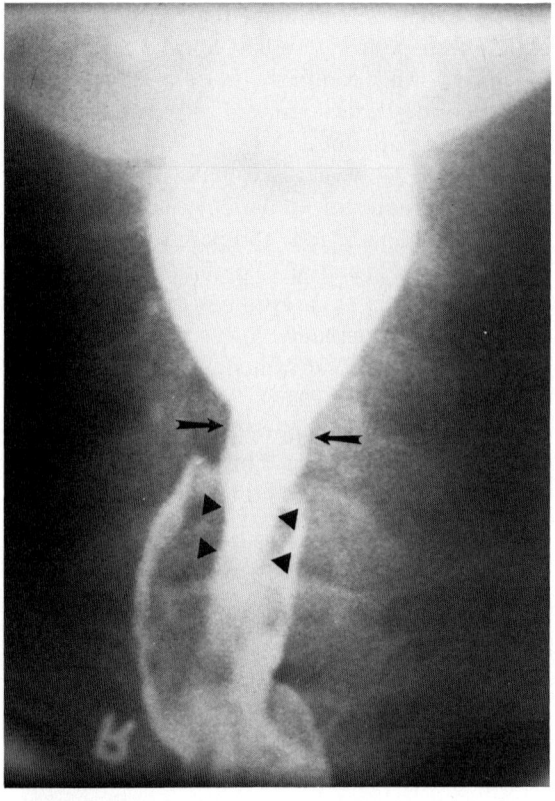 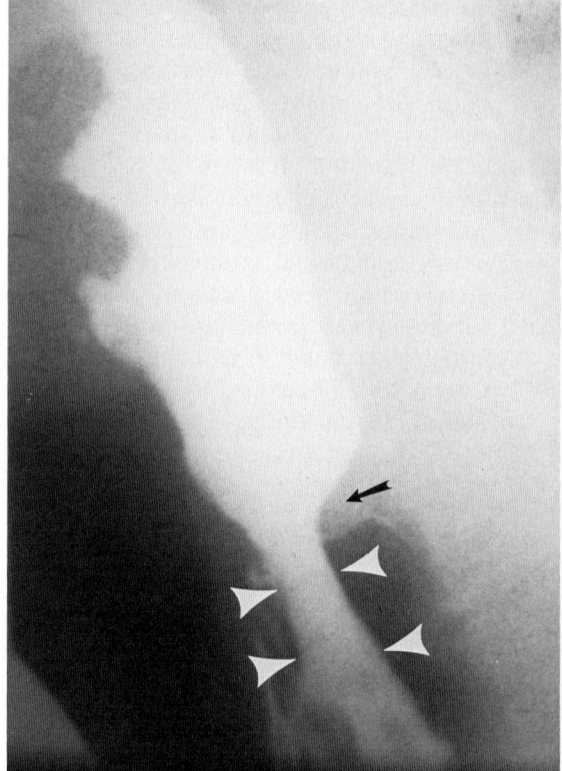

FIGURE 6.4. Achalasia with prominence of the cricopharyngeus. In the frontal (A) and lateral (B) views there is prominence of the cricopharyngeus (arrows) with a jet effect (arrowheads) indicating luminal compromise. Note the partially air-filled, partially barium-filled, dilated esophagus below the narrowed cricopharyngeus. (Reproduced with permission from Jones B, Donner MW, Rubesin SE, Ravich WJ, Hendrix TR. Pharyngeal findings in 21 patients with achalasia. *Dysphagia* 1987;2(2):87–92.)

ings in both oral and pharyngeal phases. Oral findings in the neurogenic group included drooling, atrophy, asymmetry, inability to transfer the bolus, inability to control bolus, weak tongue movements, and in the pharynx, multiple decompensations such as retention in valleculae and piriform sinuses, aspiration, failure of the epiglottis to tilt, and loss of pharyngeal contraction.

At our institution, a diagnosis of psychogenic dysphagia is reserved for patients with a strong psychological overlay and/or fear of swallowing and either a negative workup or findings on the VFSS suggestive of this disorder (as described earlier).

A manometric study in 1995 of 19 patients with completely normal results from videofluorographic swallowing study (VFSS) and abnormal pressures in the pharynx raises the question of whether a negative VFSS is adequate to exclude pharyngeal abnormality (52). In 14 of 19 patients, there was at least 1 abnormality (5 patients) or multiple abnormalities (9 patients), including high UES resting pressures, high residual pressures, weak pharyngeal contraction, pharyngeal spasm, prolonged contraction/relaxation times, reduced compliance of the UES, and UES-pharyngeal incoordination.

Further studies are necessary to define the role of VFSS and manometry in the diagnosis and workup of dysphagia in general and psychogenic dysphagia in particular.

References

1. Edwards DAW. History and symptoms of esophageal disease. In: Vantrappen G, Hellemans J, eds. *Diseases of the Esophagus.* New York: Springer-Verlag; 1974.
2. Jones B, Ravich WJ, Donner MW, Kramer SS, Hendrix TR. Pharyngoesophageal interrelationships: observations and working concepts. *Gastrointest Radiol* 1985;10:225–233.
3. Murakami Y, Fukuda H, Kirchner JA. The cricopharyngeus muscle. *Acta Otolaryngol (suppl) (Stockh)* 1972;311:1–19.
4. Creamer B, Schlegel J. Motor responses of the esophagus to distension. *J Appl Physiol* 1957;10:498–504.
5. Enzmann DR, Harell GS, Zboralske FF. Upper esophageal responses to intraluminal distention in man. *Gastroenterology* 1977;72:1292–1298.
6. Gerhardt DC, Shuck BS, Bordeaux RA, Winship DH. Human upper esophageal sphincter: response to volume, osmotic and acid stimuli. *Gastroenterology* 1978;75:268–274.
7. Rosenberg SJ, Harris LD. A single physiologic mechanism for changing strength of both esophageal sphincters (abstract). *Gastroenterology* 1971;60:798.
8. Hunt PS, Connell AM, Smiley TBN. The cricopharyngeal sphincter in gastric reflux. *Gut* 1970;11:303–306.
9. Stanciu C, Bennett JR. Upper oesophageal sphincter yields pressure in normal subjects and in patients with gastroesophageal reflux. *Thorax* 1974;29:459–462.
10. Vakil NB, Kahrilas PJ, Dodds WJ, Vanagunas A. Absence of an upper esophageal sphincter response to acid reflux. *Gastroenterology* 1989;84:606–610.
11. Torrico S, Ren J, Sui Z, Hofmann C, Shaker R. Upper esophageal sphincter function during gastroesophageal reflux events. *Gastroenterology* 1998;114(4):G3481.
12. Medda BK, Lang IM, Layman R, Hogan WJ, Dodds WJ, Shaker R. Characterization and quantification of a pharyngo-UES contractile reflex in cats. *Am J Physiol* 1994;167(*Gastrointest Liver Physiol* 30):G972–G983.
13. Shaker R, Ren J, Xie P, Lang IM, Bardan E, Sui Z. Characterization of the pharyngo-UES contractile reflex in humans. *Am J Physiol* 1997;273(*Gastrointest Liver Physiol* 36):854–858.
14. Shaker R, Ren J, Zamir Z, Sarna A, Liu J, Sui Z. Effect of aging, position, and temperature on the threshold volume triggering pharyngeal swallows. *Gastroenterology* 1994;107:396–402.
15. Ulualp SO, Toohill RJ, Kern M, Shaker R. Pharyngo-UES contractile reflex in patients with posterior laryngitis. *Laryngoscope* 1998;108(9):1354–1357.
16. Shaker R, Dodds WJ, Ren J, Hogan WJ, Arndorfer RC. Esophagoglottal closure reflex: a mechanism of airway protection. *Gastroenterology* 1992;102:857–861.
17. Shaker R, Ren J, Medda B, Lang I, Cowles V, Jaradeh S. Identification and characterization of the esophagoglottal closure reflex in a feline model. *Am J Physiol* 1994;266(*Gastrointest Liver Physiol* 29):G147–G153.
18. Shaker R, Ren J, Kern M, Dodds WJ, Hogan WJ, Li Q. Mechanisms of airway protection and UES opening during belching. *Am J Physiol* 1992;262(*Gastrointest Liver Physiol* 25):G621–G628.
19. Shaker R, Ren J, Hogan WJ, Liu J, Podvrsan B, Sui Z. Glottal function during postprandial gastroesophageal reflux. *Gastroenterology* 1993;104(4):A581.
20. Ren J, Shaker R, Dua K, Trifan A, Podvrsan B, Sui Z. Glottal adduction response to pharyngeal water stimulation: evidence for a pharyngoglottal closure reflex. *Gastroenterology* 1994;106(4-2):A558.
21. Henderson RD. Reflux induced cricopharyngeal dysphagia—pathologic change in muscle biopsies (abstract). Paper presented at: Second International Conference on Diseases of the Esophagus; May 19–21, 1983; Chicago.
22. Cook T, Blumbergs P, Cash K, Jamieson G, Shearman D. Structural abnormalities of the cricopharyngeus muscle in patients with pharyngeal (Zenker's) diverticulum. *J Gastroenterol Hepatol* 1992;7:556–562.
23. Lerut T, van Racmdonck D, Guelinckx P, Dom R, Geboes K. Zenker's diverticulum: Is a myotomy of the cricopharyngeus useful? How long should it be? *Hepatogastroenterology* 1992;39:127–131.
24. Chernow B, Johnson LF, Janowitz WR, Castell DO. Pulmonary aspiration as a consequence of gastro-esophageal reflux: a diagnostic approach. *Dig Dis Sci* 1979;24:839–844.
25. Kennedy JH. Silent gastro-esophageal reflux: an important but little known cause of pulmonary complications. *Dis Chest* 1962;42:42–65.

26. Overholt RH, Ashraf MM. Esophageal reflux as trigger in asthma. *N Y State J Med* 1966;66:3030–3032.
27. Mays EE. Intrinsic asthma in adults: association with gastro-esophageal reflux. *JAMA* 1976;236:2626–2628.
28. Danus O, Casar C, Larrain A, Pope CE. Esophageal reflux—an unrecognized cause of recurrent obstructive bronchitis in children. *J Pediatr* 1976;89:220–224.
29. Christie DL, O'Grady LR, Mack DV. Incompetent lower esophageal sphincter and gastro-esophageal reflux in recurrent acute pulmonary disease of infancy and childhood. *J Pediatr* 1978;93:23–27.
30. Berquist WE, Rachelefsky GS, Kadden M, Siegel SC, Katz RM, Fonkalsrud EW, Ament ME. Gastro-esophageal reflux-associated recurrent pneumonia and chronic asthma in children. *Pediatrics* 1981;68:29–35.
31. Goldberg M, Noyek AM, Pritzker KP II. Laryngeal granuloma secondary to gastro-esophageal reflux. *J Otolaryngol* 1978;7:196–202.
32. Larrain A, Lira E, Otero M, Pope CE II. Posterior laryngitis: a useful marker of esophageal reflux (abstract). *Gastroenterology* 1981;80:1204.
33. Cherry J, Margulies SI. Contact ulcers of the larynx. *Laryngoscope* 1968;78:1937–1940.
34. Olson N. The problem of gastroesophageal re-flux. *Otolaryngol Clin North Am* 1986;19:119–133.
35. Ward PH, Harrison DG. Reflux as an etiological factor of carcinoma of the laryngopharynx. *Laryngoscope* 1988;98:1195–1199.
36. Price JC, Jansen CJ, Johns ME. Esophageal reflux and secondary malignant neoplasia at laryngo-esophagectomy. *Arch Otolaryngol Head Neck Surg* 1990;116:163–164.
37. Cunningham Jr ET, Ravich WJ, Jones B, Donner MW. Vagal reflexes referred from the upper aerodigestive tract: an infrequently recognized cause of common cardiorespiratory responses. *Ann Intern Med* 1992;116:575–582.
38. Cherry J, Siegel CI, Margulies SI, Donner MW. Pharyngeal localization of symptoms of gastro-esophageal reflux. *Ann Otolaryngol* 1970;79:912–915.
39. Brady AP, Stevenson GW, Somers S, Hough DM, Di Giandomenico E. Premature contraction of the cricopharyngeus: a new sign of gastro-esophageal reflux disease. *Abdom Imaging* 1995;20:225–229.
40. Ravich WJ, Jones B, Kramer SS, Donner MW. Unexplained pharyngeal dysphagia—the role of esophageal disease (abstract). *Gastroenterology* 1983;84:1282.
41. Cook IJ, Gabb M, Panagopoulos V, Jamieson GG, Hains JD, Dodds WJ, Dent J, Shearman DJ. Zenker's diverticulum: a defect in upper esophageal sphincter compliance. *Gastroenterology* 1989;96:A98.
42. Cook IJ, Blumbergs P, Cash K, Graham S, Jamieson GG, Hains JD, Shearman DJ. Zenker's diverticulum: evidence for a restrictive cricopharyngeal myopathy. *Gastroenterology* 1989;96:A98.
43. Shaw DW, Cook IJ, Simula ME, Jamieson GG, Holloway RH, Gabb M, Dent J. Restoration of normal upper esophageal sphincter compliance following cricopharyngeal myotomy in patients with Zenker's diverticulum. *Gastroenterology* 1990;95:A122.
44. Dohlman G, Mattsson O. The role of the cricopharyngeal muscle in cases of hypopharyngeal diverticula. *AJR Am J Roentgenol* 1959;81:561–569.
45. Knuff TE, Benjamin SB, Castell DO. Pharyngoesophageal (Zenker's) diverticulum: a reappraisal. *Gastroenterology* 1982;82:734–736.
46. Jones B, Donner MW, Rubesin SE, Ravich WJ, Hendrix TR. Pharyngeal findings in 21 patients with achalasia of the esophagus. *Dysphagia* 1988;2:87–92.
47. Dudnick RS, Castell JA, Castell DO. Abnormal upper esophageal sphincter function in achalasia. *Am J Gastroenterol* 1991;87(12):1712–1715.
48. Zhang ZG, Diamant NE. Repetitive contractions of the upper esophageal body and sphincter in achalasia. *Dysphagia* 1994;9(1):12–19.
49. Ravich WJ, Wison RS, Jones B, Donner MW. Psychogenic dysphagia and globus: reevaluation of 23 patients. *Dysphagia* 1989;4:35-38.
50. Ott DJ, Ledbetter MS, Koufman JA, Chen MY. Globus pharyngeus: radiographic evaluation and 24-hour pH monitoring of the pharynx and esophagus in 22 patients. *Radiology* 1994;191(1):95–97.
51. Barofsky I, Ravich W, Buchholz D, Jones B. Oral findings on video swallowing study in neurogenic and psychogenic dysphagia (abstract). Paper presented at: 25th Annual Meeting and Postgraduate Course of the Society of Gastrointesti-

nal Radiologists; Bermuda; March 24–29, 1996.
52. Olsson R, Castell JA, Castell DO, Ekberg O. Solid-state computerized manometry improves diagnostic yield in pharyngeal dysphagia: simultaneous videoradiography and manometry in dysphagia patients with normal barium swallows. *Abdom Imaging* 1995;20(3):230–235.

7
Common Structural Lesions

BRONWYN JONES

Webs

Webs are mucosal folds that are usually thin, but occasionally thick; they most commonly occur on the anterior wall of the cervical esophagus (1–4). These may be incidental and nonobstructive or deeper and circumferential, causing narrowing of the lumen. Radiographically they are seen as discrete, shelflike defects 1 to 2 mm thick (Figure 7.1).

Depending on the degree of narrowing, the patient may or may not complain of dysphagia. Sometimes, severe luminal narrowing may produce a "jet effect," a flow phenomenon that can simulate a long stenosing lesion (Figure 7.2) (5). Such a jet effect has also been reported in narrowing in the esophagus (6) and can be seen transiently with spasm (Jones, unpublished observation).

A truly linear, horizontal web should not be confused with the notchlike, triangular, changing appearance of the postcricoid impression, also seen on the anterior wall of the cervical esophagus, just below the level of the cricopharyngeus. This impression is thought to result from a prominent submucosal venous plexus (7).

An oblique or vertical weblike linear filling defect may also be seen in the lateral piriform sinus. This is thought to be puckering of mucosa rather than a true web (8). Whether this is a pathological finding is controversial, for it has been seen frequently in asymptomatic volunteers as well as in patients with dysphagia. Such a linear filling defect can also be seen in patients with pharyngeal paresis and may result from bunching of mucosa.

Clinically, symptoms occur with larger or solid boluses. Similarly, radiographic detection of webs is directly related to bolus size; even a large web can be missed, unless a large bolus is swallowed. Radiographic detection rate is also low unless dynamic imaging is utilized, since the defect may be visible on only one or two frames during each swallowing sequence. A solid bolus such as a barium-impregnated tablet or marshmallow may be helpful in determining whether the web is clinically significant. (Remember, however, that if the marshmallow becomes impacted, the patient may require a Heimlich maneuver!) The symptoms due to a web can be dramatically relieved by endoscopy, which ruptures the web. The endoscopist may not appreciate the presence of the web at all as the endoscope ruptures it.

The relationship of webs and iron-deficiency anemia is controversial. In 1921 Vinson reported a number of patients with anemia who had postcricoid dysphagia (9). This association has subsequently become known as the Plummer-Vinson syndrome. Kelly (10) and Paterson (11) observed that these patients may also have atrophy of the tongue, pharynx, and cervical esophagus. The term Paterson-Kelly syndrome was then coined. In 1939 Waldenstrom and Kjellberg observed that patients with this syndrome had iron deficiency anemia (12). The term "sideropenic dysphagia" was therefore introduced. Waldenstrom's group

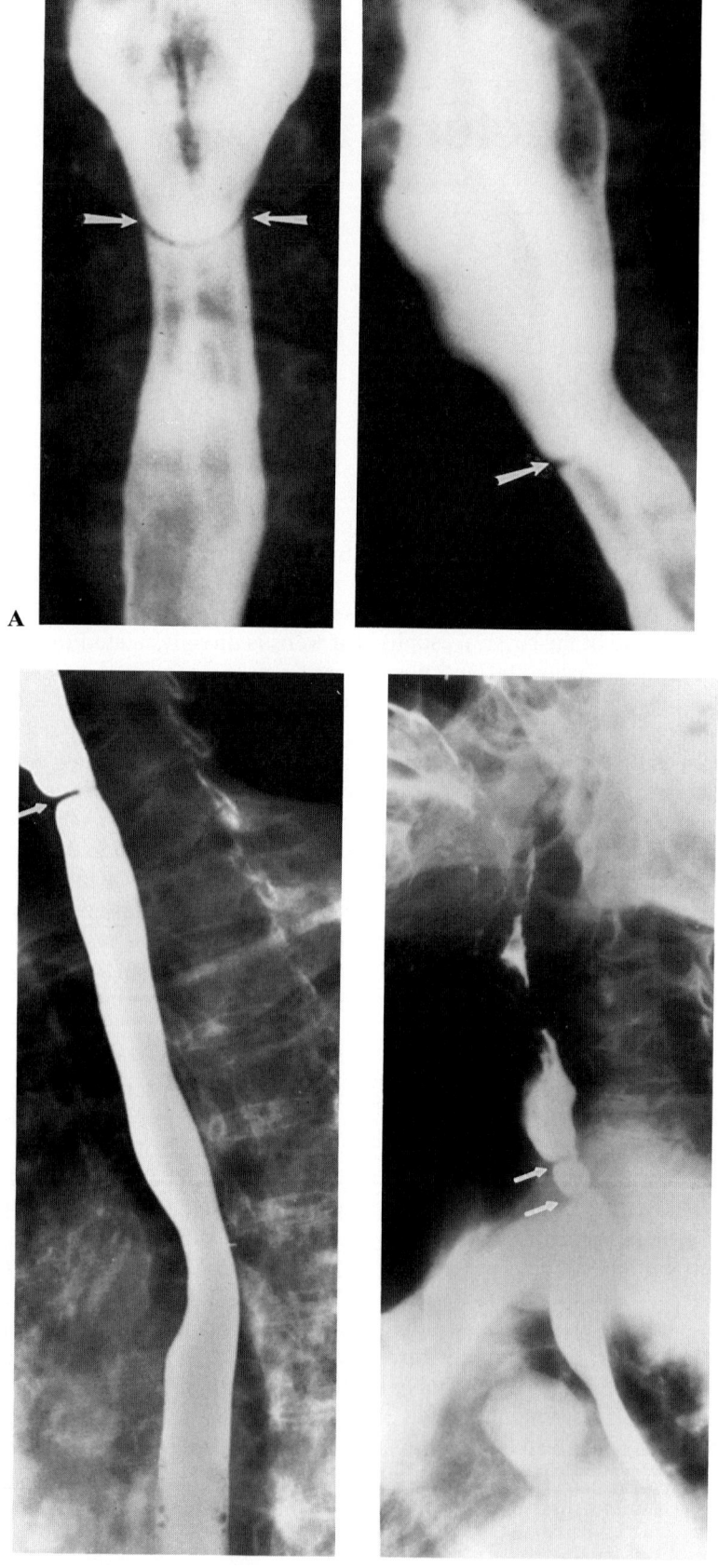

7. Common Structural Lesions

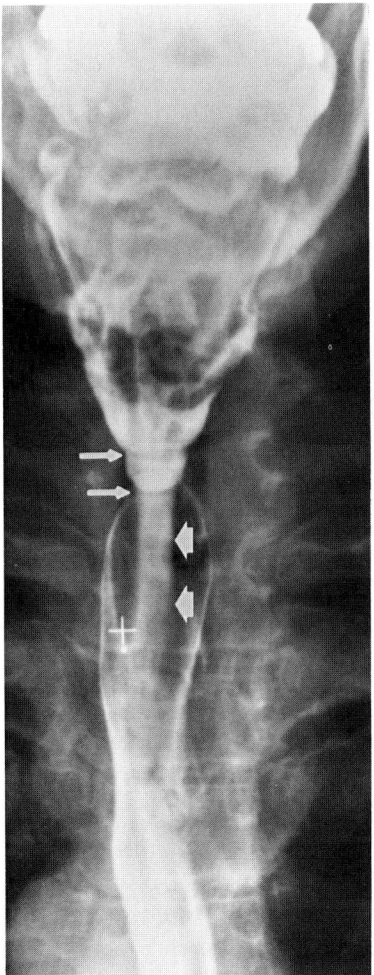 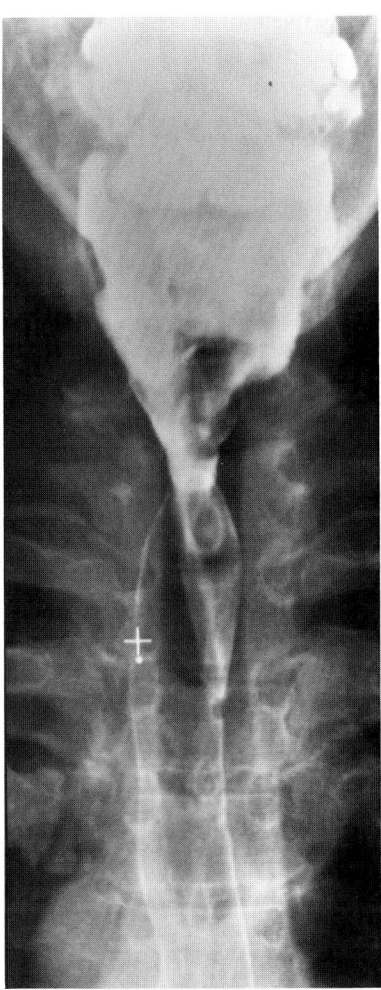

FIGURE 7.2. Jet phenomenon. There are several fine, horizontal linear defects within the barium column due to a focal collection of webs in a patient with benign mucosal pemphigoid (arrows). The jet of contrast (arrowheads) below the luminal narrowing indicates decreased luminal diameter. Note, however, that air in the cervical esophagus demonstrates that the lumen below the narrowing is significantly wider (arrowheads). (Reproduced with permission from Jones B, Donner MW. Examination of the patient with dysphagia. *Radiology* 1988;167: 319–326.)

A **B**

was the first to demonstrate hypopharyngeal and cervical esophageal webs as a cause of dysphagia in these patients. In recent times, with increased attention to iron supplements and improved nutrition, the association between webs and anemia has dramatically decreased and webs are found commonly in patients without iron deficiency anemia.

There is also controversy in the literature over whether Plummer-Vinson syndrome should be classified as a premalignant condition with an increased risk of developing pharyngeal or esophageal carcinoma. In one study, 9 of 58 patients with Plummer-Vinson syndrome with cervical esophageal webs developed carcinoma of the hypopharynx or esophagus (13). In most

FIGURE 7.1. Webs: three films demonstrate slightly different appearances of webs. (A) A thin, translucent filling defect is seen on the frontal and lateral projections (arrows). While it does not appear to narrow the lumen, such a thin web may have only a pinhole opening. In such a case, there may be a "jet phenomenon." (B) A thicker, almost horizontal filling defect is present on the anterior wall of the cervical esophagus (arrow). This appears to be narrowing the lumen by approximately 50%. (C) Two webs, or very focal strictures, partially obstruct the lumen in the cervical esophagus (arrows).

cases, the tumor was found above the web, not at the level of the web.

Webs may also be caused by scarring from unusual blistering inflammatory diseases involving the pharynx or esophagus, such as epidermolysis bullosa dystrophica (14) and benign mucous membrane pemphigoid (Figure 7.2) (15,16) or other skin diseases such as lichen planus. There has also been a report linking webs in the esophagus and another skin disease, psoriasis, but this association remains to be proven (17). Patients with chronic graft-versus-host disease can develop desquamative esophagitis and webs as a result of scarring (18). Gastroesophageal reflux has been implicated in the formation of webs in the lower esophagus (19). However, webs are common as an isolated finding without any underlying associated disorder.

Pouches and Diverticula

Lateral Pharyngeal Pouches

Lateral pharyngeal pouches form in an area of weakness in the thyrohyoid membrane where the membrane is penetrated by the superior laryngeal artery (20).

These pouches are common, and the incidence increases with increasing age. They are also common in neuromuscular disorders affecting the pharynx. Pouches may be symptomatic or asymptomatic, probably depending on whether they retain bolus after the swallow (21). The retained bolus may empty into the piriform sinuses after swallow (Figure 7.3) and may even result in overflow aspiration. Curtis et al. studied a large group of patients with lateral pharyngeal pouches and attempted to correlate these with gastroesophageal reflux (21).

Zenker's Diverticulum

A hypopharyngeal (Zenker's) diverticulum occurs at the pharyngoesophageal junction. This kind of diverticulum was actually first described in 1769 by Ludlow as a "preternatural dilatation" of the pharynx (22). Zenker's diverticulum is thought to be a type of pulsion (and false) diverticulum in which there is protrusion of mucosa and submucosa through the posterior muscle layers of the pharynx through an anatomically weak area. The most common site is between the oblique and horizontal fibers of the cricopharyngeal muscle through a triangular area known as Killian's triangle or dehiscence. This area is only one of the several possible sites of weakness and potential herniation at the pharyngoesophageal junction level (23).

Another less common site for a herniation is through Laimer's triangle, bordered superiorly by the cricopharyngeal muscle and inferiorly by the circular and longitudinal fibers of the cervical esophagus.

Zenker's diverticulum always originates from the posterior wall of the pharynx (Figure 7.4). As it enlarges, it tends to flop to one side, more commonly to the left. The diverticulum bulges inferiorly as it enlarges, thereby retaining food debris (hence halitosis is a presenting symptom), and it usually fills preferentially to the cervical esophagus. As the neck is higher than the diverticulum itself, it tends to collect ingested particulate matter (e.g., peas and corn kernels), and the patient may regurgitate undigested particles several hours after eating. On soft tissue views of the neck, an air-fluid level will often be seen (Figure 7.5).

These diverticula often empty back into the pharynx after swallow, resulting in a double swallow or even repetitive swallows in an attempt to clear the pharynx. There is also the potential for overflow aspiration when the diverticulum empties back into the pharynx (Figure 7.4F).

Below the diverticulum the cricopharyngeus almost always appears prominent, and a large diverticulum may compress and displace the cervical esophagus. It is important not to confuse barium trapped in the sphincter segment between a prominent posterior pharyngeal stripping wave and a prominent cricopharyngeus with a true diverticulum.

The pathogenesis of Zenker's diverticulum remains unclear, although incoordination between pharyngeal contraction and cricopharyngeal opening may be a contributing factor (24,25).

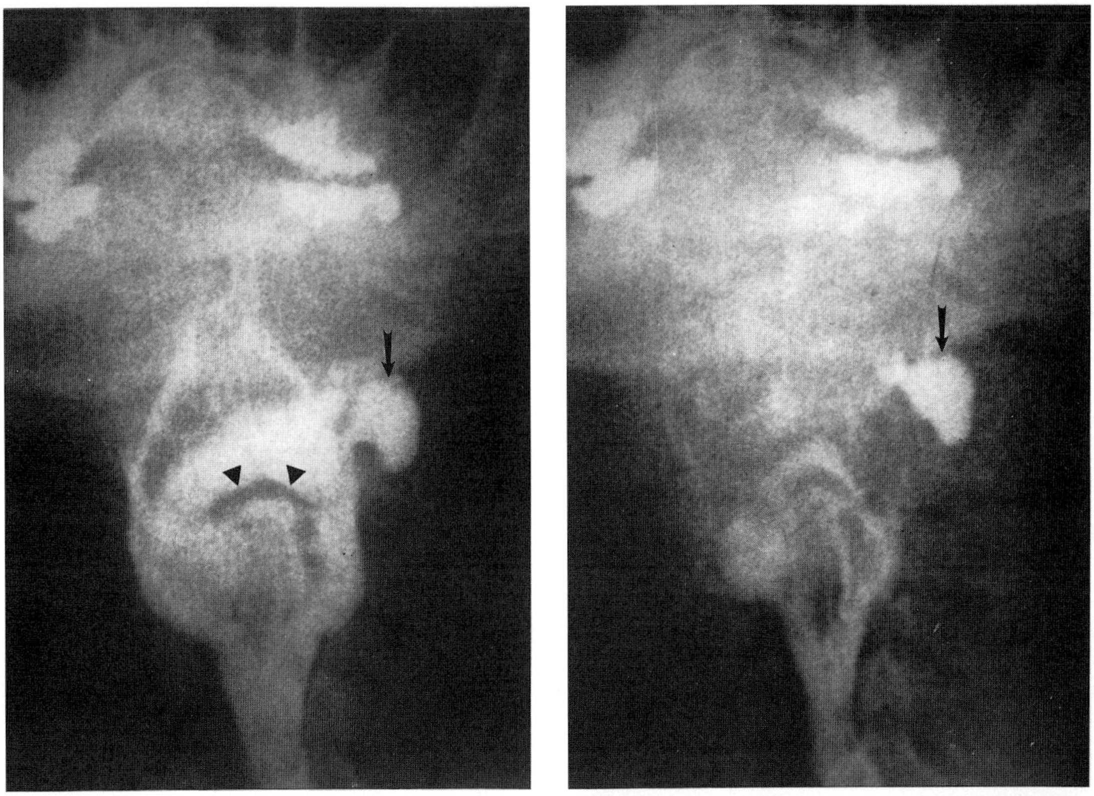

7. Common Structural Lesions

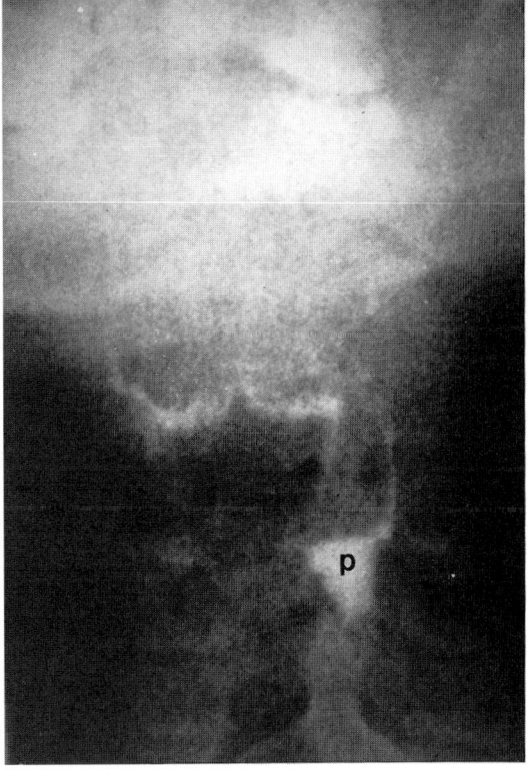

FIGURE 7.3. Late-emptying pouch. A series of three still frames from a cinepharyngoesophagogram. (A) A large, left lateral pharyngeal pouch is seen during swallowing (arrows). The inverted epiglottis is seen as a "seagull-shaped" filling defect (arrowheads). (B) The pouch remains filled after swallowing. (C) After swallowing, the pouch empties into the left piriform sinus (p).

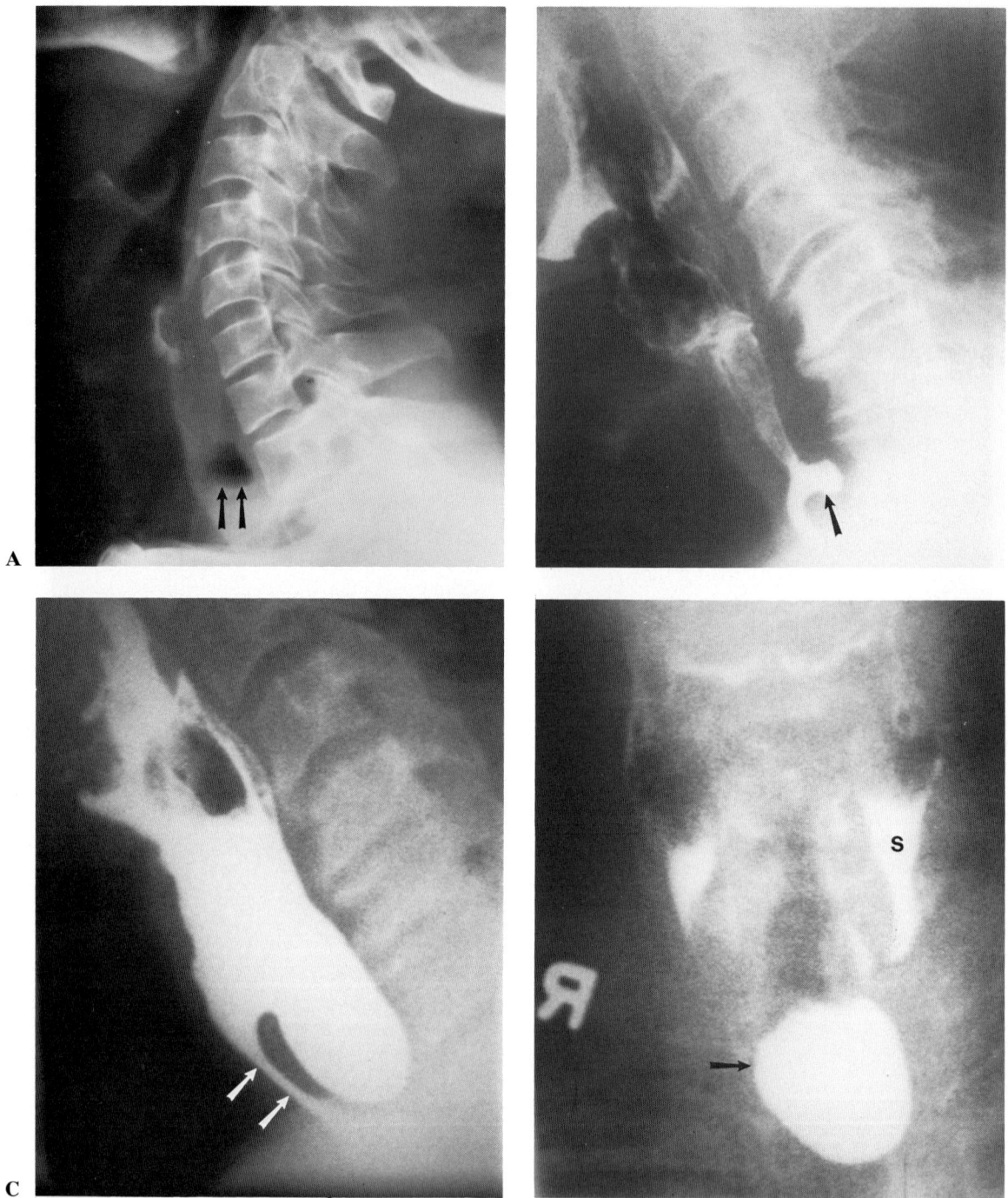

FIGURE 7.4. A spectrum of Zenker's diverticula. (A) Lateral soft tissue view of the neck demonstrates an air-fluid level seen at about the level of the cricopharyngeus muscle (arrows). This represents a partially fluid, partially air-filled Zenker's diverticulum. (B) Stop-frame from a cinepharyngoesophagogram reveals a very small Zenker's diverticulum (arrow) remaining filled after the bolus has passed by. Note also the severe degenerative change in the cervical spine. (C) Lateral and (D) frontal films from a patient with a moderately large Zenker's diverticulum show the diverticulum filled during swallowing and its wide open neck. Stasis and halitosis occur because the neck is wide open and above the main body of the diverticulum. Note the displacement and narrowing of the cervical esophagus below the diverticulum (arrows). After swallowing (D), there is residual filling of the diverticulum (arrow) and some retention in the piriform sinuses (s).

7. Common Structural Lesions

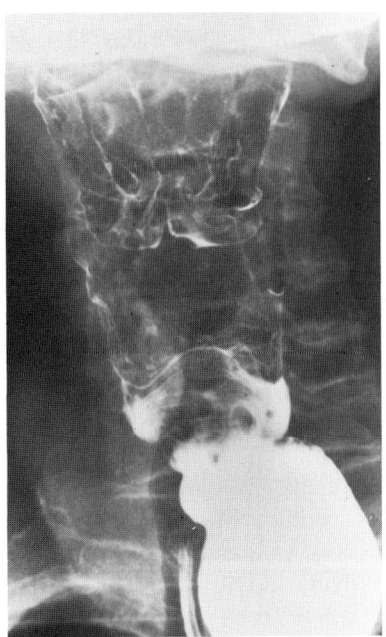

FIGURE 7.4. *Continued* (E) A very large Zenker's diverticulum has flopped to the left owing to lack of space. Some patients learn to empty these large diverticula by exerting pressure on the sac. (F) Two frames from a cinepharyngoesophagogram reveal a large Zenker's diverticulum, this time on the right side, remaining filled with contrast after swallowing (arrowhead). There is also a lateral buccal pouch on the left (arrowheads). (G) Stop-frame several frames later shows that the diverticulum is emptying back into the piriform sinuses (arrows), which could result in overflow aspiration. The regurgitated material will often produce a second swallow to clear the pharynx.

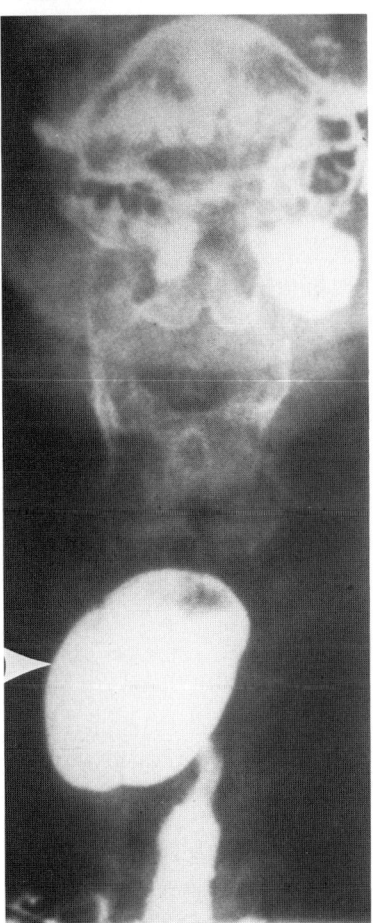

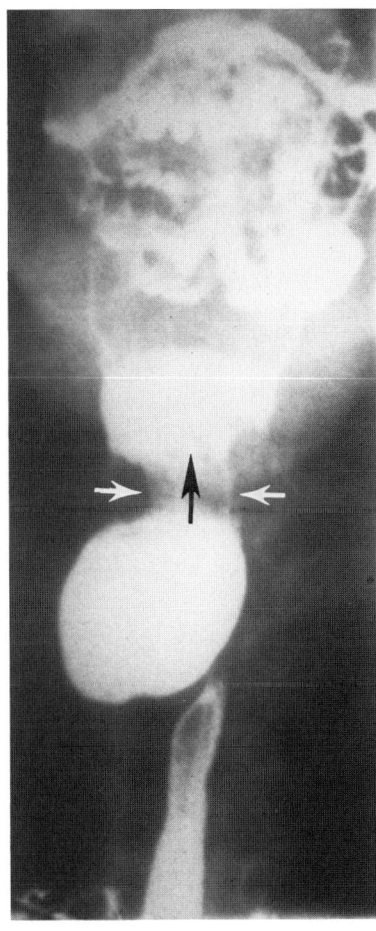

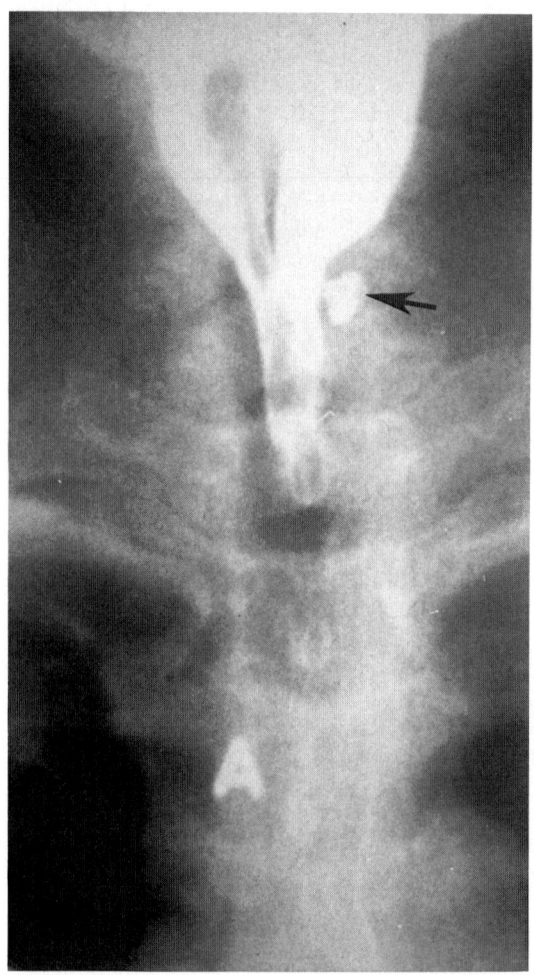

FIGURE 7.5. Lateral pharyngeal diverticulum at the pharyngoesophageal junction. Film from a cinepharyngoesophagogram reveals a diverticulum with a well-defined neck at the pharyngoesophageal junction on the left side (arrow). This would appear to be a true diverticulum. (Reproduced with permission from Jones B, Donner MW. Pharyngeal diverticula. In: Thompson WM, ed. *Common Problems in Gastrointestinal Radiology*. Chicago: Year Book Medical Publishers; 1989.)

Some manometric and cineradiographic studies have demonstrated premature sphincter closure in some patients with Zenker's diverticulum. Many studies, however, were performed in patients with fully developed diverticula, at which point pharyngeal contraction and cricopharyngeal relaxation do not appear to be out of synchronization.

In 1989 Cook et al. reported a high intrabolus pressure in patients with Zenker's diverticulum (26), and this high pressure has been relieved in patients with Zenker's who have had cricopharyngeal myotomy (27).

Gastroesophageal reflux may play a role in the development of Zenker's diverticulum (28,29). In our experience, almost all patients with Zenker's diverticulum have esophageal disorders such as gastroesophageal reflux, segmental spasm, acid-induced spasm, hiatal hernia, or Schatzki's ring (see Chapter 6).

Further studies are necessary, including those of the early stages of development, before the pathophysiology will be understood.

Treatment depends on symptoms and the size of the diverticulum. Many patients learn to live with the condition and empty the diverticulum by applying gentle manual pressure over it. Other adjust their dietary intake to exclude foods that might lodge in the diverticulum. Surgery may be necessary for symptomatic diverticula, especially when progressive enlargement occurs. Surgical treatment varies from simple diverticulopexy (i.e., the diverticulum is tacked up so that it drains by gravity) to excision alone to excision with cricopharyngeal myotomy. Recurrence following surgery is common, especially if cricopharyngeal myotomy is not performed with the original surgery.

Suggestions for laser endoscopic diverticulectomy and/or laser endoscopic cricopharyngeal myotomy as an alternative to surgery appeared as long ago as 1977 (30). More recently, dilatation of the cricopharyngeus alone was reported to result in the disappearance of a small Zenker's in each of two patients (31).

Lateral Diverticula at the Pharyngoesophageal Segment Level

Although much less common than the posterior Zenker's diverticulum, lateral diverticula also occur at the pharyngoesophageal junction (Figure 7.5) (32). These are thought to be situated at the level of a lateral slit near the outer and lateral border of the cricoid cartilage. The anomaly occurs at the insertion of the cricopharyngeal muscle and corresponds to the passage of the inferior laryngeal nerve. Diverticula with both narrow and wide necks have been described at this level. Outpouching with wide openings may represent merely pouches or bulges due to pharyngeal paresis; those with narrow necks appear to be true diverticula.

Pharyngeal Carcinoma (see also Chapter 10)

The most common tumor of the pharynx is squamous cell carcinoma: benign tumors are uncommon. Predisposing factors include alcohol and tobacco. As discussed earlier, patients with Plummer-Vinson syndrome also may have an increased risk of developing pharyngeal cancer.

Detection of small tumors requires exquisite radiographic technique. High-quality, double-contrast views are essential, since even large tumors may be obscured by the barium bolus during swallowing (32). Some infiltrative tumors may result in a focal area of decreased distensibility without producing a discrete mass. Double-contrast views during pharyngeal insufflation by a modified Valsalva maneuver or enunciation of "eee" may be helpful in demonstrating subtle lesions. Most advanced pharyngeal carcinomas can be confidently diagnosed on double-contrast radiographs of the pharynx (33).

The most common site of tumor involvement in the oro- and hypopharynx is the palatine tonsil. However, one should also carefully evaluate all structures in the area including the base of the tongue, epiglottis, piriform sinuses, and valleculae. Carcinoma of the base of the tongue usually can be detected as an ulcerating or exophytic lesion that distorts the normally smooth surface. A tumor from the posterior wall of the pharynx may produce an ulcerating or exophytic mass or local fixation of the area (Figure 7.6). Tumors of the lateral portion of the piriform sinus tend to be exophytic, whereas a medially located tumor is more often infiltrating. Thickening of the prevertebral soft tissues on lateral plain films of the neck usually indicates extensive tumor infiltration. Computed tomography is more sensitive than contrast pharyngography in delineating extension to the soft tissues of the skull base (see Chapter 9), but areas of fixation should be viewed with suspicion.

The pharynx may also be involved secondarily by spread of carcinoma of the larynx. Other conditions may be confused with tumor, especially around the tonsillar and tongue base area. For example, hypertrophy of the palatine or lingual tonsil may be indistinguishable radiographically from a polypoid tumor on the lateral view. Endoscopy and biopsy may be necessary for definitive diagnosis.

Patients with pharyngeal carcinoma (and squamous cell carcinoma of the head and neck in general) have an increased risk of developing a second separate primary esophageal carcinoma; in several studies the risk of a synchronous or metachonous esophageal cancer was 8–10%, and some authors advocate double-contrast radiography of all patients with head and neck cancer (34,35). Therefore, it is imperative to obtain a good double-contrast examination of the esophagus in all patients with head and neck cancer. If the oral, pharyngeal, or laryngeal tumor is interfering with swallowing so that aspiration is a problem, one should resort to a tube esophagogram to demonstrate the esophagus adequately (36) (see Chapter 3).

Radiation (see also Chapter 10)

Radiotherapy was commonly used in the past in children for the treatment of hypertrophied adenoids or tonsils, enlargement of the thymus gland, and even some skin lesions such as acne and hemangiomas. A delayed complication of such radiotherapy is an increased risk of thyroid carcinoma, and possibly of parotid tumors. Adult patients with head and neck cancer also commonly receive radiation therapy, either as the sole treatment or as an adjuvant to surgery. Complications in such patients include radionecrosis and soft tissue necrosis, as well as pain, fibrosis, and xerostomia (37).

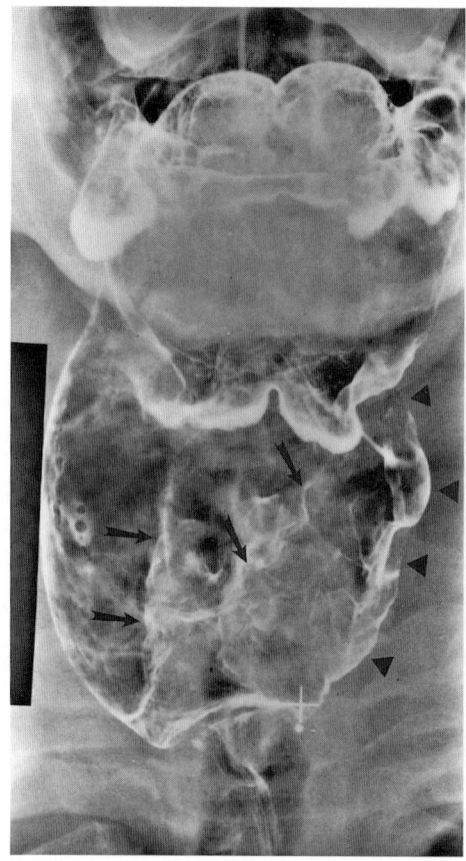 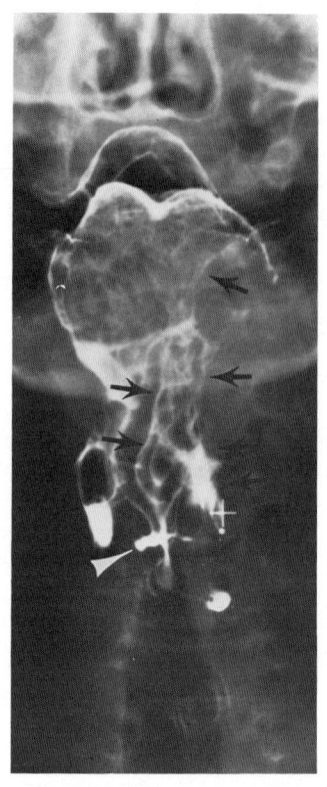

FIGURE 7.6. Multiple examples of carcinoma. (A) There is a large soft tissue mass originating in the left piriform sinus, crossing the midline to involve the right piriform sinus and involving the entrance to the larynx (arrows). This insufflation view shows the involvement of the lateral wall of the pharynx which is infiltrated and does not distend (arrowheads). (B) Frontal and (C) lateral views of a large tumor involving the left and posterior wall of the pharynx with a large soft tissue mass crossing almost to the midline (arrows). The bulk of the tumor mass is interfering with laryngeal closure and there is aspiration with contrast in the larynx (arrowhead). (D) Frontal and (E) lateral views of another large tumor, originating from the left piriform fossa. The tumor is seen crossing the midline on the frontal view (arrows), and extending along the aryepiglottic fold to involve the base of the epiglottis, resulting in a "double epiglottis." The mass is beginning to invade the entrance of the larynx, and there has been laryngeal penetration.

Radiation to the neck area for thyrotoxicosis and tuberculous lymphadenitis has resulted in pharyngeal malignancy; most of the reported cases are situated in the hypopharynx, the postcricoid area being the commonest site, with some cases reported in the piriform fossa or cervical esophagus (38).

The effects of acute radiation on pharyngeal function have not been well studied; this would be a very interesting area of investigation. Chronic effects, although not well appreciated, have been studied to some extent. Ekberg and Nylander studied a group of 13 patients with head and neck cancer who had received radiotherapy prior to resection of the tumor: abnormal radiographic findings, present in 12 of the 13, consisted of paresis, dysfunction, dysfunction of the laryngeal vestibule, and cricopharyngeal incoordination (39). Interestingly, static films were unremarkable and dynamic imaging (at that time cineradiography) was

7. Common Structural Lesions

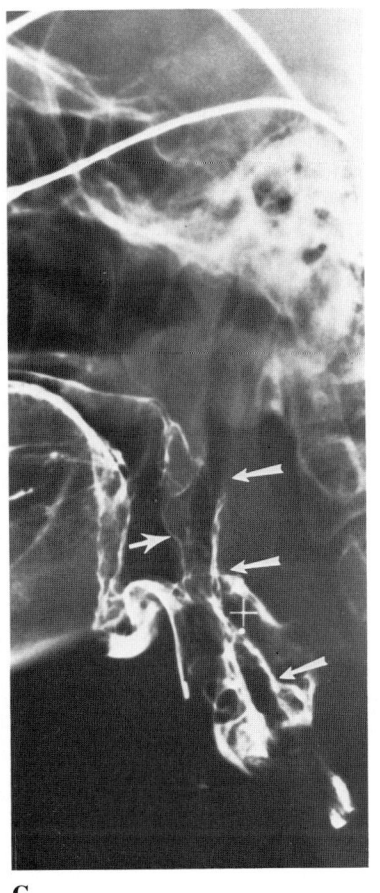 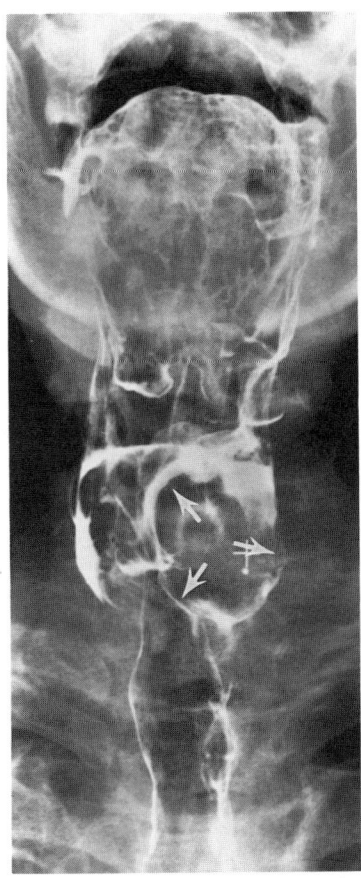 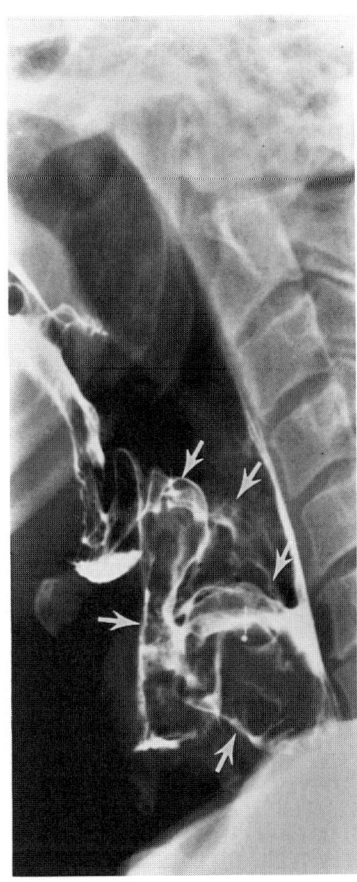

C D E

FIGURE 7.6. *Continued*

necessary to perceive abnormalities. Further studies are needed, especially directed at determining the effects of radiotherapy alone on swallowing.

The esophagus is relatively radiation sensitive and is by necessity included in the portals of mediastinal irradiation. The relatively uncommon problem of clinically symptomatic radiation esophagitis is thought to be related to the very high cell turnover rate in the esophagus. A radiation dose in excess of 4500 to 6000 rads over 4 to 6 weeks is critical (40,41). The effect of radiotherapy, however, is potentiated if combined with a chemotherapeutic regimen such as adriamycin (42).

Although symptoms may occur during the course of therapy, odynophagia is more common 4 to 6 weeks after completion of therapy. The most common finding on barium swallow is abnormal motility with loss of primary peristalsis within the radiation portal and irregular, nonpropulsive tertiary waves distally; spasm and delayed emptying are also common (40). Stricturing occurs 6 to 8 months posttherapy (43) or earlier with combination therapy. The time frame for other long-term sequelae, such as fistula formation or pseudodiverticulosis, is unpredictable (37).

Trauma

The larynx and pharynx can be damaged by both penetrating and closed trauma. Serious complications may go undetected over a long period of time. Imaging studies may be particularly relevant in caring for the patient with perforating injuries from a gunshot or knife wound.

Damage produced by endoscopy (44) may involve the piriform sinus and the tissue adjacent to the cricopharyngeus muscle; perforation is a potential complication during endoscopy in patients with Zenker's diverticulum.

During resuscitation attempts, perforations in the area of the larynx and pharynx can be produced by emergency endotracheal intubation (45). Pneumatic rupture of the pharynx or esophagus can occur when individuals use their teeth to open cans or bottles containing carbonated liquids. Damage can also occur when people try to open fire extinguishers under pressure or when they inflate rubber inner tubes, balloons, or hoses by mouth (46).

In addition, blunt trauma in car accidents with hyperextension of the cervical spine and compression of the neck by the steering wheel can lead to perforation with resultant pneumomediastinum (Figure 7.7). Films of the neck in two projections, contrast examination, and

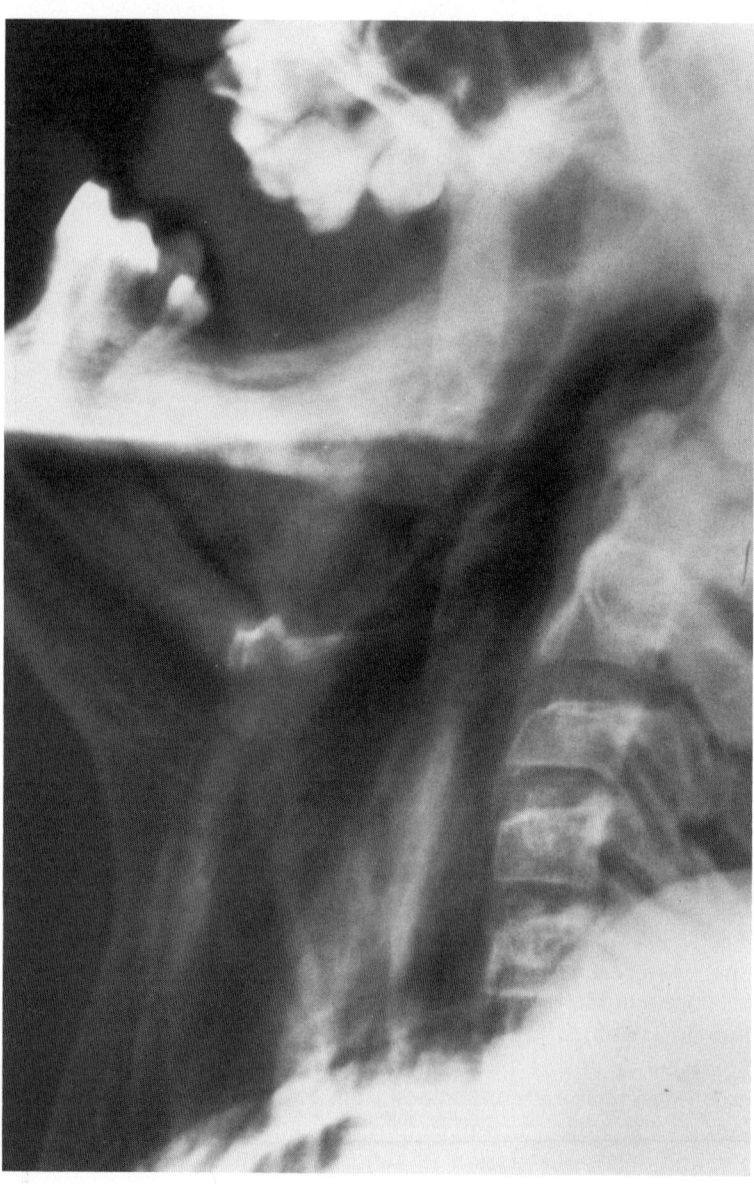

FIGURE 7.7. Trauma to the neck from a motor vehicle accident. There is extensive air dissection of the neck muscles, the muscles of mastication, and prevertebral soft tissues following laryngeal and tracheal laceration.

7. Common Structural Lesions

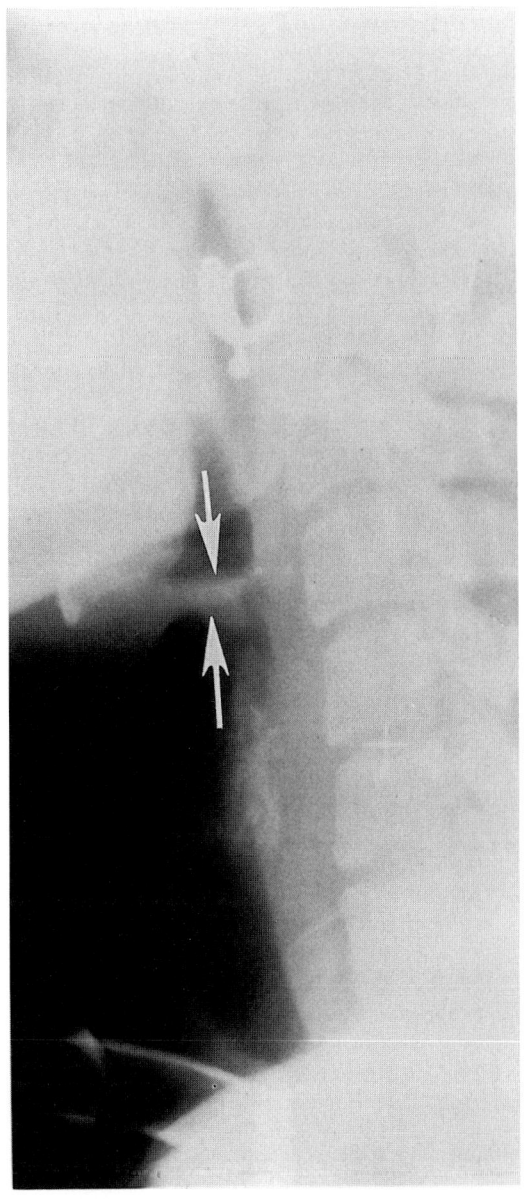 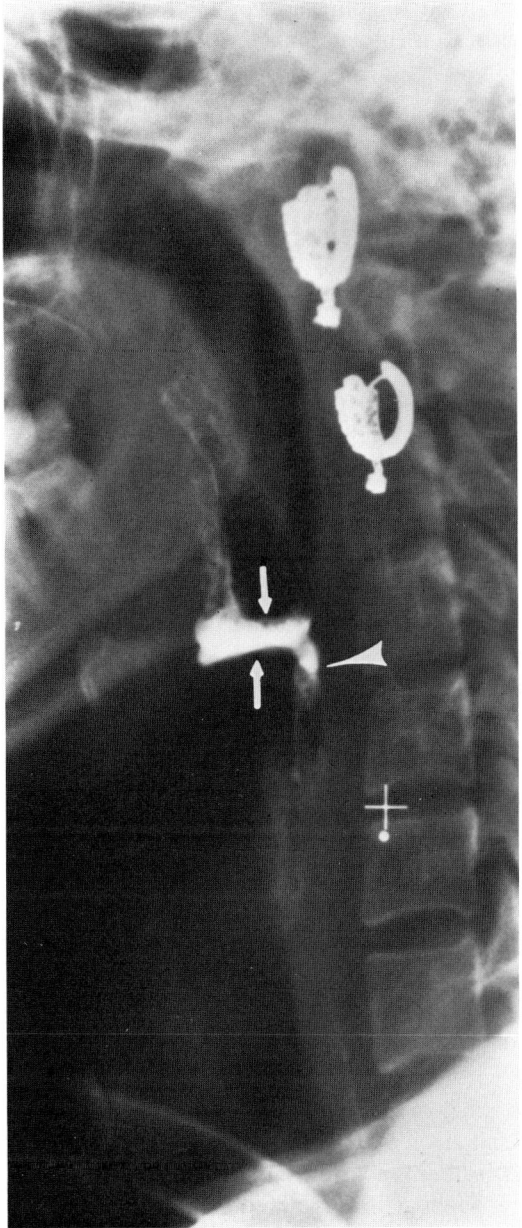

FIGURE 7.8. Scarring of the epiglottis and pharynx due to lye ingestion. (A) An abnormal broad soft tissue band, extending horizontally across the pharynx (arrows), consists of epiglottis scarred in the horizontal position and tethered to the posterior wall of the pharynx; this resulted in almost complete occlusion of the lumen. The patient required a tracheostomy to breathe. Note, also, thickening of the prevertebral soft tissues due to scarring (arrowhead). (B) After swallowing of a small amount of barium, the broad "web" is outlined (arrows). Note that minimal contrast has passed below the obstructing lesion (arrowhead).

computed tomography can be helpful in such cases. Remember to balance the risk of *aspiration* versus the risk of *perforation*. A nonionic contrast medium such as Omnipaque may be useful.

Foreign Bodies

Foreign bodies, such as fish and chicken bones, as well as dental prostheses, can become lodged in the walls of the pharynx and occasionally lead to perforation and abscess formation (47). Most foreign bodies are swallowed by children in their first decade of life. Objects swallowed include coins, nuts, pebbles, nails, and rings. These smaller objects can lodge in the region of the cricopharyngeal sphincter or may be aspirated into the lungs. In these patients, one must consider complications (e.g., retropharyngeal abscess or osteomyelitis of the cervical spine).

Ingestion of Chemicals

Lye solutions, acids, and other corrosive substances may be swallowed accidentally or in suicide attempts (48). Initially, considerable impairment of swallowing is caused by severe edema, ulcerations, and pain. Subsequently, extensive scar formation can be demonstrated radiologically (Figure 7.8).

Early reports of caustic injury stressed esophageal injury (49), with little attention being given to mouth and pharyngeal damage. Scott et al. reported on five patients in whom the damage to mouth and/or pharynx overshadowed other findings (50). Findings included thickening or fixation of the soft palate, destruction of the tongue, fixation or scarring of the epiglottis, lack of pharyngeal constriction, and aspiration (often silent), presumably due to damage to laryngeal sensation.

References

1. Clements JL, Cox GW, Torres WE, Weens HS. Cervical esophageal webs—a roentgen-anatomic correlation. *AJR Am J Roentgenol* 1974;121:221–231.
2. Nosher JL, Campbell WL, Seaman WB. The clinical significance of cervical esophageal and hypopharyngeal webs. *Radiology* 1975;117:45–47.
3. Ekberg O. Cervical oesophageal webs in patients with dysphagia. *Clin Radiol* 1981;32:633–641.
4. Ekberg O, Nylander G. Webs and web-like formations in the pharynx and cervical esophagus. *Diagn Imaging* 1983;52:10–18.
5. Shauffer IA, Phillips HE, Sequeira J. The jet phenomenon: a manifestation of esophageal web. *AJR Am J Roentgenol* 1977;129:747–748.
6. Taylor AJ, Stewart ET, Dodds WJ. The esophageal "jet" phenomenon revisited. *AJR Am J Roentgenol* 1990;155(2):289–290.
7. Pitman RG, Fraser GM. The post-cricoid impression on the esophagus. *Clin Radiol* 1965;16:34–39.
8. Ekberg O, Birch-Iensen M, Lindstrom C. Mucosal folds in the valleculae. *Dysphagia* 1986;1:68–72.
9. Vinson PO. Hysterical dysphagia. *Minn Med* 1921;5:107–108.
10. Kelly AB. Spasm of entrance to oesophagus. *J Laryngol* 1919;34:285–289.
11. Paterson DR. Clinical type of dysphagia. *J Laryngol* 1919;32:289–291.
12. Waldenstrom J, Kjellberg SR. The roentgenological diagnosis of sideropenic dysphagia (Plummer-Vinson's syndrome). *Acta Radiol (Stockh)* 1939;20:618–638.
13. McNab Jones RF. The Paterson-Brown-Kelly syndrome: its relationship to iron deficiency and postcricoid carcinoma. *J Laryngol Otol* 1961;71:529–561.
14. Agha FP, Francis IR, Ellis CN. Esophageal involvement in epidermolysis bullosa dystrophica: clinical and roentgenographic manifestations. *Gastrointest Radiol* 1983;8:111–117.
15. Sharon P, Greene ML, Rachmilewitz D. Esophageal involvement in bullous pemphigoid. *Gastrointest Endosc* 1978;24:122–123.
16. Agha FP, Raji MR. Esophageal involvement in pemphigoid: clinical and roentgen manifestations. *Gastrointest Radiol* 1982;7:109–112.
17. Harty RF, Boharski MG, Harned RK, Agha FP. Psoriasis, dysphagia, and esophageal webs or rings. *Dysphagia* 1988;2:136–139.
18. McDonald GB, Sullivan KM, Schuffler MD, Shulman HM, Thomas ED. Esophageal abnormalities in chronic graft-versus-host disease in humans. *Gastroenterology* 1981;80:914–921.

19. Weaver JW, Kaude JV, Hamlin DJ. Webs of the lower esophagus: a complication of gastroesophageal reflux? *AJR Am J Roentgenol* 1984; 142:289–292.
20. Bachman AL, Seaman WB, Macken KL. Lateral pharyngeal diverticula. *Radiology* 1968;91:774–782.
21. Curtis DJ, Cruess DF, Crain M, Sivit C, Winters Jr. C, Dachman AH. Lateral pharyngeal outpouchings: a comparison of dysphagic and asymptomatic patients. *Dysphagia* 1988;2:156–161.
22. Ludlow A. A case of obstructed deglutition from a preternatural dilatation of and bag formed in the pharynx. *Med Observ Inq* 1769;3:85–101.
23. Perrott JW. Anatomical aspects of hypopharyngeal diverticula. *Aust NZ Surg* 1962;31:307–317.
24. Dohlman G, Mattsson O. The role of the cricopharyngeal muscle in cases of hypopharyngeal diverticula. *AJR Am J Roentgenol* 1959; 81: 561–569.
25. Knuff TE, Benjamin SB, Castell DO. Pharyngoesophageal (Zenker's) diverticulum: a reappraisal. *Gastroenterology* 1982;82:734–736.
26. Cook IJ, Gabb M, Panagopoulos V, Jamieson GG, Hains JD, Dodds WJ, Dent J, Shearman DJ. Zenker's diverticulum: a defect in upper esophageal sphincter compliance. *Gastroenterology* 1989;96:A98.
27. Shaw DW, Cook IJ, Simula ME, Jamieson GG, Holloway RH, Gabb M, Dent J. Restoration of normal upper esophageal sphincter compliance following cricopharyngeal myotomy in patients with Zenker's diverticulum. *Gastroenterology* 1990;95:A122.
28. Smiley TB, Caves PK, Porter DC. Relationship between posterior pharyngeal pouch and hiatus hernia. *Thorax* 1970;25:725–731.
29. Delahunty JE, Margulies SE, Alonso UA, Knudson DH. The relationship of reflux esophagitis to pharyngeal pouch (Zenker's diverticulum). *Laryngoscope* 1971;81:570–577.
30. van Overbeek JJM. *The Hypopharyngeal Diverticulum. Endoscopic Treatment and Manometry.* Thesis; Assen; 1977.
31. Ravich W, Neumann S, Jones B. Dilatation as treatment of pharyngo-esophageal segment (PES) prominence with hypo-pharyngeal (Zenker's) diverticulum. *Dysphagia* 2000;15(2): 103.
32. Ekberg O, Nylander G. Lateral diverticula from the pharyngoesophageal junction area. *Radiology* 1983;146:117–122.
33. Semenkovick JW, Balfe DM, Weyman PJ, Heiken JP, Lee JKT. Barium pharyngography: comparison of single and double contrast. *AJR Am J Roentgenol* 1985;144:715–720.
34. Goldstein HM, Zornoza J. Association of squamous cell carcinoma of the head and neck with cancer of the esophagus. *AJR Am J Roentgenol* 1978;131:791–794.
35. Thompson WM, Oddson TA, Kelvin F, et al. Synchronous and metachronous squamous cell carcinomas of the head, neck, and esophagus. *Gastrointest Radiol* 1978;3:123–127.
36. Levine MS, Kressel HY, Laufer I, Herlinger H, Goren R. The tube esophagogram: a technique for obtaining a detailed double-contrast examination of the esophagus. *AJR Am J Roentgenol* 1984;142:293–298.
37. Larson DL, Lindberg RD, Lane E, Goepfert H. Major complications of radiotherapy in cancer of the oral cavity and oropharynx—a 10 year retrospective stuudy. *Am J Surg* 1983;146:531–536.
38. Goolden AWG. Pharyngeal malignancy following irradiation of the neck. *Br J Radiol* 1972; 45:795.
39. Ekberg O, Nylander G. Pharyngeal dysfunction after treatment for pharyngeal cancer with surgery and radiotherapy. *Gastrointest Radiol* 1983;8:97–104.
40. Goldstein HM, Rogers LF, Fletcher GH, Dodd GD. Radiological manifestations of radiation-induced injury to the normal upper gastrointestinal tract. *Radiology* 1975;117:135–140.
41. Rogers LF, Goldstein HM. Roentgen manifestations of radiation injury to the gastrointestinal tract. *Gastrointest Radiol* 1977;2:281–291.
42. Chabora BM, Hofan S, Wittes R. Esophageal complications in the treatment of oat cell carcinoma with combined irradiation and chemotherapy. *Radiology* 1977;123:185–187.
43. Lepke RA, Lipshitz HI. Radiation-induced injury of the esophagus. *Radiology* 1983;148: 375–378.
44. Meyers MA, Ghahremani GG. Complications of fiberoptic endoscopy. *Radiology* 1975;115: 293–300.
45. Wolff AP, Kuhn FA, Ogura JH. Pharyngealesophageal perforations associated with rapid oral endotracheal intubation. *Ann Otol* 1972;81: 258–261.
46. Forer M, Flynn P, Hughes CF, Szasz J. Pneumatic rupture of the posterior pharyngeal wall. *Aust NZ J Surg* 1986;56:89–91.

47. Nayak SR, Kirtane MV, Shah AK, Karnik PP. Foreign bodies in the cricopharyngeal region and oesophagus. *J Postgrad Med* 1984;30:214–218.
48. Chitrov FM, Mumladze RB. Special aspects of injury and surgical treatment of the mouth cavity walls and pharynx following thermal burns. *Acta Chir Plast* 1983;25:34–43.
49. Hardin JC. Caustic burns of the esophagus; a ten-year analysis. *Am J Surg* 1956;91:742–748.
50. Scott JC, Jones B, Eisele DW, Ravich WJ. Caustic ingestion injuries of the upper aerodigestive tract. *Laryngoscope* 1992;102(1):1–8.

8
Ultrasound Imaging and Swallowing

BARBARA C. SONIES, GLORIA CHI-FISHMAN, AND JERI L. MILLER

Ultrasound technology has advanced substantially, providing clinicians and researchers with vastly expanded noninvasive opportunities to study the dynamics of the oral pharyngeal system and the muscles and other soft tissues of the oropharynx during swallowing. In the current climate of cost containment and efficiency, ultrasound imaging presents a viable alternative to videofluorography to examine the oropharyngeal swallow. Because ultrasound imaging is uniquely suited for investigating soft tissue structures, it is used to view the abdomen, fetus, heart, bladder, genitalia, breast, and to visualize tumors and masses throughout the body (1–3). Ultrasound can be used to identify normal and abnormal oropharyngeal tissues such as the thyroid and salivary glands, tongue, palate, and floor of the mouth in various diseases, infections, and genetic conditions (4,5). Because of its inherent advantages (Table 8.1), ultrasound has been successfully adapted for viewing the oral cavity during swallowing (6–9). Real-time ultrasound is totally noninvasive, dynamic, and has no known bioeffects and minimal risk to the patient. Studies can therefore be performed repeatedly or for extended periods of time without risk of future tissue change from effects of long-term radiation. This property is especially relevant when one is studying infants and children who are at greater risk than adults for showing the cumulative effects of ionizing radiation. The air interface at the surface of the tongue is a nearly perfect reflector of sound, thus clearly displaying the lingual musculature and vessels both at rest and during oral motion. Ultrasound imaging is ideally suited to identifying the various soft tissues that compose the upper aerodigestive tract. In addition, the transduction properties of sound waves allow these soft tissues to be distinguished from ingested fluids, semisolids, and solid materials. Since no contrast material is needed to visualize the oropharynx and the bolus during swallowing, any type of food commonly ingested by the patient can be used during a study. The ultrasound examination is conducted with the adult or child patient seated in a comfortable position, while an infant is held on the mother's lap. All ultrasound systems are portable, have built-in video systems, online computerized image processing and measurement programs, a computer keyboard, display screen, and hard copy printout capacity. Ultrasound is easy to use and provides reliable diagnostic information. Because of these advantages, ultrasound technology is well suited to evaluate individuals of any age from infancy to senescence, and any neurological, systemic, genetic, traumatic, developmental, or progressive condition that affects oral physiology.

Ultrasound examinations, like all other imaging techniques, require that the examiner have basic knowledge of the appearance of the anatomical structures of the oropharynx, imaging procedures, and operation of the system. Ultrasound images of the oropharynx can be obtained in various planes: sagittal, parasagittal, coronal, and transverse (9,10). The flexibility of multiple viewing planes allows the

TABLE 8.1. Ultrasound imaging of swallowing.

> Advantages
>   Dynamic, multiple plane images
>   Noninvasive
>   No risks
>   No long-term bioeffects
>   Regular foods used
>   Safe, comfortable procedure
>   Portable
>   Easy to use instantaneous output
>   Repeated studies without time limits
>   Useful to compare progress in treatment
>   Biofeedback technique
>   Lingual and oral muscular compensations visualized
>   Built-in data recording, video display, and computerized measurements
>   Multiple recording formats (CD, optical disk, video, hard copy)
>   Three-dimensional imaging
>   No patient preparation time needed
>   Patient studied when awake or asleep
> Limitations
>   Limited scanning region
>   Bone not visualized
>   Limited detection of aspiration
> Swallowing applications
>   Diagnose oral preparation and oral pharyngeal bolus transport
>   Determine tongue-hyoid interactions
>   Determine swallowing duration
>   Study bolus volume and viscosity
>   Examine the motions of the lateral pharyngeal wall
>   Evaluate effects of reduced saliva
>   Evaluate effects of neuromuscular conditions
>   Evaluate symmetry
>   Examine postsurgical and postradiation effects
>   Examine gross vocal fold activity
>   Evaluate infants during suck/suckle feeding on breast or bottle
>   Examine swallowing in elderly, infirm
>   Determine effects of developmental delay
>   Evaluate immediate, short- and long-term effects of therapeutic interventions
>   Evaluate effects of medication
>   Evaluate effects of vascular changes on swallowing

examiner to study the activity of the oropharynx from several positions, to determine compensatory motions, and to evaluate tongue/muscular patterns used in bolus preparation and transport during swallowing. Technological advances in ultrasound include three-dimensional (3D) imaging and power Doppler displays of blood flow (11). These specialized techniques can be applied to further our understanding of swallowing and oral motor function.

Ultrasound, like all other techniques used to examine swallowing, has limitations in addition to advantages. The physical properties of sound transmission do not allow high-frequency sound waves to pass through substances such as bone. Most of the oral cavity is encased in bone, creating an echo-free area or dark shadow when bones are present within the scanning region (e.g., mandible, maxilla, hyoid). Motions of the hyoid bone are essential to understanding swallowing dynamics. The displacement of the echo-free shadow created by hyoid activity during swallowing can be easily tracked on ultrasound, turning this potential limitation into an advantage. The viewing region of most transducers is 60 to 120°. Consequently, structures residing outside the viewing range cannot be seen until the transducer has been repositioned. Because of the limited field of view of most currently available transducers, the multiple phases of the swallow cannot be viewed simultaneously. The esophageal swallow is not suited for study using ultrasound. Although pooling of secretions and residue in the valleculae may be detected on ultrasound, aspiration is not visible.

The remainder of this chapter will discuss, in more detail, principles of ultrasound imaging, equipment, sonoanatomy, applications of ultrasound for studies in adults, infants, and children, special procedures, new techniques, and advanced technologies used in the application of ultrasound imaging of the oropharynx and larynx.

Basics of Ultrasound

Ultrasound consists of high-frequency sound waves ranging from 1 to 40 MHz for medical imaging. Ultrasound is based on the transmission and reflection of these waves at interfaces between two substances of different impedances. The transmission of ultrasound for oropharyngeal imaging is achieved by a transducer that generates and receives reflected sound waves. The reflection of these acoustic waves is the central premise of ultrasound imaging. The signals generated by the transducer are transmitted through the structure until an interface with another material is encountered. The echoes produced at and within these boundaries are responsible for the major organ outlines observed in oropharyngeal ultrasound images. Some echoes, however, are not reflected back to the transducer but are transmitted through the next tissue or scattered at interface boundaries throughout the medium. These scattered diffuse reflections comprise the gray, specklelike patterns observed in ultrasound images (12).

Any commercially available real-time ultrasound system can be used to study swallowing. Advancements in ultrasound transducer design and scanning methods allow greater choices for viewing oral, pharyngeal, and laryngeal anatomy. The selection of an appropriate scanning system and transducer array is important when imaging the curved and irregular shaped structures of the oropharynx. The image format, resolution depth, and scan line capabilities will influence the size and extent of detail that can be obtained. For example, selection of the frequency range of the transducer will influence both the depth to which structures can be viewed and the image resolution. If a high frequency is selected, the image resolution will increase but the depth of the image will be reduced. Selection of a lower frequency will increase the depth of view but reduce the image resolution. Choice of the shape of the transducer will influence the viewing region of the structures studied. Sector, convex, or curvilinear transducers will produce wedge- or pie-shaped images and thus are ideal for viewing the tongue from the anterior blade to the base of the tongue and upper pharynx. A real-time sector scanner with a convex, curvilinear, or phased-array transducer with a frequency in the range of 3.5 to 7.5 MHz is advised for viewing the oropharynx. A linear transducer produces a rectangular image and is most suited for viewing the laryngeal region.

Placement of the transducer is also critical for obtaining clear images of the oropharyngeal anatomy. To best view the oral cavity, floor muscles, tongue, hyomuscular region, palate, and upper pharynx, the transducer must be placed submentally (in the soft tissue area just behind the chin) with the beam then angled upward (Figure 8.1C). Depending on the orientation of the midline of the transducer, this placement will create either a sagittal or coronal image. By rotating the transducer 90° from the initial placement, both sagittal and

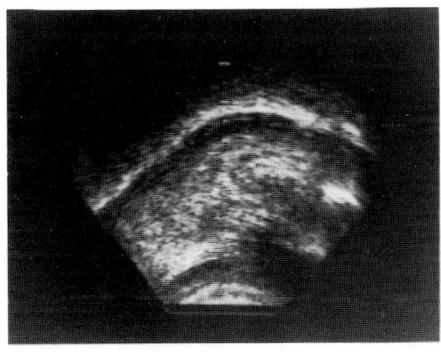 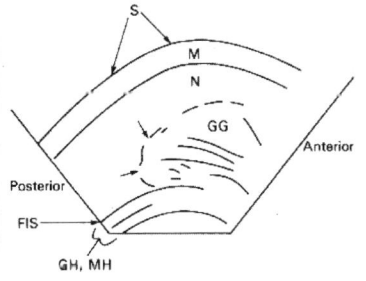 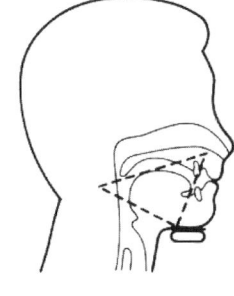

FIGURE 8.1. Midline sagittal scan of mid tongue. The submental transducer placement and anatomic area scanned are shown on the right panel of the figure. The following are shown on the schematic of the ultrasound scan in the center panel: mucosa (M), tongue surface (S), genioglossus muscle (GG), floor intermuscular septum (FIS), geniohyoid muscle (GH), mylohyoid muscle (MH), arrows → termination of fibers of GG, intersecting network of vertical and horizontal lingual muscle fibers (N). (ATL Ultrasound System, Bothel, Washington.)

coronal views of the tongue and oral cavity can be obtained (6,10). To view the larynx, airway, and vocal folds in the transverse plane, a linear transducer is placed on the neck at the level of the thyroid notch (13,14). Views of the lateral pharyngeal wall are obtained by placing a linear or convex transducer near the ramus of the mandible along the side of the neck.

Advanced ultrasound units provide new possibilities for the identification and quantification of normal and pathological oropharyngeal tissues, the observation of muscular configurations, and the visualization of coordinated movements of integrated structures within the oropharynx (6,7,9). Computerized systems with television monitors allow real-time viewing of an endless number of swallows. Video playback and digital recording systems can provide an economical means of storing large amounts of visual data for later analysis. Today's commercial ultrasound systems also allow the acoustic information received by the transducer to be converted and presented to the operator in various displays. The most common displays in swallowing are brightness mode (B-mode), time-motion mode (M-mode), or new forms of Doppler imaging displays (color or power Doppler).

B-Mode

Gray-scale images are produced by sound waves that are directed through the oropharyngeal region. The reflected echoes are converted to electrical voltages that are then displayed on a viewing screen as a linear series of closely spaced dots (scan lines) of varying brightness levels. The brightness of these dots corresponds to the intensities of the returned echoes and the locations of the echo generating structures. The resulting image is therefore described as a B-mode (brightness-modulated) ultrasound display. Traditional B-mode ultrasound displays anatomy in two dimensions (Figure 8.2) while recording dynamic images of oropharyngeal movements during swallowing.

M-Mode

M-mode (time-motion) provides a visual presentation of movement rates, amplitudes, and motion patterns of a selected reflecting tissue interfaces. The operator positions a cursor along a single line of sight on the image. If interfaces along this line of sight move, a display of the motions is depicted on a viewing screen. This M-mode display provides a two-dimensional representation of the speed, distance, and

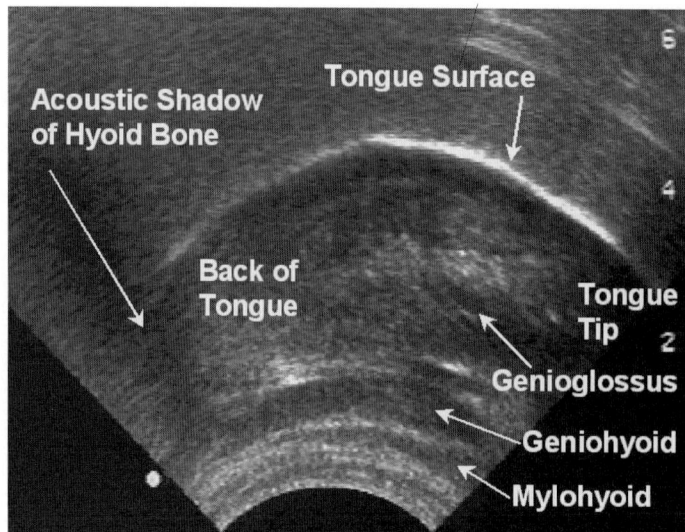

FIGURE 8.2. Midline sagittal scan of the tongue from tip to dorsum. The acoustic shadow of the hyoid is indicated by an arrow at the left. The white curved line is the surface of the tongue. The genioglossus, geniohyoid, and mylohyoid muscles are seen.

8. Ultrasound Imaging and Swallowing

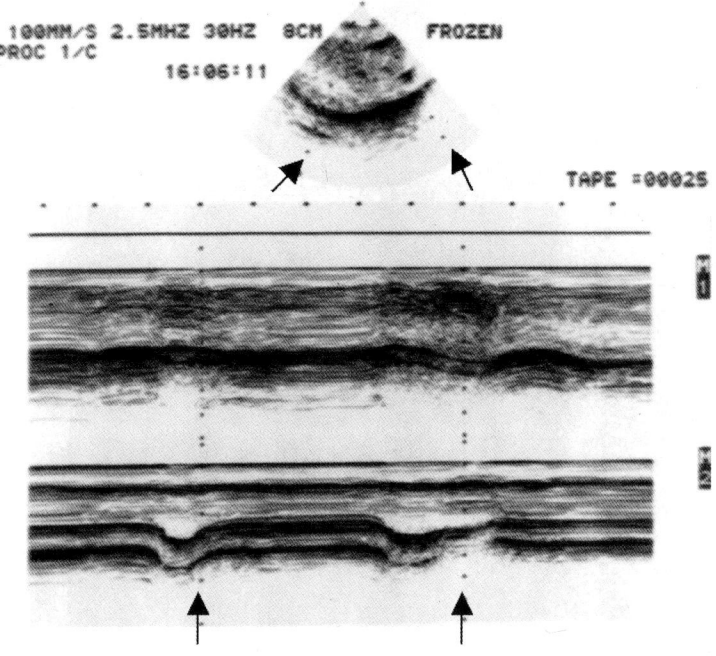

FIGURE 8.3. M-mode scan of the tongue with a B-mode scan at the top of the figure. The arrows indicate the motion of the surface of the tongue at the tip and blade during oral preparatory motion.

type of motion of tissue interfaces (Figure 8.3). Advances in duplex (double) screen ultrasound systems provide simultaneous views of both M-mode and B-mode. Duplex B/M mode-imaging allows the morphology of swallowing structures to be examined while simultaneously recording the timing and displacement patterns of movement of individual soft tissue regions.

Doppler

Doppler ultrasound is traditionally used to analyze the direction and timing of blood flow through the cardiovascular system. Based on the Doppler shift spectra, movements marked by a selected Doppler beam orientation within a sampling volume can be used to measure the displacement motion of oropharyngeal tissues. Sonies, Wang, and Sapper (15) developed a computerized image acquisition and processing system that allowed simultaneous gathering of B-mode ultrasound images with Doppler spectra data on hyoid bone movement during swallowing. Controlled water bolus swallows of normal subjects and patients with swallowing disorders were compared for swallow duration, hyoid bone movement trajectories, and hyoid bone velocities. This duplex Doppler imaging method can assist in discriminating between normal and abnormal movements of the hyoid bone and the surrounding muscles during swallowing.

Other imaging modes based on Doppler techniques now provide additional information about the cardiovascular supply to the oropharyngeal region. Imaging modes based on Doppler techniques can provide information about the vascularization of the oropharyngeal region. Color Doppler flow (CDF) and power Doppler flow (PDF) ultrasound are noninvasive methods for clinically detecting and measuring blood flow patterns in structures such as the tongue and oropharynx (16). Color-coded images that depict the position and magnitude of blood flow are superimposed onto traditional B-mode images (Figure 8.4). The resulting combined image provides real-time viewing of vascular distributions within gated anatomical regions. Color and power flow Doppler techniques rapidly detect small degrees of blood flow and accurately

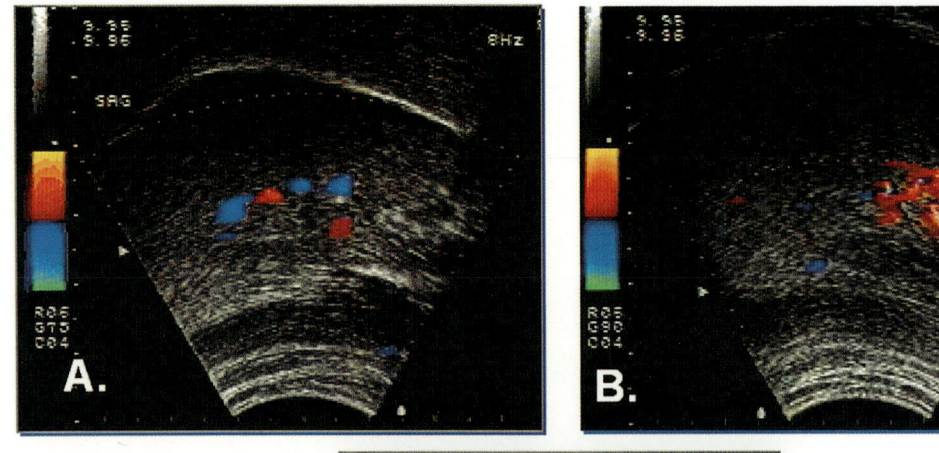
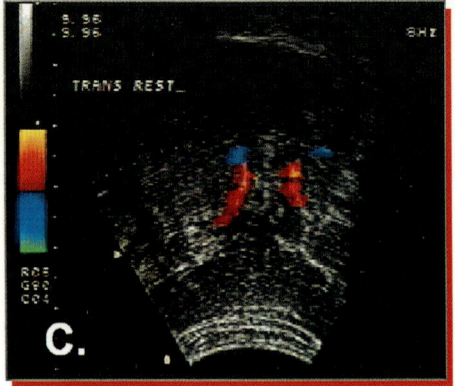

FIGURE 8.4. Color Flow Doppler imaging of the sublingual arteries and veins. Red indicates flow toward the transducer and blue indicates flow away from the transducer. (A) Midsagittal view of the tongue at rest with uniform blood flow seen in both directions; (B) rush of blood flow at tip displayed in red after the swallowing contraction; (C) coronal scan of the tongue showing symmetric blood flow in both directions.

identify the magnitude of flow direction. Both methods are similar to the more invasive angiographic techniques used in diagnostic radiology to explore circulation patterns in cardiovascular tissues. Preliminary oropharyngeal applications of CDF and PDF techniques have identified regional lingual vessels and alterations in hemodynamic patterns in response to physiological tasks (17). In normal adults, notable changes in arterial returns are seen following isometric contraction and swallowing tasks. Further, decreased patterns of blood flow to lingual tissues have been observed in a small group of postoperative anterior and floor-of-the-mouth oral cancer patients (18). These preliminary studies suggest CDF and PDF ultrasonography may be useful in evaluating not only lingual hemodynamics in individuals with oropharyngeal cancers but also the responses of these patients to interventions such as surgery, drug treatments, or chemotherapy.

Normal Ultrasound Anatomy

Sagittal View

The major oral soft tissues are visible from a posterior midline sagittal position (Figure 8.2). The muscles and fascial boundaries of the tongue and floor of the mouth (genioglossus, geniohyoid, and mylohyoid) can be seen (8). The surface of the tongue and the lingual mucosal covering are depicted as a broad, curved white line. The transducer was angled 15° posteriorly to visualize the hyoid bone and upper pharynx. Since ultrasound does not pass through bone, an acoustic echo-free shadow is present at the site of insertion of the geniohyoid and mylohyoid, which represents the middle of the body of the hyoid bone and the hyomuscular region.

Coronal View

The normal lingual anatomy can be viewed from the coronal plane by turning the transducer 90° from the midline sagittal placement. The tongue has a mushroom-shaped appearance, with the triangular genioglossus muscle in the center (Figure 8.5A). Since the tongue is grossly separated into halves, asymmetry can be readily appreciated. Some lingual muscle asymmetries are nonpathological, whereas others may reflect paresis, tissue invasion, or neuromuscular conditions. The mandibular bone casts a slightly curved, echo-free shadow on both sides of the tongue musculature. Inferiorly, the floor intermuscular septum separates the tongue from the geniohyoid, mylohyoid, and anterior digastric muscles of the floor of the mouth that are located below the tongue body.

Transverse View

The larynx can be seen in cross section in Figure 8.6A. The vocal folds are abducted, and the glottis can be seen. To obtain this transverse view, a 5MHz linear array transducer is positioned on the neck at the thyroid notch. Since the images are not static, the motion of the vocal folds can be captured in real time on videotape for poststudy analysis. The edge of the epiglottis is present at the front or top of the image. The thyroid cartilage, trachea, valleculae, and piriform sinuses are discernible. Since the laryngeal area is so clearly visible on this scanning view, the examiner can detect whether residue remains in the pharynx after a swallow, whether there are resting asymmetries or masses in the laryngeal structures, and whether the airway is protected by vocal fold adduction during the swallow. During the swallow, the glottis cannot be seen because the epiglottis has lowered over the top of the airway (see Figure 8.6B). Glottic closure can also be viewed during throat clearing, swallowing, and any swallow maneuvers used to produce adduction (Figure 8.6C).

Imaging Applications for Adults

In adults, the viewing region visualized during swallowing is limited to the oral cavity and upper pharynx (9,10). All swallowing studies

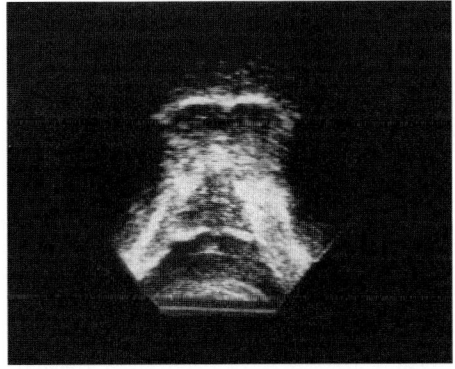
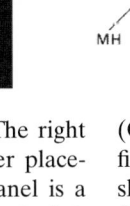
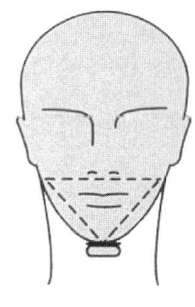

A   B,C

FIGURE 8.5. Coronal scan of the tongue. The right panel is a diagram of submental transducer placement and the area scanned. The center panel is a schematic of the coronal ultrasound scan on the left panel indicating tongue surface (S), genioglossus (GG), geniohyoid (GH), mylohyoid (MH), median fibrous septum (MFS), lateral muscles (LM), inner shadow of mandible or jaw (J), paramedian septum (PS), cervical fascia (CF).

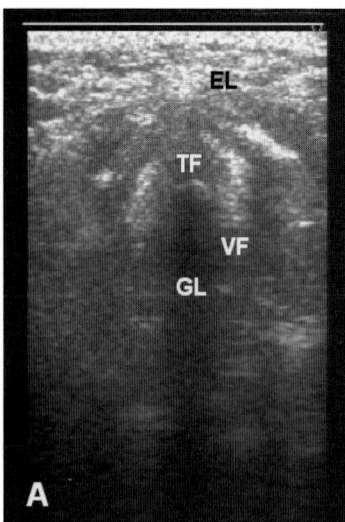 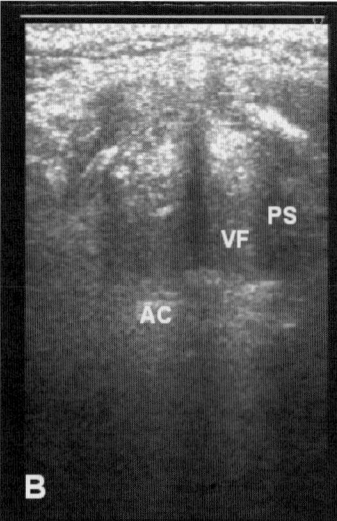 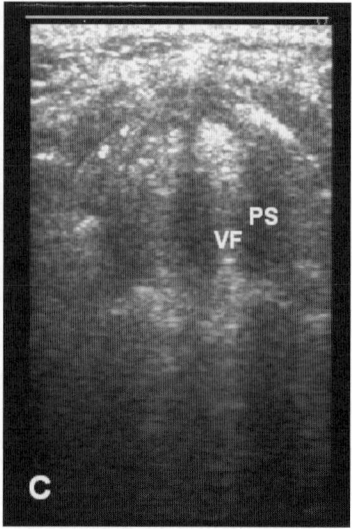

FIGURE 8.6. Transverse B-mode scans of larynx using a linear array transducer. Panel A illustrates the larynx during normal breathing. The ventricular folds (VF), true folds (TF), epiglottic ligament (EL), piriform sinus (PS) and glottis (GL) are seen. Panel B shows partial laryngeal adduction during throat clearing, and the arytenoids cartilage (AC), and Panel C shows more complete laryngeal adduction during coughing.

can be videotaped for immediate review, follow-up, and comparison with subsequent studies, and to determine whether changes occur after treatment. Correct placement of the transducer is essential to obtain the most accurate anatomical images. In the sagittal plane the transducer should be placed submentally and angled backward approximately 10° to simultaneously capture the upper surface of the tongue and the hyoid shadow. The coronal plane is best suited for viewing lingual accommodation of the bolus, depth of the central tongue groove, lingual symmetry, and lateral motion of the lingual borders (19). Studies can be conducted without liquid or food, since a swallow can be stimulated by the natural oral lubrication from saliva (9,20). The effects of bolus size and viscosity can be studied in either the sagittal or coronal view. Ultrasound imaging is not limited to descriptive studies. It should be emphasized that to perform discrete displacement measures on a moving structure, the head and transducer must be stabilized and measurement errors determined.

Tongue and Hyoid Scanning During Swallowing

Tongue

In clinical swallowing studies, the outline of the surface of the tongue is one of the most salient sonographic characteristics. The patterns of tongue surface motion reveal how the tongue changes its shape to accommodate and transport the bolus and initiate the pharyngeal swallow. The movement of the bolus, as it is transported over the tongue surface from front to base, is also clearly depicted. As shown in Figure 8.7, during oral bolus transport, functional segments of the tongue (anterior, mid, dorsal, posterior, root) systematically and serially elevate and anchor against the hard palate from front to back, propelling the bolus toward the oropharynx. At the peak of the pharyngeal swallow, the tongue makes firm, full contact with the entire hard palate (21,22), and the air-tissue interface on the surface of the tongue will disappear.

In addition to descriptive examination of deglutitive tongue motion, lingual displacement can be quantified. Chi-Fishman (21,22), for example, used the "radial grid" method originally developed for tongue shape analysis during speech (23,24) to track the swallow-related displacement of functional tongue segments and then contrasted the derived velocity profiles as a function of bolus type.

Hyoid Bone

On midsagittal views, the hyoid shadow should appear at one side of the image as a dark triangular shadow about 45° from midline. This position allows the complete dynamic excursion of the hyoid to be visualized for the entire duration of the swallow. Prior to a swallow, there is no hyoid activity. Figure 8.7 shows the initial phase of the swallow: the bolus has moved slightly posteriorly over the blade of the tongue, and the hyoid has begun to move slightly anteriorly from its resting position. As the swallow continues, the hyoid bone reaches its maximum anterosuperior displacement

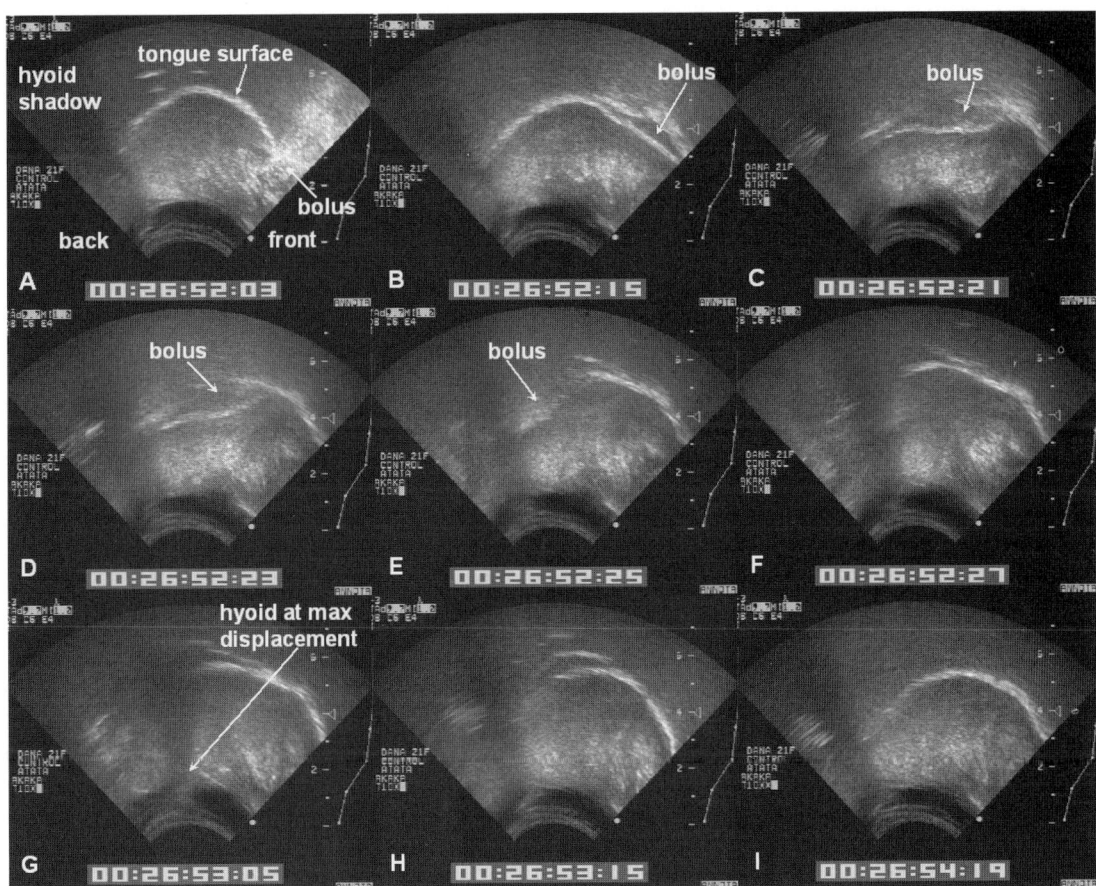

FIGURE 8.7. Movement patterns of the tongue and hyoid during a 10-cc water swallow. In sequence, the following activities are illustrated: (A) resting state of tongue and hyoid before the swallow with water bolus kept in the front of the mouth; (B) loading of bolus onto anterior tongue surface with hyoid remaining in resting state; (C) anchoring of anterior tongue segment against the palate (bolus now behind elevated tongue) and start of hyoid excursion; (D) anchoring of mid tongue segment against the palate, continued bolus propulsion and hyoid excursion; (E) anchoring of dorsal tongue segment against the palate; (F) anchoring of posterior tongue segment against the palate as bolus propulsion and hyoid movement continue; (G) peak of the swallow with hyoid at maximum displacement and tongue-palate in full contact; (H) tongue and hyoid retraction after the swallow; (I) tongue and hyoid back at rest.

under the mandible. Another triangular, echo-free region (the epiglottis) may be seen briefly moving into view during the swallow just posterior to the shadow cast by the maximally displaced hyoid. Maximal displacement of the hyoid bone, in conjunction with laryngeal elevation and epiglottis inversion/closure, protects the airway. Temporally, maximal displacement of the hyoid corresponds well with full tongue-palate contact and bolus passage over the epiglottis into the hypopharynx. When the hyoid bone returns to its resting position, the oropharyngeal swallow is complete (20).

Dynamic movement of the hyoid shadow on midsagittal ultrasound provides a ready means for quantitative analysis of swallowing physiology. Specifically, durational measures that can be made from videotaped hyoid motion include bolus loading time, bolus transport time, hyoid retraction time, and total swallow time (6–8,15). In addition, frame-by-frame and point-by-point tracking of hyoid shadow displacement throughout a swallow can be performed to examine differences in the derived velocity profiles due to bolus properties (i.e., variations in volume and viscosity) and swallowing tasks (i.e., single swallow vs continuous drinking). Using a custom computer program, we have developed a method of systematically measuring the changing position of the hyoid shadow where its posterior-inferior border intersects with the anterior-superior point of the hyomuscular region (i.e., the point of convergence of the floor-of-mouth muscles).

Abnormal and Compensatory Motions of Tongue and Hyoid

In patients with swallowing disorders, the motions of the hyoid bone and tongue seen on ultrasound are often the most revealing of deglutitive pathophysiology. Tongue and hyoid movement abnormalities may consist of several patterns: incomplete anterior excursion of the hyoid, inability of the hyoid to move superiorly, jerky or spasmodic motions of hyoid and/or tongue, excessive activity of the tongue dorsum, lack of tongue and/or hyoid movement, and use of geniohyoid and mylohyoid muscles to compensate for loss of tongue/hyoid motion. Abnormal motions are most common in the initiation phase of the oropharyngeal swallow as the hyoid moves from rest to its anterosuperior position (20,25,26).

Neurologically impaired patients and patients with xerostomia (salivary hypofunction) have been found to have different patterns of swallowing based upon the amount of natural lubrication in the oral cavity as seen on ultrasound (20,27). Although dry or unstimulated swallows are characteristically longer than stimulated swallows, the patient with xerostomia may be unable to produce even a single dry swallow. Patients with neuromuscular conditions (e.g., amyotrophic lateral sclerosis, Parkinson's, postpolio) or paresis caused by cranial nerve neuropathy often use the floor-of-the-mouth muscles (e.g., geniohyoid and mylohyoid) in a compensatory maneuver to initiate a swallow (28). This pattern of compensation can be clearly seen in the floor of the mouth or base of the tongue on both sagittal and coronal ultrasound scans. Alterations in tongue motion caused by oral soft tissue masses or swelling can also be seen. The backward bunching of the posterior surface of the tongue typical of Parkinson's patients and some forms of dystonia can be visualized, along with tremors and fasciculations of the body, tip, or base of the tongue. A recent study (29) using simultaneous ultrasound and polysomnography revealed unusually long periods of posterior lingual positioning, followed by a compensatory swallow during episodes of sleep-induced apnea.

Compensatory maneuvers and gestures do not necessarily indicate swallowing abnormality. For example, ultrasound reveals that in normal aging there are multiple hyoid gestures prior to completion of a swallow that are not observed in young persons (20).

Laryngeal Scanning During Swallowing

A linear transducer can be used to obtain transverse images of the anatomy and physiology of the larynx before, during, and after a swallow. These images are ideal for tracking the activity of the vocal folds (see Figure 8.6). When the folds adduct during a swallow, the airway is

TABLE 8.2. Applications of vocal fold imaging.

Visualize asymmetry and paralysis of the vocal folds
Visualize adduction and abduction of the vocal folds
Examine airway protection
Visualize residue in the pyriform sinuses
Examine motion of the ventricular folds
View laryngeal tumors and masses
Visualize the motion of the epiglottis and thyroepiglottic ligament
Compare phonatory motion and swallowing motion
Visualize the cough response and throat clearing
Biofeedback for laryngeal adduction exercises

protected from entry of foreign material. Visualization of vocal fold movement permits the examiner to determine symmetry of vocal cord closure, as well as whether residue has pooled in the laryngeal vestibule. If residue is detected on the vocal folds or in the valleculae, the pooled material may penetrate into the trachea after the swallow. It is, therefore, possible to make predictions regarding the potential threat of aspiration. The epiglottis can be seen as it lowers to protect the airway. In addition, laryngeal elevation, protective laryngeal maneuvers (e.g., supraglottic, supersupraglottic, Mendohlson), coughing, throat clearing, and responses to residue in the laryngopharynx are clearly visible (Figure 8.6B,C; Table 8.2).

Lateral Pharyngeal Wall Scanning During Swallowing

Ultrasound can be used to image regions of the pharyngeal walls and to assess the intricate anatomical and temporal relationships of the oropharyngeal musculature during swallowing. B-mode anatomical images can be recorded and displayed simultaneously with M-mode traces of echo reflections along selected lines of sight by using split-screen duplex (30). One screen shows anatomical structures of the lateral pharyngeal wall from the superior to midpharynx, while the other side of the screen displays displacement of the structures over time (Figure 8.8). Clinical studies have demonstrated that the movements of the lateral pharyngeal wall do not vary in movement patterns with 5 and 10 mL bolus volumes (31). However, the duration of lateral pharyngeal wall displacements was increased during volitional execution of swallow maneuvers (e.g., supersupraglottic and Mendelsohn maneuvers). B/M-mode imaging can be used to obtain useful spatial and temporal information on the actions of the pharyngeal musculature during bolus propulsion, swallowing maneuvers, and postural changes.

Imaging Applications for Pediatrics

Prior to B-mode ultrasound imaging, the intraoral organization of feeding and swallowing in infants and children had been difficult to assess accurately and noninvasively. Even though intraoral aspects of swallowing are now observed radiographically, these examinations are conducted in environments that differ from normal feeding contexts. In bottle-fed infants, the taste and texture of the infant formula are altered by the addition of radiopaque contrast material. Everyday seating systems or postures are often difficult to replicate. More important, videofluorographic examinations expose both the mother and the child to ionizing radiation.

B-mode sonography, however, by virtue of its safety and ease of use, is a unique method for observing oral-motor performance and reflex behaviors without the use of contrast material. In fact, much of what is known about sucking physiology has been derived from early ultrasound studies that described the coordination of the tongue, cheeks, palate, and pharynx during sucking responses (32–35).

During nutritive sucking, placement of the ultrasound transducer on the cheek provides clear views of lateral compression and elongation of a nipple by posterior and vertical motions of the tongue. With the transducer under the chin, middorsal lingual compression of the nipple against the palate can be observed. These ultrasound observations provide crucial information about the adequacy of overall tongue movements in nipple

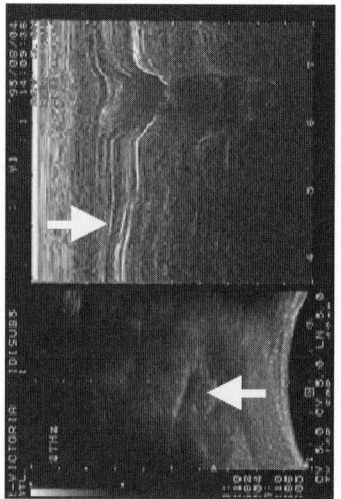
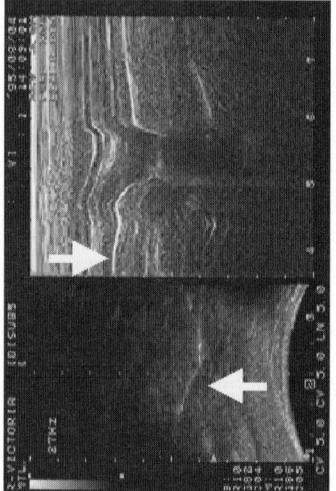
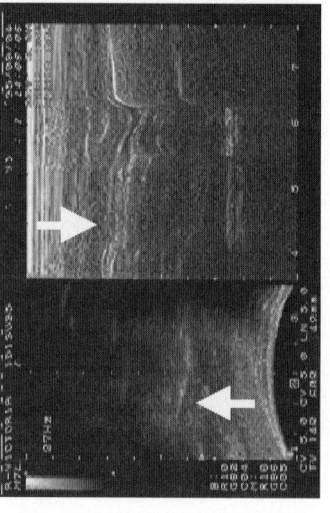

FIGURE 8.8. Lateral pharyngeal wall (LPW) motion displayed on simultaneous B- and M-mode ultrasound for dry, 5 ml and ml bolus swallows. Arrows on left side of each panel indicate location of the LPW wall on B-mode scans; arrows on right side of each panel indicate displacement of the same tissue area during the swallow in M-mode.

8. Ultrasound Imaging and Swallowing

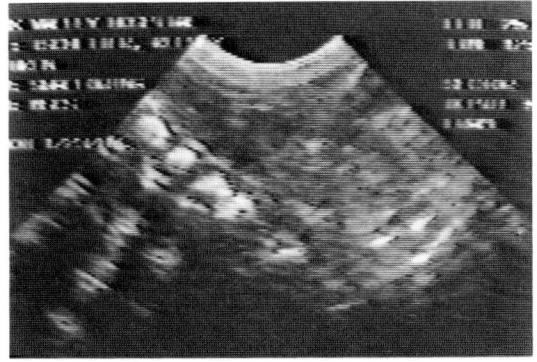

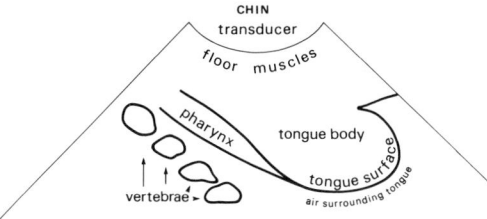

FIGURE 8.9. Top portion shows an ultrasound scan with a schematic of the infant anatomy below. The image is inverted because of the infant's position in the mother's arms. Four cervical vertebrae, the tongue body and tongue surface are seen.

compression and fluid extraction, the flexibility of the tongue in adapting to different feeding conditions (e.g., breast, bottle), and the functionality of the lateral margin of the tongue in nipple sealing and fluid channeling. In addition, B-mode imaging permits the examiner to identify the presence or absence of a midline depression in the posteromedial aspect of the tongue (32,34,36,37) and to determine the ratio of sucking to swallowing as a potential index of the maturation of sucking skills (36). Furthermore, ultrasonography can be performed during nonnutritive sucking via the use of a pacifier to allow the examiner to evaluate lingual movement patterns and integration and to predict the adequacy of tongue activity for oral feeding (38,39). Since infants progress through various early feeding gestures that require movement of the tongue in several directions (suckle, suck), ultrasound can assist in assessing developmental feeding patterns from multiple imaging planes (40,41). These important aspects of feeding and swallowing physiology are not readily identifiable from x-ray imaging, nor can they be properly evaluated through noninstrumental clinical testing or observations.

Integrated movements of the oropharynx can be monitored by using small B-mode transducers that do not disrupt infant feeding actions. Unlike in adults, a complete view of the oral region extending from the tongue tip to the upper margins of the larynx and lower pharynx is obtained (Figure 8.9). Other advantages are listed in Table 8.3. Velopharyngeal closure to prevent nasal regurgitation and laryngeal elevation to prevent tracheal penetration can be identified. The peristaltic actions of the cervical esophagus can be viewed in small infants (36).

The infant can be studied in the most comfortable feeding position, usually cradled in the mother's arms. Submental transducer placement is easy to achieve in this position while the infant is bottle-fed with regular formula (Figure 8.10). The infant can be studied while awake or while asleep. A variety of oral reflexes can be viewed while the baby is sleeping, and the ability to handle natural oral secretions can be examined (42). Since infants do not need to be compliant for this simple procedure, ultrasound can be used safely for any length of time or until a swallow response emerges.

A truly unique application of ultrasound is in the examination of intrauterine development of swallowing. B-mode imaging has been used to observe swallowing responses as early as the

TABLE 8.3. Use of ultrasound imaging of the oropharynx for infants.

Repeated use to monitor treatment effects and developmental change
Determine developmental organization of suck, suckle, and swallow
Safe, comfortable, noninvasive
No long-term bioeffects
Regular formula; normal food
Natural feeding positions
Compare nutritive and nonnutritive sucking
Evaluate effects of oral stimulation
Compare movements during sleep and wakefulness
Evaluate breast vs bottle feeding
Intrauterine studies

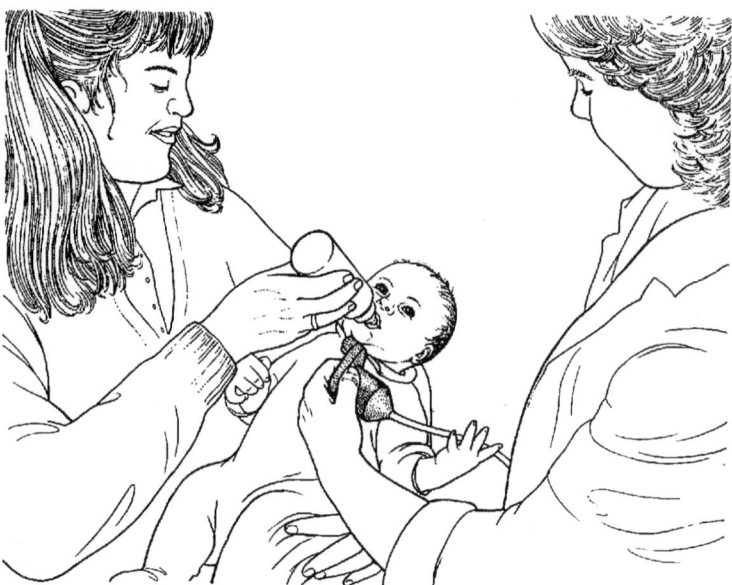

FIGURE 8.10. Infant ultrasound scanning position. The infant is held in the mother's arms with the sonographer holding the transducer beneath the infant's chin.

tenth to the fourteenth week of gestational life (43,44). Sucking and oral motor responses reportedly follow at 15 to 18 weeks of gestation (43). Advances in 2D and 3D ultrasound imaging now provide the means to study in utero structures and functions of the upper aerodigestive tract in both normal and pathological conditions and to permit correlations of postnatal swallowing dysfunctions with abnormalities identified in the embryo (45). A reconstructed 3D fetal face in utero is seen in Figure 8.11.

Multi-Instrumental Applications

Ultrasound imaging can be readily combined with several other instruments to increase the scope of the diagnostic and/or research infor-

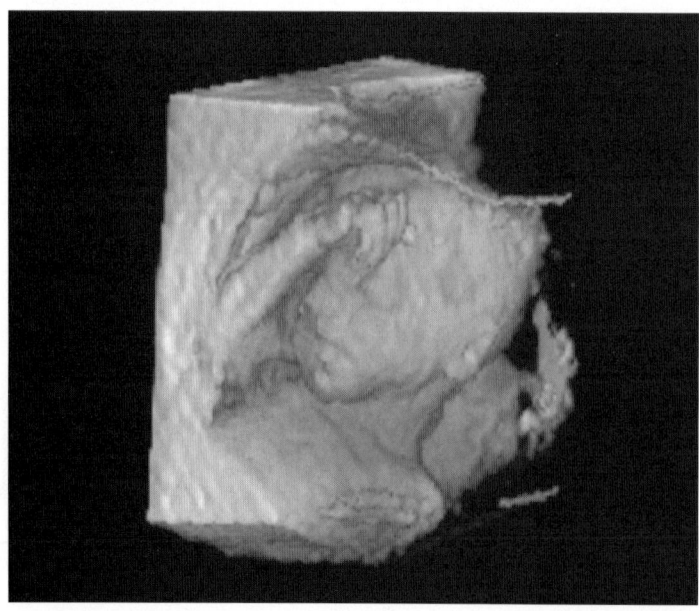

FIGURE 8.11. Three-dimensional in utero view of the fetal face, head, arm, and placenta. (Courtesy of 3D Echotech, Broomfield, Colorado.)

mation acquired on deglutitive physiology/pathophysiology.

For Adults

Synchronized ultrasound imaging and submental surface electromyography (EMG) are useful in studying normal and abnormal swallowing. Sonies et al. (46), in a study of 15 healthy volunteers and 6 patients with dysphagia, found the two instruments to be comparable in measurements of swallow durations. In addition, ultrasound and EMG corresponded well in revealing deglutitive pathophysiological details, including excessive oral and pharyngeal swallow initiation gestures and oral bolus transport gestures. Furthermore, a strong relationship ($r = 0.99$) was identified between maximum contraction of the submental muscle complex on EMG and maximum displacement of the hyoid bone on ultrasound.

Concurrent use of ultrasound imaging and electropalatography (EPG) has been shown to have distinct benefits in the study of deglutition (21,22). An electropalatographic device provides noninvasive real-time visualization of linguopalatal contact through the miniature sensors of a thin, custom-made artificial palate. During swallowing, while EPG supplies lateral and medial tongue-palate contact information, ultrasound shows posterior tongue action as well as precontact and postcontact lingual movements. Combined ultrasound-EPG imaging has clinical applicability in providing biofeedback to patients with oral dysphagia during training or retraining of systematic tongue-palate contact patterns and tongue shape changes.

For Infants and Children

The coordination of sucking and swallowing with respiration is an important issue in infant feeding. Several studies have approached this

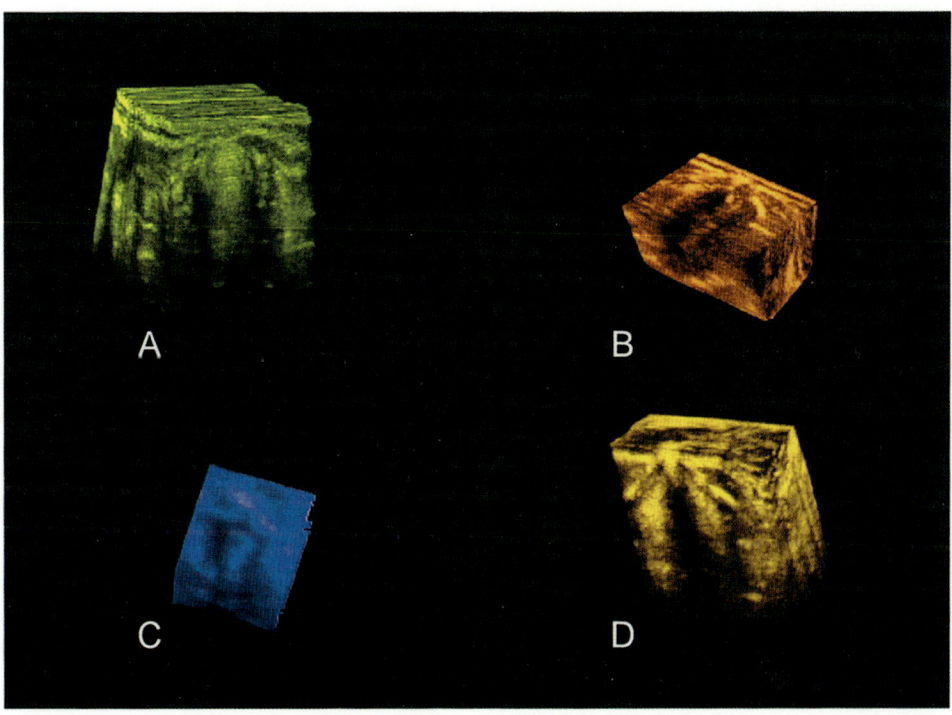

FIGURE 8.12. Three-dimensional views of the larynx. (A) lowered epiglottis and glottal closure; (B) transverse view with open glottis; (C) glottis and ventricular folds; (D) rotated segment displaying open glottis.

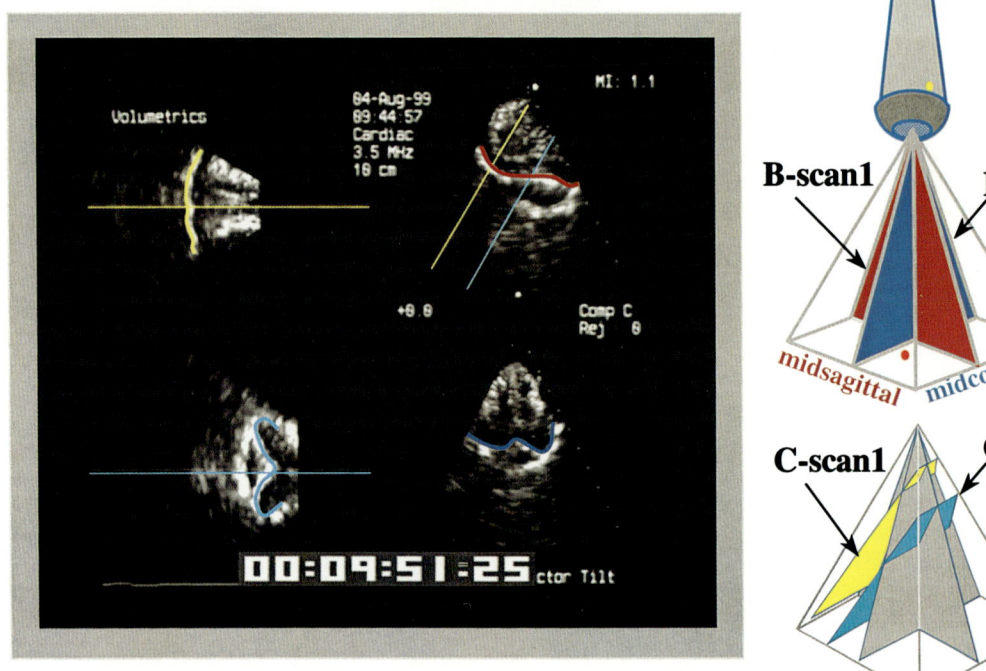

FIGURE 8.13. On-line multiplane display of scans and transducer scanning planes during real-time volumetric ultrasound imaging. Two B-scans, one midsagittal (top right, with tongue surface outlined in red) and one midcoronal (bottom right, with tongue surface outlined in dark blue), are in view. B-scans are perpendicular to the transducer face and adjustable anywhere within the pyramidal volume. Two C-scans, one posterior diagonal-coronal (top left, with tongue surface outlined in yellow) and one anterior diagonal-coronal (bottom left, with tongue surface outlined in light blue), are also in view. C-scans are parallel to the transducer face and fully adjustable in spacing and tilt. This setup permits real-time, dynamic recording and viewing of the same swallow from four different perspectives at once during data acquisition.

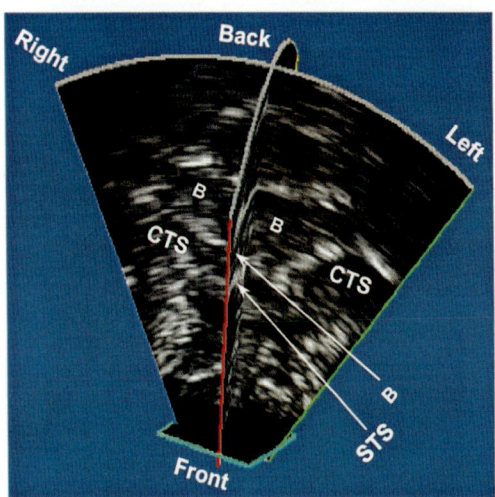 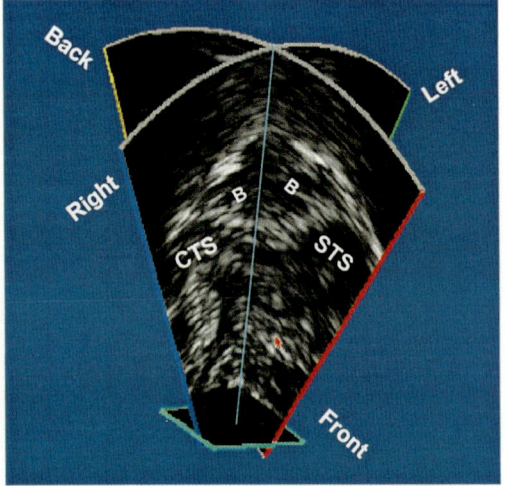

FIGURE 8.14. Off-line biplane views of a 10-cc water swallow at two different angles. The two planes illustrated are midsagittal and midcoronal. In both panels, the coronal tongue surface (CTS) and the sagittal tongue surface (STS) are seen; the bolus (B) is above the surface of the tongue and at the intersection of these planes. These biplane views permit systematic interrogation of the volumetric data and detailed analysis of the dynamic interactions between the tongue and the bolus.

topic by combining ultrasound imaging methods with simultaneous respiratory measurement systems during nutritive and non-nutritive sucking (33,36). The interactions between swallowing and ventilation have also been studied in normal older children and in children with spastic cerebral palsy during cup drinking, by means of concurrent B-mode ultrasound and respiratory inductance plethysmography (47–49). In the same studies the investigators also used simultaneous masseter and infrahyoid surface EMG and found that coordinated analysis of ultrasound and EMG data increased the validity of swallow detection.

Several investigators have combined ultrasound imaging with pressure recordings during sucking (50,51). These approaches were useful in understanding the integration between intraoral organization and biomechanical properties of infant sucking behaviors.

Advanced Ultrasound Technologies

Reconstructive Three-Dimensional Ultrasound Imaging

Advances in technology now provide ways to reconstruct 2D ultrasound images acquired serially into static 3D volumes. Because this method requires that the transducer be physically moved and that the changes in its position be systematically tracked, movement of the anatomical structure is restricted during image acquisition. Newer ultrasound systems are in development that promise rapid 3D reconstruction. Any offline reconstruction may result in some loss of image detail due to pixel averaging. Nonetheless, while dynamic swallowing activity cannot be adequately depicted, reconstructive ultrasound is useful in obtaining 3D perspectives of the tongue, pharynx, and larynx (Figure 8.12) in the static state of swallow-related maneuvers (e.g., preswallow lingual accommodation of different bolus sizes).

Real-Time Volumetric Ultrasound Imaging

Technological advancements in ultrasound have brought us a new system that provides true volumetric imaging at high speed. The system was designed and developed on the principles of pulse-echo phased-array and parallel-receive-mode processing at Duke University (52,53). Unlike the conventional linear phased-array transducer with a single row of elements, the transducer for this real-time 3D (RT3D) system contains over 400 elements arranged in a 2D matrix array. The matrix array, when coupled with 16:1 (receive:transmit) parallel processing, permits a pyramid-shaped volume to be imaged dynamically and displayed in real time without reconstruction. This presents an advantage over static, reconstructive 3D imaging. As revealed in a pilot study by Chi-Fishman et al. (54), this system permits a swallow to be viewed in multiple planes simultaneously during data acquisition (Figure 8.13), providing different perspectives of deglutitive tongue action and tongue-bolus interactions at once. Offline dynamic data interrogation can be performed in biplanes at varying angles by combining any two orthogonal parasagittal and paracoronal slices of the volumetric data set as one geometric unit (see examples in Figure 8.14; see color insert). Quantitative analysis includes tongue surface mapping and volume measurements. In sum, RT3D ultrasound imaging has the distinct advantage of providing more realistic details of lingual anatomy and more comprehensive visualization of swallow dynamics than previously possible. Moreover, RT3D ultrasound imaging possesses the potential for modeling the oropharyngeal swallowing mechanisms for clinical evaluation and management of dysphagia.

Summary

Ultrasound imaging is an excellent technique for studying swallowing. It should be used along with a baseline videofluorographic study. It can be used without fluorographic studies to determine whether developmentally delayed infants can transport material from the mouth through the pharynx. Since it is harmless and noninvasive, there is no limitation on the length of a study or the number of studies conducted. Thus, it is a good technique for determining the effects of treatment or the progression of a condition. It is easy to use in noncompliant persons and for those who react negatively to oral contrast material. Most equipment is portable and can be used at the bedside, if necessary. Studies are videotaped to provide permanent records of function for both clinical and research purposes. Ultrasound imaging provides much of the same information as fluorography but is not as easy to interpret because the bones are not visible. However, since the oral soft tissues and muscles are clearly seen, compensatory or aberrant swallowing patterns are easily detected. The emergence of noninvasive laryngeal and pharyngeal wall imaging provides newer ultrasound applications for the study of swallowing.

Ultrasound offers the possibility to study safely and noninvasively the intraoral and oropharyngeal responses across a spectrum of food stimuli and postural and sensory conditions. Many questions regarding oral-motor development, swallowing-ventilatory interactions, postural effects, bolus influences, and responses to therapeutic myofunctional treatments remain possibilities for future research efforts investigated through this technique.

Continued developments in transducer designs may allow fine detailed resolution of oropharyngeal regions in even the smallest of neonates. In addition, image processing and high-resolution, high-definition ultrasound may provide important information on the normal and altered development of oral-motor and swallowing skills in vivo and a means to monitor high-risk populations for early identification and intervention. The use of combined technologies, 3D imaging, and volumetric analyses may provide more quantitative approaches to the examination of normal and disordered swallowing behaviors and to the investigation of the integration of respiratory or postural conditions on swallowing abilities. These sonographic data may give much needed insights into neuromotor integrity, learning, and skill development that may serve to guide both diagnostic and therapeutic interventions.

References

1. Heckmatt JZ, Pier N, Dubowitz V. Real-time ultrasound imaging of muscles. *Muscle Nerve* 1988;11:56–65.
2. Fischer AQ, Carpenter DW, Hartlage PL, Carroll JE, Stephens S. Muscle imaging in neuromuscular disease using computerized real-time sonography. *Muscle Nerve* 1988;11:270–275.
3. Ishikawa H, Ishill F, et al. Evaluation of grayscale ultrasonography in the investigation of oral and neck mass lesions. *J Oral Maxillofac Surg* 1983;41:775–781.
4. Garel C, Elmaleh M, Francois M, Narcy P, Hassan M. Ultrasonographic evaluation of the tongue and the floor of the mouth: normal and pathological findings. *Pediatr Radiol* 1994;24:554–557.
5. Ueda D, Yano K, Okuno A. Ultrasonic imaging of the tongue, mouth, and vocal cords in normal children—establishment of basic scanning positions. *J Clin Ultrasound* 1993;21:431–439.
6. Shawker TH, Sonies B, Stone M, Baum BJ. Real-time ultrasound visualization of tongue movement during swallowing. *J Clin Ultrasound* 1983;11:485–490.
7. Shawker TH, Sonies B, Hall TE, Baum BF. Ultrasound analysis of tongue, hyoid, and larynx activity during swallowing. *Invest Radiol* 1984;19:82–86.
8. Shawker TH, Stone M, Sonies BC. Sonography of speech and swallow. In: Sanders RC, Hill MC, eds. *Ultrasound Annual*. New York: Raven Press; 1984:237–260.
9. Shawker TH, Sonies BC, Stone M. Soft-tissue anatomy of the tongue and floor of the mouth—an ultrasound demonstration. *Brain Lang* 1984;21:335–350.
10. Gritzman N, Frühwald F. Sonographic anatomy of tongue and floor of the mouth. *Dysphagia* 1988;3:196–202.
11. Watkin KL, Miller JL. 3D ultrasonic imaging of the tongue-volume rendering, surface modeling and volume estimation [abstract]. *Dysphagia* 1997;12:108.
12. Hedrick WR, Hykes DL, Starchman DE. *Ultrasound Physics and Instrumentation*. St. Louis, MO: CV Mosby; 1995.
13. Keneko T, Numata T, Suzuki H, Hino T, Komatsu K, Masuda T. Newly developed ultrasound laryngographic equipment and its clinical application.

In: Fujimura D, ed. *Social Physiology: Voice Production, Mechanism and Function.* New York: Raven Press; 1988:271–278.
14. Raghavendra BN, Horri SC, Reede DL, Rumancik WM, Persky M, Bergeron T. Sonographic anatomy of the larynx with particular reference to the vocal cords. *J Ultrasound Med* 1987;6:225–230.
15. Sonies BC, Wang C, Sapper DJ. Evaluation of normal and abnormal hyoid bone movement during swallowing by use of ultrasound duplex-Doppler imaging. *Ultrasound Med Biol* 1996;22:1169–1175.
16. Watkin KL, Miller JL. Instrumental imaging technologies and procedures. In: Sonies BC, ed. *Dysphagia: A Continuum of Care.* Gaithersburg, MD: Aspen Publishers; 1997:171–196.
17. Miller JL, Watkin KL. Color flow Doppler ultrasound of lingual hemodynamics: a preliminary study [abstract]. *Dysphagia* 1996;11:158.
18. Miller JL, Watkin KL. Color flow Doppler US of lingual vascularization in postoperative oral cancer subjects [abstract]. *Dysphagia* 1997;2:114.
19. Hamlet SL, Stone M, Shawker T. Posterior tongue grooving in deglutition and speech: preliminary observations. *Dysphagia* 1988;3:65–68.
20. Sonies BC, Parent L, Morrish K, Baum BJ. Durational aspects of the oral-pharyngeal swallow in normal adults. *Dysphagia* 1988;3:1–10.
21. Chi-Fishman G, Stone M, McCall GN. Lingual action in normal sequential swallowing. *J Speech, Lang Hear Res* 1998;41:771–785.
22. Chi-Fishman G. *Tongue-Palate Interaction in Discrete and Sequential Swallowing.* Dissertation Abstracts International 1997;58:01B (University Microfilms No. 9719724).
23. Morrish KA, Stone M, Shawker TH, Sonies BC. Distinguishability of tongue shape during vowel production. *J Phonet* 1985;13:189–203.
24. Stone M, Sonies BC, Shawker TH, Weiss G, Nadel L. Analysis of real-time ultrasound images of tongue configuration using a grid-digitizing system. *J Phonet* 1983;11:207–218.
25. Stone M, Shawker T. An ultrasound examination of tongue movement during swallowing. *Dysphagia* 1986;1:78–83.
26. Sonies BC, Stone M, Shawker T. Speech and swallowing in the elderly. *J Gerodontol* 1984;3:115–123.
27. Caruso AJ, Sonies BC, Atkinson JC, Fox PC. Objective measures of swallowing in patients with primary Sjögren's syndrome. *Dysphagia* 1989;4:101–105.
28. Sonies BC, Dalakas MC. Progression of oral-motor and swallowing symptoms in the post-polio syndrome. *Ann NY Acad Sci* 1995;753:87–95.
29. Siegel H, Sonies BC, Graham B, et al. Obstructive sleep apnea: a study by simultaneous polysomnography and ultrasound imaging. *Neurology* 2000;54(9):1872.
30. Watkin KL, Miller JL. Lateral pharyngeal wall motion during swallowing: analysis of B/M-mode ultrasound imaging [abstract]. *Dysphagia* 1996;11:161.
31. Miller JL, Watkin KL. Lateral pharyngeal wall motion during swallowing using real time ultrasound. *Dysphagia* 1997;12:125–132.
32. Smith WL, Erenberg A, Nowak A, Franken EA. Physiology of sucking in the normal term infant using real-time US. *Radiology* 1985;156:379–381.
33. Weber F, Woolridge MW, Baum JD. An ultrasonographic study of the organization of sucking and swallowing by newborn infants. *Dev Med Child Neurol* 1986;28:19–24.
34. Bosma JF, Hepburn LG, Josell SD, Baker K. Ultrasound demonstration of tongue motions during suckle feeding. *Dev Med Child Neurol* 1990;32:223–229.
35. Bosma JF. Development and impairments of feeding in infancy and childhood. In: Groher ME, ed. *Dysphagia Diagnosis and Management.* (2nd ed.). Boston: Butterworth-Heinemann; 1992:107–142.
36. Bullock F, Woolridge MW, Baum JD. Development of co-ordination of sucking, swallowing and breathing: ultrasound study of term and preterm infants. *Dev Med Child Neurol* 1990;32:669–678.
37. Lau C, Schanler J. Oral motor function in the neonate. *Clin Perinatol* 1996;23:161–178.
38. Nowak AJ, Smith WL, Erenberg A. Imaging evaluation of artificial nipples during bottle feeding. *Arch Pediatr Adolesc Med* 1994;148:40–42.
39. Nowak AJ, Smith WL, Erenberg A. Imaging evaluation of breast-feeding and bottle-feeding systems. *J Pediatr* 1995;126:S130–S134.
40. Smith WL, Erenberg A, Nowak A. Imaging evaluation of the human nipple during breast-feeding. *Am J Dis Child* 1988;142:76–78.
41. Thach BT, Stark AR. Spontaneous neck flexion and airway obstruction during apneic spells in preterm infants. *J Pediatr* 1979;95:26–54.
42. Sonies BC, Solomon BI, Miller JL. Pediatric ultrasound. Paper presented at: American Speech-Language and Hearing Association Annual Convention; 1996; Seattle.

43. Humphrey T. Reflex activity in the oral and facial area of the human fetus. In: Bosma JF, ed. *Oral Sensation and Perception: Second Symposium*. Springfield, IL: Charles C Thomas Publisher; 1970:195–233.
44. Ianniruberto A, Tajani E. Ultrasonographic study of fetal movements. *Semin Perinatol* 1981; 5:175–181.
45. Sonies BC, Miller JL, Macedonia C. Ultrasound evaluation of the development of the fetal upper aerodigestive tract: establishing clinical indicators of deglutitive function. 2000; unpublished raw data.
46. Sonies BC, Gottlieb E, Solomon BI, Matthews K, Huckabee ML. Simultaneous ultrasound and EMG study of swallowing [abstract]. *Dysphagia* 1997;12:106.
47. Casas MJ, Kenny DJ, McPherson K. Swallowing/ventilation interactions during oral swallow in normal children and children with cerebral palsy. *Dysphagia* 1994;9:40–46.
48. Casas MJ, McPherson KA, Kenny DJ. Durational aspects of oral swallow in neurologically normal children and children with cerebral palsy—an ultrasound investigation. *Dysphagia* 1995;10:155–159.
49. Kenny DJ, Casas MJ, McPherson KA. Correlation of ultrasound imaging of oral swallow with ventilatory alterations in cerebral palsied and normal children: preliminary observations. *Dysphagia* 1989;4:112–117.
50. Selley WG, Ellis RE, Flack FC, Brooks WA. Coordination of sucking, swallowing and breathing in the newborn: its relationship to infant feeding and normal development. *Br J Disord Commun* 1990;25:311–327.
51. Wein B, Böckler R, Klajman S. Temporal reconstruction of sonographic imaging of disturbed tongue movements. *Dysphagia* 1991;6: 135–139.
52. Smith SW, Pavy JG Jr, von Ramm OT. High-speed ultrasound volumetric imaging system, I: transducer design and beam steering. *IEEE Trans Ultrasonics, Ferroelectrics, Frequency Control* 1991;38:100–108.
53. von Ramm OT, Smith SW, Pavy JG Jr. High-speed ultrasound volumetric imaging system, II: parallel processing and image display. *IEEE Trans Ultrason Ferroelectrics, Frequency Control* 1991;38:109–115.
54. Chi-Fishman G, Sonies BC, Ohazama CJ, Freidlin RZ. Real-time 3-D ultrasound imaging of lingual action during swallowing [abstract]. *Dysphagia* 2000;15(2):106.

9
Cross-Sectional Imaging of Dysphagia

STUART W. POINT, KAREN M. HORTON, R. NICK BRYAN,
EMMETT T. CUNNINGHAM, JR., AND S. JAMES ZINREICH

For the past 30 years, videopharyngography has been successfully utilized for evaluation of patients with a variety of swallowing abnormalities. However, this radiological examination has two major limitations. First, although the videopharyngogram is a sensitive physiological technique that provides valuable functional information, it is limited in its ability to assess structure and detailed anatomy. Small pathological lesions may easily elude detection by this technique. In addition, owing to limited resolution, poor soft tissue contrast, and the inability to visualize extraluminal extension of tumors, only gross anatomical localization of larger lesions is possible. Second, the functional abnormalities identified with videopharynography are often nonspecific. Many conditions can produce the same symptoms and the same abnormalities on videopharyngography. Therefore, these patients often require additional imaging techniques (i.e., CT or MR) to demonstrate the precise neuroanatomical cause of the physiological swallowing abnormalities.

Until approximately 25 years ago, actual identification and delineation of pathological lesions resulting in dysphagia was extremely difficult. However, with continuing technical advancements in computed tomography (CT) and magnetic resonance imaging (MRI), it is now possible to directly and noninvasively image many lesions and conditions that result in dysphagia. Thus, radiologists now play a crucial role in the evaluation of patients with a variety of swallowing complaints.

In general, there are two main indications for such cross-sectional imaging in the dysphagic patient: (1) to confirm and stage a mass in or near the upper aerodigestive tract that is interfering with swallowing and (2) to diagnose a lesion of the peripheral or central nervous system that has resulted in a physiological swallowing disorder.

The objective of this chapter is to describe the CT and MRI appearance of the gross anatomical structures directly involved in swallowing and the pertinent anatomy related to the neural control of swallowing. In addition, major anatomical categories of disease will be outlined and a brief differential diagnosis discussed. Representative pathological cases that are amenable to study by up-to-date cross-sectional imaging techniques will be included.

Cross-Sectional Imaging Techniques

Although endoscopy is considered to be the imaging modality of choice for evaluation of the pharyngeal and esophageal mucosa, it provides very limited information of aspects that are crucial for accurate diagnosis and staging, namely, intramural or extraluminal spread of disease. For this reason, cross-sectional imaging techniques such as CT and MR have come to play a vital role in the evaluation of patients with swallowing disorders.

Computed Tomography

Computed tomography produces images with contrast due to differences in electron density (usually expressed as the linear attenuation coefficient). Consequently, the CT scan is a simultaneous display of regional soft tissue, fat, air, and bone densities. The bone contrast and detail are exquisite and superior to images produced by any other imaging technique. In addition, CT is very sensitive to pathological calcifications. There is excellent contrast between fatty and nonfatty soft tissues, but otherwise there is little soft tissue discrimination on conventional CT. However, the development and now widespread availability of spiral CT and more recently multidetector CT has greatly improved evaluation of the neck and mediastinum in patients with dysphagia.

Spiral CT was introduced in the early 1990s. It combines subsecond scanning with a rapid infusion of iodinated contrast material (1,2). This decreases motion artifact, allows narrow collimation, and improves evaluation of tissue enhancement (3). Spiral CT data are acquired as a volume set, which can then be viewed and manipulated in three dimensions with the proper software. The 3D volume set can be manipulated by using different orientations and cut planes and by adjusting window level, center, brightness, and opacity to best demonstrate anatomy and pathology (4). Three-dimensional software can also be utilized to better visualize vasculature (CT angiography) (5). This is a distinct advantage over traditional axial images.

Multidetector CT (MDCT) is now available and offers the latest advancements in CT technology by combining multiple rows of detectors and faster gantry rotation speeds (6,7). In MDCT, the x-ray tube still emits a single radiation beam. However, instead of one row of detectors, there are multiple rows (8). First-generation MDCT scanners offered 2 rows of detectors. Modern second-generation MDCT scanners offer between 8 and 32 detector rows. Therefore, the multidetector scanner can be up to 8 times faster than a 1-second, single-slice spiral scan. Once acquired, the data can be processed at rates of around 2 slices per second. The incremental spacing used can be as little as 0.5 mm, which improves the quality of the 3D images (9). This technology not only allows routine exams to be performed faster, but can also be used to develop new applications, especially related to CT angiography.

Magnetic Resonance Imaging

Contrast in MRI is secondary to differences in the number of protons in tissue and the biophysical state of these protons. Therefore, there are multiple tissue parameters that can be imaged by MRI, including proton density (T1) and longitudinal and transverse (T2) relaxation times (the latter two relating to the biophysical state of the protons). In addition MRI is intrinsically sensitive to the movement of protons and therefore can image flowing blood. These MRI parameters result in soft tissue contrast resolution superior to that obtainable from CT (10–12). This affords a clearer display of the deep soft tissues, including the various regional muscle groups and surface mucosa, as well as the intracranial neuroanatomical structures relating to swallowing (13). Other advantages of MRI include unrestricted multiplanar slice orientation, diminished artifacts related to metal dental amalgam and bone, and the lack of ionizing radiation (14). Although MRI results in better soft tissue discrimination than CT, there are several disadvantages associated with MRI. These include longer acquisition times, which makes MRI more sensitive to patient motion artifacts. Moreover, MRI is also less reliable in the detection of calcium and the evaluation of bony margins (15). Finally, pacemakers, intracranial aneurysm clips, and other devices are contraindications for MRI.

Anatomy and Pathology Related to Swallowing

The first major indication for cross-sectional imaging in the evaluation of patients with swallowing disorders is to confirm and stage masses in or near the upper aerodigestive tract that interfere with swallowing. This requires a thorough knowledge of cross-sectional anatomy. This chapter emphasizes the structures that can be identified by current cross-sectional imaging techniques, notes clinically important anatomical relationships, and highlights anatomical points critical for evaluation of pathological lesions. After a discussion of each anatomical region, a brief review of pathological entities occurring in that region is provided.

Oral Cavity

Anatomy

The oral cavity includes the hard palate (forming the roof of the mouth), floor of the mouth, gingivobuccal surface, buccal space, retromolar trigone, and anterior two thirds of the tongue (Figures 9.1–9.3). The buccinator muscle forms the muscular substance of the cheek. The buccinator space is just lateral to the muscle and is continuous with the infratemporal fossa above. The parotid duct passes through this space, piercing the muscle and emerging on the buccal mucosa adjacent to the second maxillary molar.

The lingual surface of the mandible serves as an important attachment for the extrinsic muscles of the tongue and muscles of the floor of the mouth. The tongue is made up of paired intrinsic and extrinsic muscles, which are seen in exquisite detail with MRI (16,17). The intrinsic tongue muscles are arranged in three planes at right angles to each other on each side of the median raphe, a structure well seen on CT and MRI, definable by its fat content. The longitudinal group is divided into inferior and superior bands, the superior band being the more superficial. Its fibers extend from the tongue tip, fanning out as the fibers insert posteriorly into the tongue base. The transverse fibers radiate from the median raphe to help form the aponeurosis on the sides of the tongue. These transverse fibers can be confused with a mass on axial CT images (18). The vertical fibers extend from the dorsal aponeurosis to attach on the deep inferior portion of the tongue.

The extrinsic muscles are named for their points of attachment and include the genioglossus, geniohyoid, hyoglossus, palatoglossus, and styloglossus. These muscles have an important relationship to the neurovascular bundle, containing the hypoglossal nerve, artery, and vein. For successful partial glossectomy, at least one of these bundles must be preserved (19,20). It has been reported that MRI with contrast enhancement is more accurate than CT for separation of tumor within the tongue from surrounding edema.

The mylohyoid muscles form the floor of the mouth, with the posterior fibers attaching to the hyoid bone. The sublingual space is situated above this muscle but communicates with the submandibular space. The submandibular gland, which is predominantly inferior to the mylohyoid muscles, has a small component that extends over the posterior edge of the muscle to enter the sublingual space.

The retromolar trigone is a small triangular mucosal region behind the third molar. Its deep relationship places it at a crossroads with the oropharynx, nasophayrnx, and floor of the mouth. Therefore, oral pathology in this area can gain access and spread into all these regions (21).

Pathology

Pathologies affecting the oral cavity are classified as congenital anomalies, infections, inflammatory lesions, benign tumors, and malignant tumors (Figure 9.4) (22).

Congenital anomalies that may cause dysphagia are further classified as vascular malformations, hemangiomas, dermoid cysts, and lingual thyroid and thyroglossal duct cysts (Figure 9.5). Vascular malformations may affect the capillaries, veins, lymph nodes, or arteries (23). Capillary malformations do not normally cause dysphagia, as they are usually located on the surface of the mucosa. Hemangiomas, venous malformations, and lymphatic or arterial malformations, however, can affect the oral cavity in a way that makes swallowing difficult or impossible. For the diagnosis of vascular lesions, the role of CT is limited to the detection of calcifications in hemangiomas or of venous malformations. The optimal radiographic method for the evaluation of vascular lesions is MRI. Hemangiomas and venous

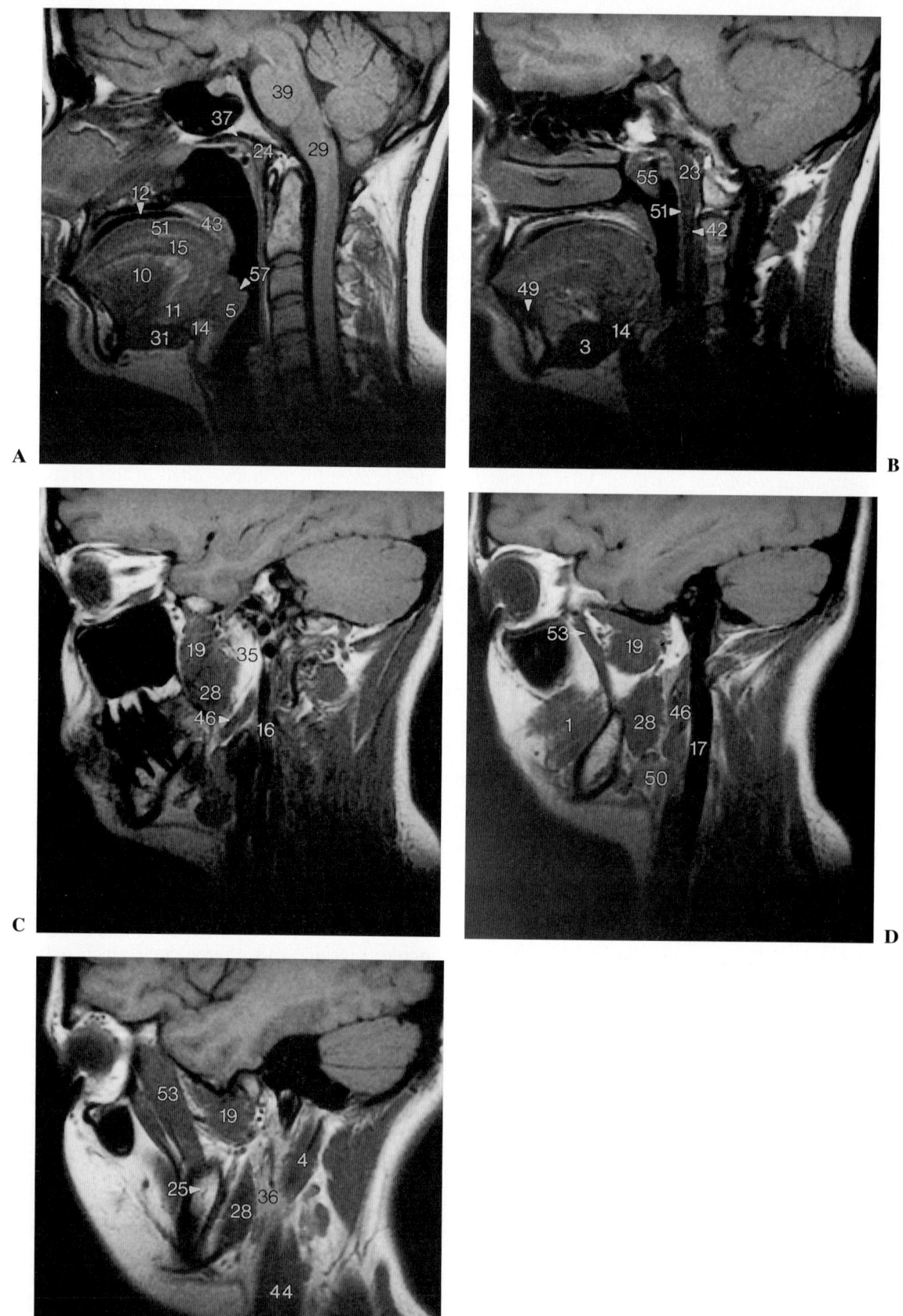

FIGURE 9.1. (A)–(E) Normal anatomy: sagittal MRI T1-weighted images extending from the midline laterally.

9. Cross-Sectional Imaging of Dysphagia

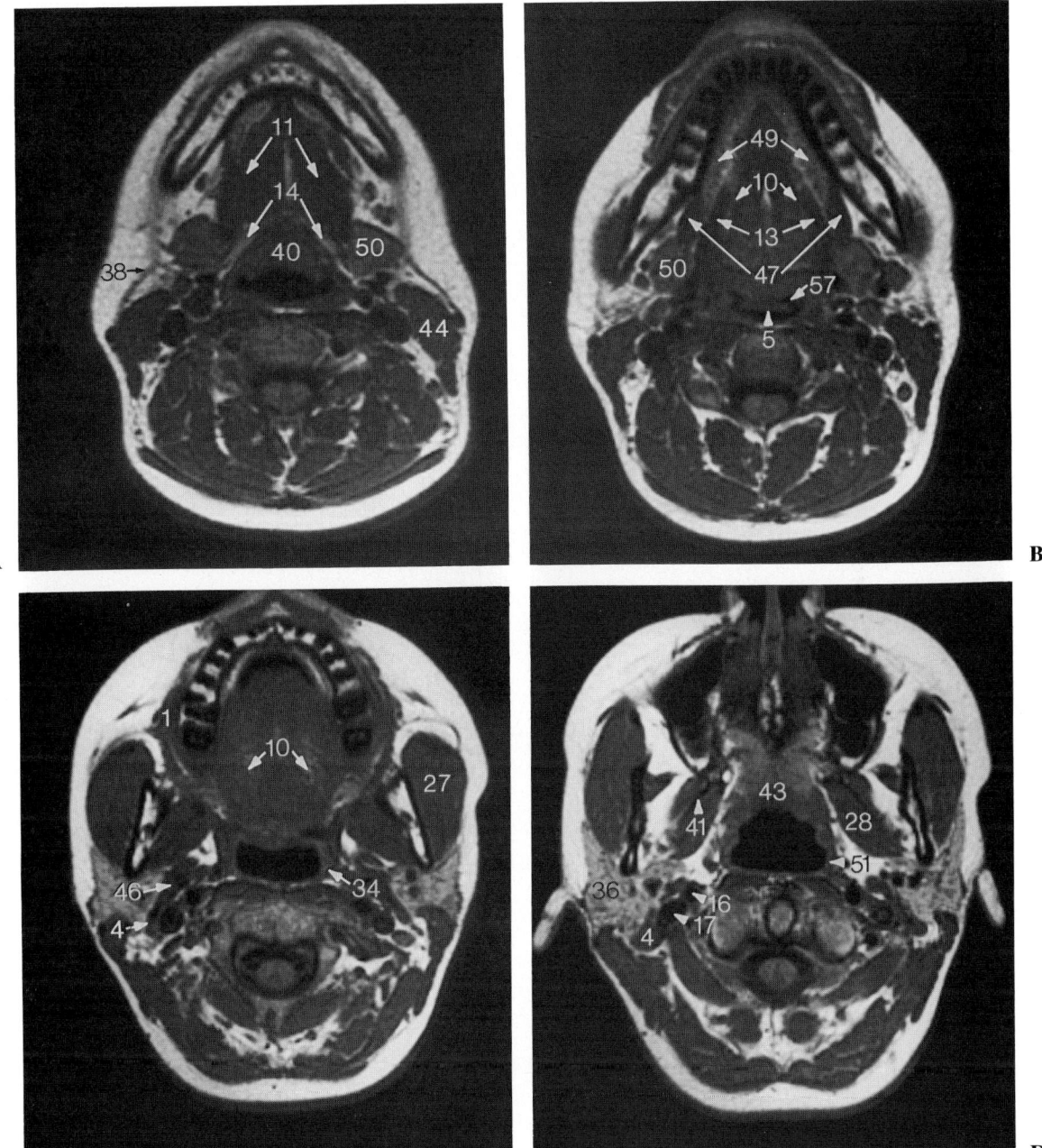

FIGURE 9.2. (A)–(F) Normal anatomy: axial MRI T1-weighted images extending from the floor of the mouth (caudal) through the nasal cavity (cranial).

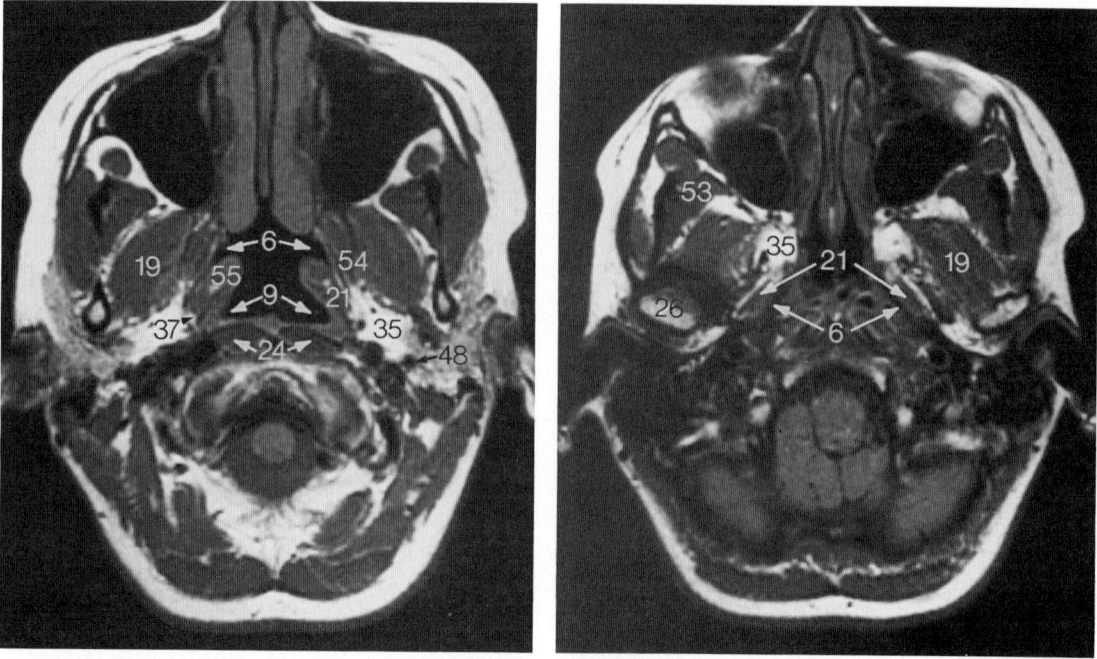

FIGURE 9.2. *Continued*

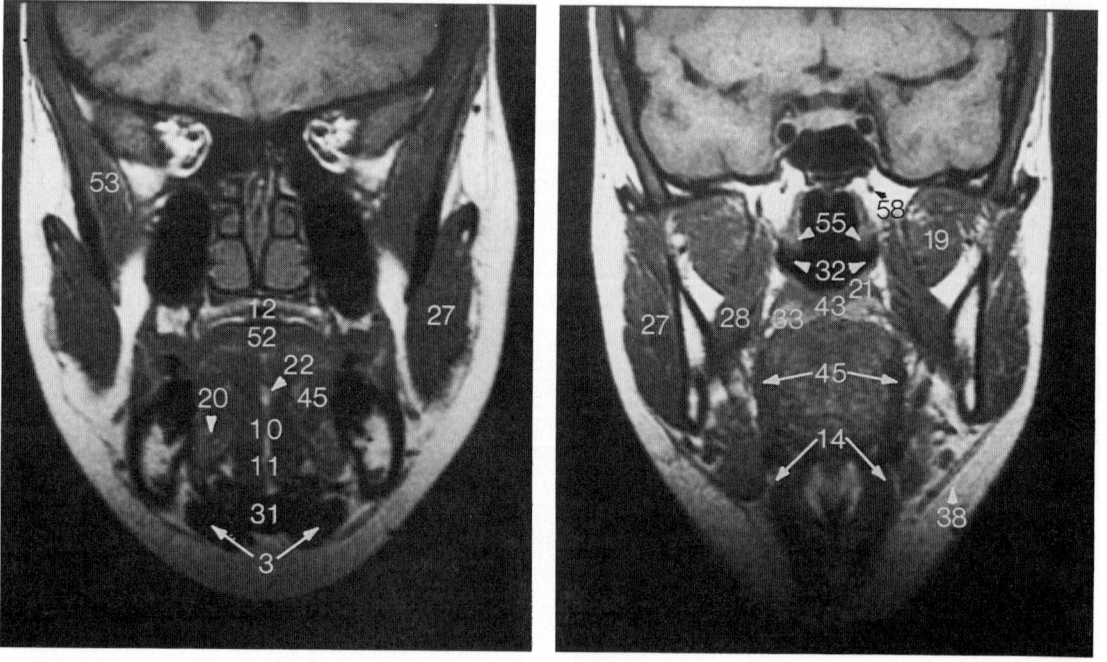

FIGURE 9.3. (A)–(F) Normal anatomy: coronal MRI T1-weighted images extending from the midline tongue (anterior) to the prevertebral space (posterior).

9. Cross-Sectional Imaging of Dysphagia

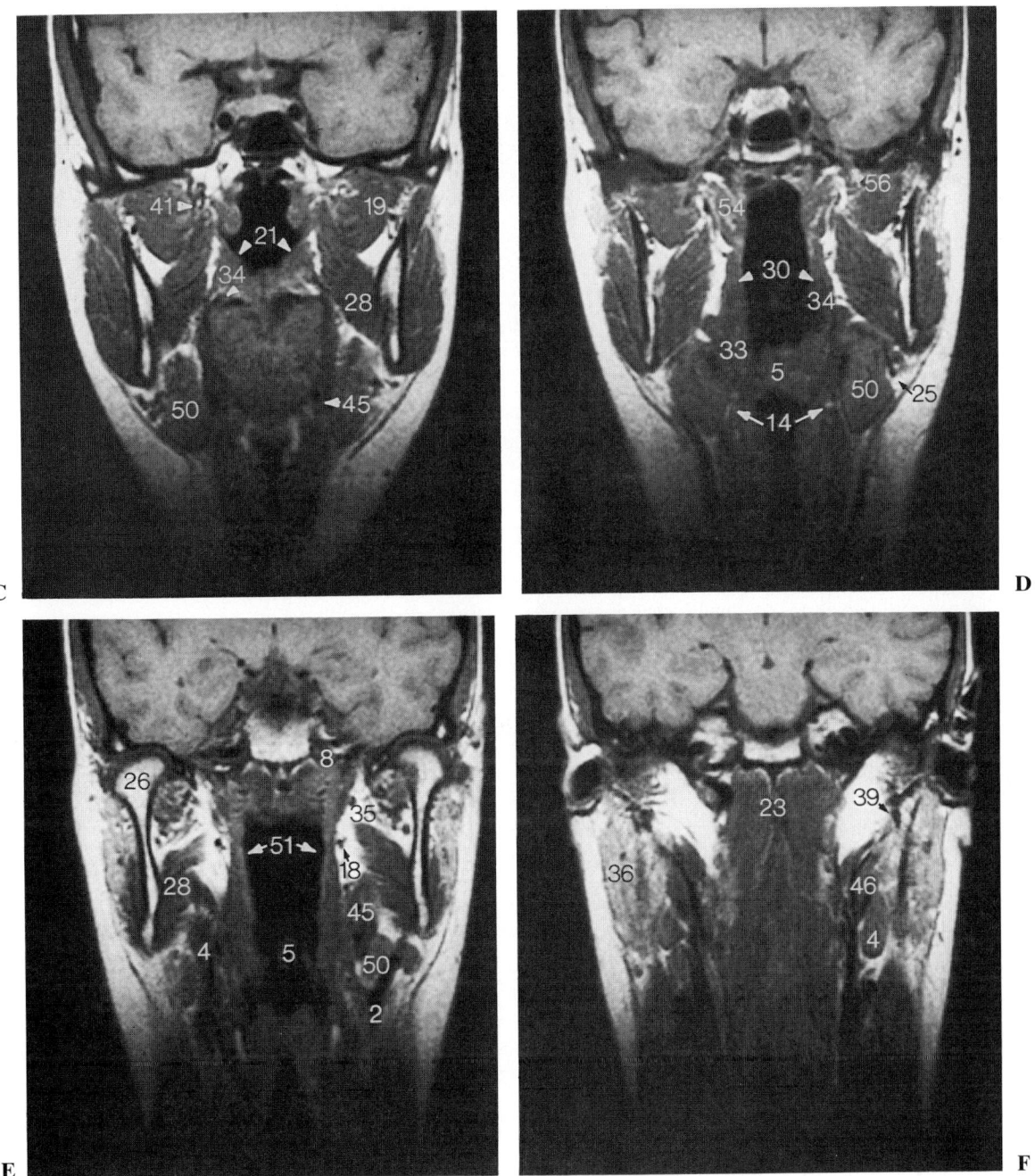

FIGURE 9.3. Continued

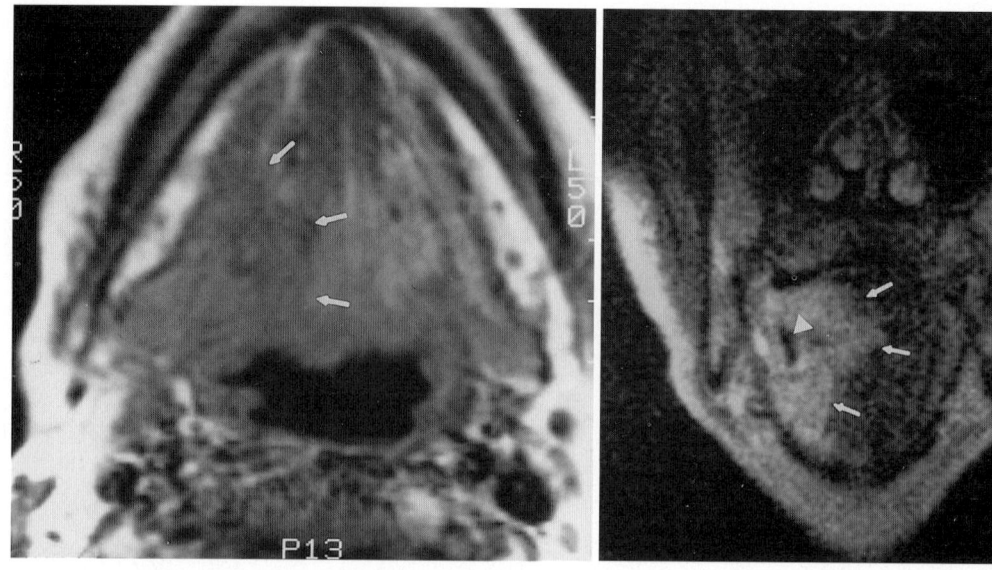

FIGURE 9.4. Right tongue base carcinoma: (A) T1-weighted axial and (B) T2-weighted coronal MR images. Note the low signal of the mass on the T1 images and high signal on the T2 images (arrows). The abnormal tissue is more clearly defined on the T2 image; however, the surrounding anatomy is better seen on the T1 image. Central area of signal loss (arrowhead in B) represents an ulcer in the lesion.

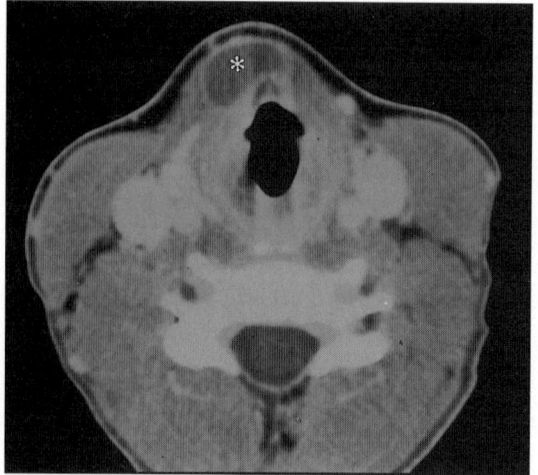

FIGURE 9.5. Thyroglossal duct cyst. Axial CT image of the neck obtained after administration of intravenous contrast material at a level just below the hyoid bone reveals a well-defined cyst (asterisk) just anterior to the larynx, compatible with thyroglossal duct cyst.

malformations are generally more iso- or hyperintense than muscle on T1-weighted images. These lesions become hyperintense on T2-weighted images and typically are enhanced following the administration of contrast material (23). Lymphatic lesions usually have a hypo- or isointense signal on T1-weighted images and a high-signal intensity (greater than that of fat) on T2-weighted images. Multiple fluid levels are commonly seen. The presence of enlarged arterial or venous components appearing as flow voids on T1- or T2-weighted MR images is characteristic of an arterial malformation.

Angiography is very useful in distinguishing among various types of vascular lesion. On angiographic images, hemangiomas usually show a typical blush, and arterial malformations are characterized by rapid flow and enlarged, tortuous arteries and veins. Lymphatic malformations do not appear on angiographic images.

Infections within the oral cavity, including the sublingual and submandibular regions, usually result from dental procedures or the presence of stenosis or calculi within the salivary gland ductal system (Figure 9.6). In some cases, infections affecting the oral cavity originate within the masticator space and subsequently spread to the oral cavity. Because of its superior ability to demonstrate both small calculi and the integrity of surrounding bony structures, contrast-enhanced CT is the preferred modality for the evaluation of oral cavity infection. MRI is used to evaluate patients for whom contrast administration is contraindicated. On CT, an abscess appears as a single, multiloculated, low-density area with or without gas collections. The abscess usually conforms to fascial spaces and demonstrates peripheral rim enhancement. The MRI appearance of an abscess is usually characterized by low T1-weighted and high T2-weighted signal intensities. Rim enhancement following the administration of contrast material is identified in mature abscesses.

The benign lesions that affect the oral cavity are pleomorphic adenomas, aggressive fibromatosis cysts, rhabdomyomas, lipomas, nerve sheath tumors, and exostoses. Only 7% of oral cavity lesions are malignant; however, approximately 90% of these lesions result from squamous cell carcinoma (24). Other malignancies that may affect this region include adenoid cystic carcinoma, adenocarcinoma, and mucoepidermoid carcinoma. Lymphoma, liposarcoma, and rhabdomyosarcoma may also be seen. At the time of initial presentation, it is estimated that 30 to 65% of patients with oral cavity squamous cell carcinoma have nodal involvement (25). Thus, all cervical lymph node chains should be included in the radiographic evaluation when this malignancy is suspected. The CT appearance of squamous cell carcinoma is characterized by a density similar to that of muscle and a variable degree of contrast enhancement. On MRI, these lesions possess increased signal intensities on T2-weighted images and frequently are enhanced to some degree after administration of gadolinium at the time of the examination.

Pharynx

The pharynx may be vertically subdivided into three components: the naso- (epi-), the oro- (meso-), and the hypopharynx (16,21). The nasopharynx extends from the base of the skull to the pharyngeal isthmus, which is demarcated anteriorly by the soft palate and posteriorly by a prominence in the posterior wall in front of the first cervical vertebral body. From this level, the oropharynx extends inferiorly to the base of the tongue and the level of the hyoid bone. Anteriorly, this compartment is bordered by the tongue; posteriorly, it is bordered by the inferior pharyngeal constrictor muscles. The hypopharynx extends from the valleculae to the pharyngoesophageal segment inferiorly.

Pharyngeal Space

Anatomy

The pharyngeal mucosal space includes the airway and is surrounded laterally and posteriorly by the pharyngobasilar fascia (PBF), being open anteriorly into the nasal and oral cavities (Figure 9.7). The PBF is a tough, fibrous aponeurosis attaching the superior pharyngeal constrictor muscle to the skull base from the

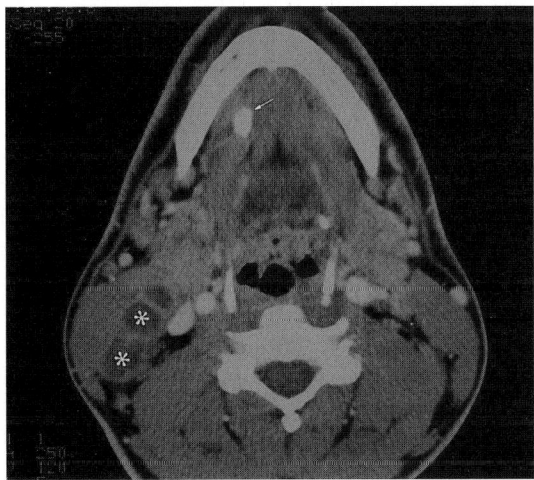

FIGURE 9.6. Sialolithiasis in sublingual space. Axial CT image at the level of the hyoid bone after administration of intravenous contrast material reveals a sialolith (small arrow) in the right sublingual space. Also, note pathological nodes (asterisks) in the right posterior cervical triangle, probably secondary to a tonsillar carcinoma.

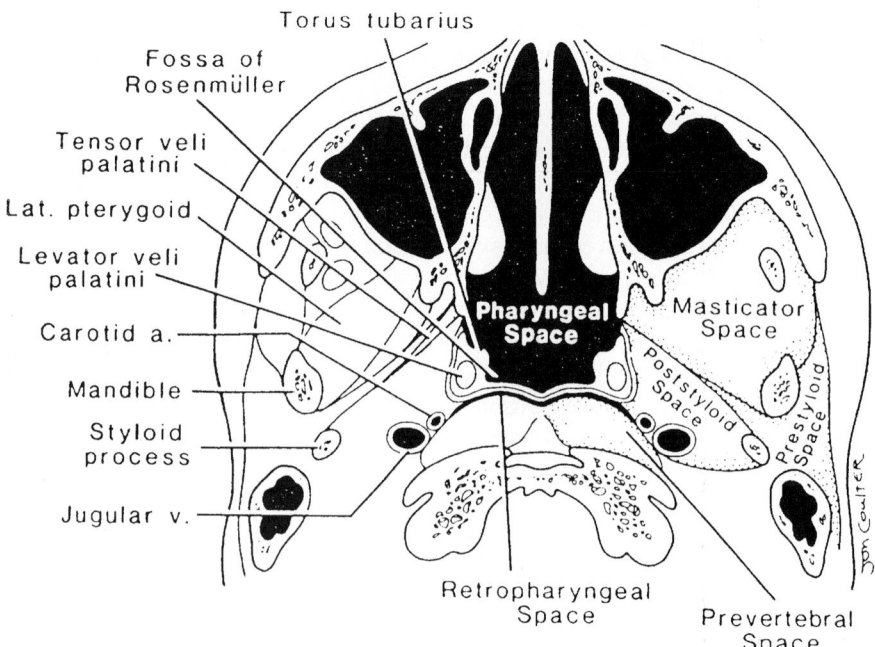

FIGURE 9.7. Anatomy of the pharynx showing the relationship of anatomical structures in defining the spaces in this region.

posterior margin of the pterygoid plate to the quadrangular surface of the temporal bone adjacent to the styloid process. The PBF, clearly seen on MRI as a thin line of low signal, is not identifiable with CT (26). This space also includes the constrictor muscles, levator veli palatini, salpingopharyngeus muscles, eustachian tube orifice, and lymphoid tissue of Waldeyer's ring. The mucosa, lymphoid tissue, and muscles blend imperceptibly on CT; however, their separate definition is possible by MRI. The overall thickness of the soft tissues in this space can vary considerably with the amount of lymphoid material and degree of muscular development.

The soft palate forms the superior border of the oropharynx, separating it from the nasopharynx. It contains the tensor and levator veli palatini muscles from the nasopharynx as well as the palatoglossus and palatopharyngeus muscles from the oropharynx. The MRI signal from the soft palate is similar to that of the surrounding structures because the soft palate is composed predominantly of fat, lymphoid tissue, and mucosa.

The oropharynx is separated from the oral cavity by the anterior pillar of the tonsil and includes the posterior third of the tongue. The anterior two thirds or oral portion of the tongue ends posteriorly at the circumvallate papillae. This boundary continues caudally along the aryepiglottic fold.

The superficial structures in the oropharynx are somewhat variable in appearance because the lymphoid tissue in the lingual and faucial tonsils. The faucial tonsils lie within a groove formed by the mucosa covering the palatoglossus muscle anteriorly and palatopharyngeus muscle posteriorly. Lymphoid tissue has almost the same attenuation as muscle on CT, but a higher signal than muscle on proton density and T2-weighted MRI.

Pathology

The majority of mass lesions in the pharynx are malignant, and 80% of these are squamous cell carcinomas (Figure 9.8) (27,28). Non-Hodgkin's lymphoma is the second most common malignancy in this area. The minority of neoplasms arise from the minor salivary glands and consist of adenocystic, adeno-, and mucoepidermoid carcinomas (16,29). Benign tumors are much less common than malignant lesions and are usually mixed tumors of minor salivary gland origin.

On CT, the density of lesions does not allow differentiation between benign and malignant processes. In this respect MRI affords a slight advantage because most carcinomas display an intermediate signal intensity on T2-weighted MR images, whereas many benign salivary gland tumors and inflammatory processes display a much higher T2 signal intensity.

Lymphoid tissue, including adenoidal hypertrophy, shows great individual variability. Prominent tonsils can be normal in children but must be viewed with suspicion in adults. Enlargement has been reported in immunodeficiency syndromes, most recently in human immunodeficiency virus (HIV)-positive individuals. Distinguishing lymphoid hyperplasia from lymphoma can be extremely difficult. Lymphoma may have less enhancement and appear more homogeneous on MRI after

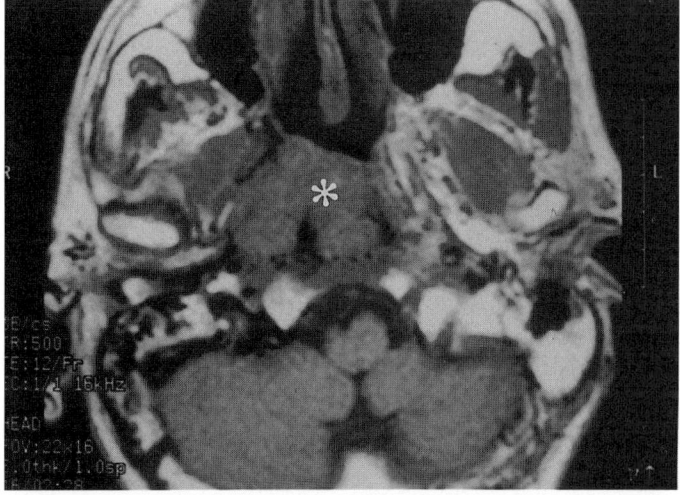

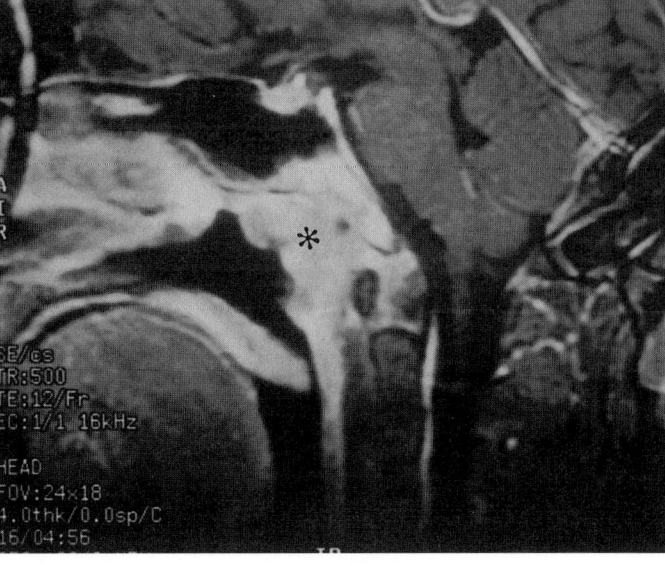

FIGURE 9.8. Nasopharyngeal mucosa–squamous cell carcinoma. (A) Axial T1-weighted MR image reveals a prominent mass (asterisk) arising from the mucosa of the nasopharynx obstructing the nasopharyngeal airway. (B) Sagittal MR image obtained after administration of intravenous contrast material reveals its diffuse enhancement.

administration of gadolinium-DTPA (diethylene triamine pentaacetic acid) (15). The clinical history may be helpful, but biopsy is often required.

Parapharyngeal Space

Anatomy

The parapharyngeal space (PPS) is found just lateral to the pharyngobasilar fascia and extends to, but does not include, the muscles of mastication. This space extends from the skull base to the hyoid bone and resembles an inverted pyramid, the lateral border being largely formed by the fascia of the medial pterygoid muscle (Figures 9.9 and 9.10) (16,29). Several muscle groups involved in deglutition are present within this space, including the tensor veli palatini muscles and the styloid group. The PPS can be divided into two compartments by drawing a line along the border of the tensor veli palatini muscle to the styloid process.

The first compartment, the *prestyloid*, is anterior and predominantly lateral to the tensor veli palatini muscle and fascia. It contains predominantly fat, but also the deep portion of the parotid gland, which gains access to this space by the stylomandibular tunnel. The course of the facial nerve (VII) through the parotid gland divides the gland into a deep and a superficial "lobe." The nerve is not routinely seen on CT or MRI but lies lateral to the retromandibular vein, which is seen with both modalities.

The second portion of the PPS is the poststyloid compartment. It is posterior and predominantly medial to the tensor veli palatini muscle. The major structures found in the poststyloid space are those included in the carotid sheath (the carotid artery, internal jugular vein, segments of cranial nerves IX, X, XI, and XII, and the cervical sympathetic nerve chain) and the lymph nodes within the deep cervical chain. The bulk of both compartments of the PPS consists of fat, and this allows easy identification of this anatomical region on CT and MRI.

In the evaluation of pharyngeal mass lesions, effects on the parapharyngeal space are key in determining the site of origin. Accurate determination of the site of origin of a lesion enables formulation of an appropriate differential. Masses arising from the masticator space displace the PPS fat posteriorly, in contrast to a lesion within the pharyngeal mucosal space, which will obliterate or deviate the fat laterally.

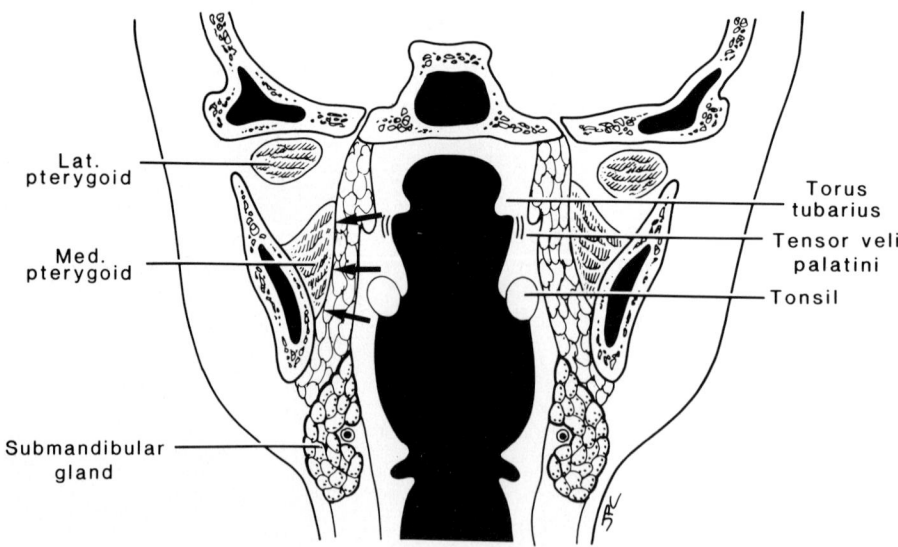

FIGURE 9.9. Coronal diagram of the anatomy of the parapharyngeal space. Note the relationship of the medial pterygoid muscle to the lateral border of the parapharyngeal space (arrows).

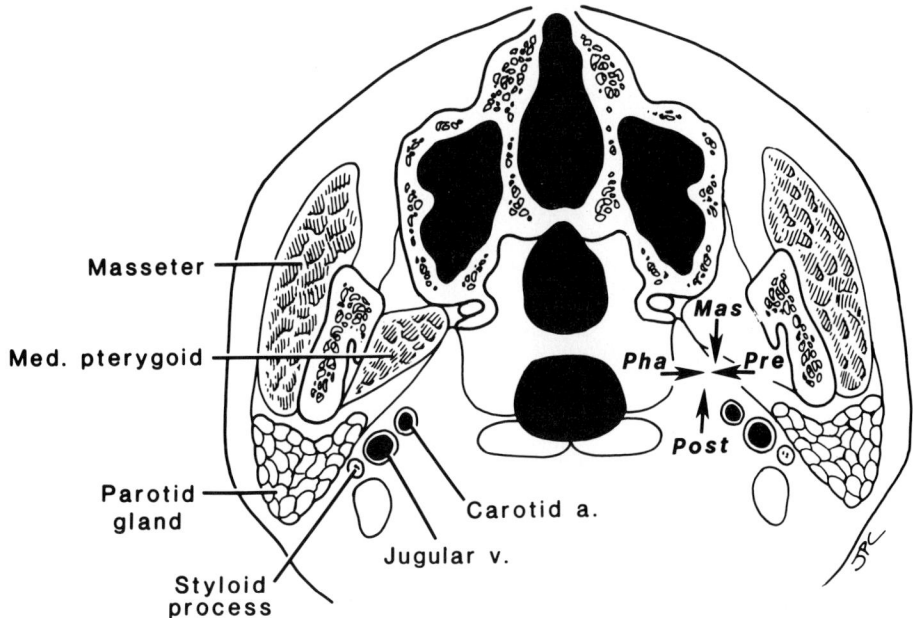

FIGURE 9.10. Axial diagram of the anatomy of the parapharyngeal space just below the level of the hard palate. Note the potential for displacement of the parapharyngeal fat by masses in the parapharyngeal and surrounding spaces (arrows). *Mas*, masticator space; *Pha*, pharyngeal mucosal space; *Pre*, prestyloid compartment; *Post*, poststyloid compartment.

The prestyloid compartment is predominantly lateral, so lesions in the area should displace the fat medially. The poststyloid compartment is posterior, so masses in this location should deviate the fat anteriorly.

Pathology

Parotid tumors of the deep lobe are by far the most common neoplasm of prestyloid compartment of the parapharyngeal space (16,27). The majority are pleomorphic adenomas (Figure 9.11). Similar tumors from minor salivary glands are also seen in this compartment (30). In evaluation of lesions in this area it is important to determine whether the lesion is intra- or extraparotid because the precise location of the pathology will determine the surgical approach. A transoral, submandibular, or cervical approach can be used for extraparotid lesions, whereas a transparotid approach is usually used for intraparotid lesions. Malignant tumors in the PPS arising from the parotid gland are less common. They may be well circumscribed and indistinguishable from benign neoplasms (31,32). Poorly defined extension into surrounding spaces, adenopathy, or associated cranial nerve involvement strongly suggests a malignant process. In particular, adenoid cystic carcinomas have a propensity for perineural spread, which allows them access to middle and posterior cranial fossae.

Inflammatory lesions, including odontogenic, tonsillar, or parotid gland infections, can extend into the prestyloid compartment of the PPS. The history is usually suggestive. Both MRI and CT are accurate in detecting the inflammatory mass and can usually define an abscess. Some authors believe that CT is more accurate in the evaluation of a drainable abscess collection (33). Congenital lesions, including cystic hygroma, lymphangioma, second branchial cleft cyst, and hemangioma, can all extend into this region. These lesions usually have a bright signal on T2-weighted MRI scans and often show septation and fluid-fluid levels. Usually MRI is the best modality for evaluation of these lesions, although CT holds a minor

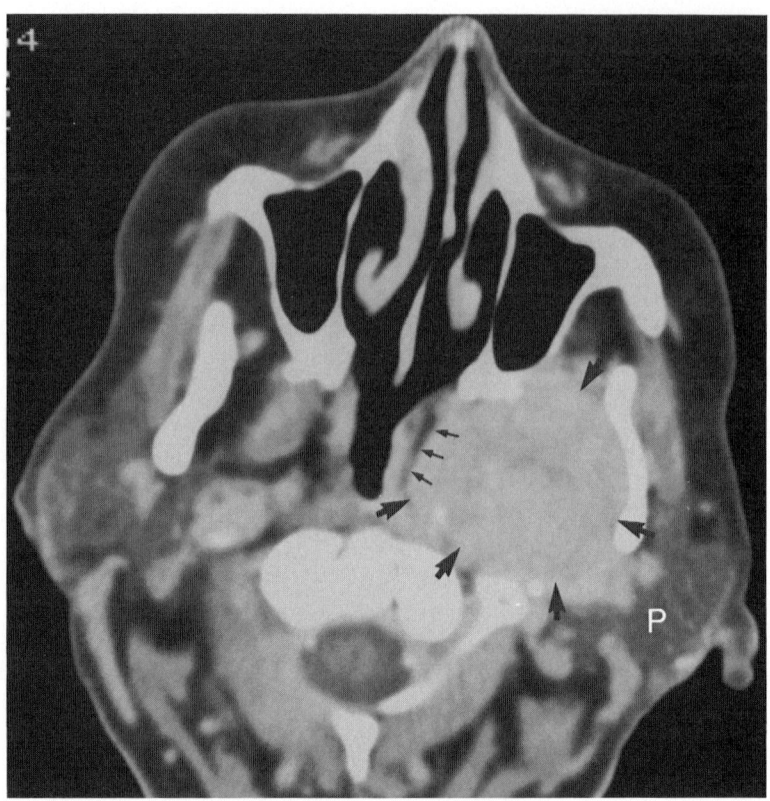

FIGURE 9.11. Pleomorphic adenoma. Enhanced axial CT scan showing a pleomorphic adenoma arising from the parotid gland (P). Note the displacement of the parapharyngeal fat medially (small arrows), consistent with a prestyloid mass.

advantage in differentiation of hemangiomas because calcifications from phleboliths are better seen.

Lesions in poststyloid portion of the PPS most commonly arise from the contents of the carotid sheath (Figure 9.12) (16,34). Schwannomas or neurofibromas can arise from any of the cranial nerves. Schwannomas are usually well circumscribed and have central imaging characteristics similar to those of fluid. Most arise from the vagus nerve. Paragangliomas (glomus tumors) (Figure 9.13) in this region often extend into the skull base and present with pulsatile tinnitus or with cranial nerve palsies. These lesions are highly vascular and show intense contrast enhancement. On MRI they have homogeneous signal intensity when under 2 cm in diameter; when larger, the presence of high-flow vessels results in a "salt and pepper" MRI appearance. Associated bony erosion may be present and is better evaluated by CT.

Masticator Space

Anatomy

The masticator space (often referred to as the infratemporal fossa) is located anterior and lateral to the parapharyngeal space and extends superomedially to the sphenoid bone. It is bounded anteriorly by the posterior maxillary sinus wall and laterally by the zygomatic arch. This space contains the medial and lateral pterygoid muscles, the masseter and temporalis muscles, the mandible, and the third branch of the fifth cranial nerve as it emerges through the foramen ovale.

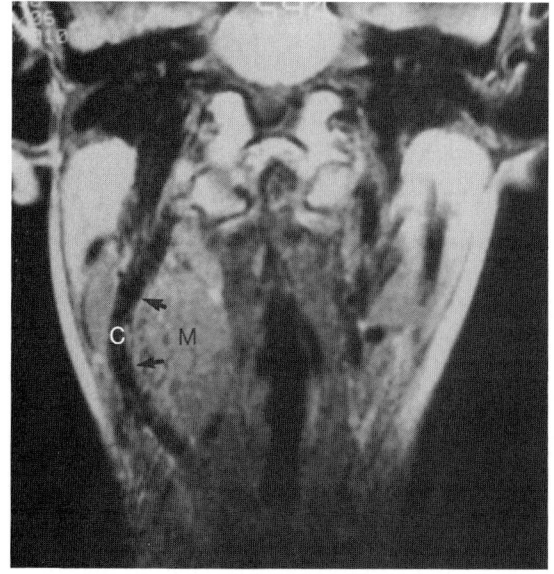
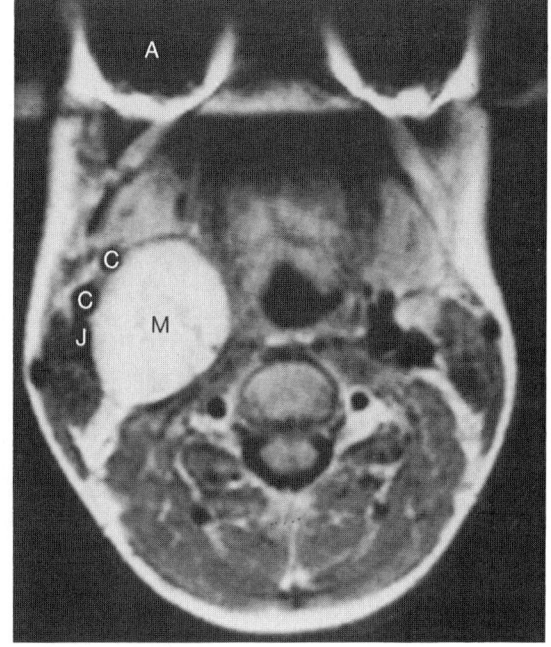

FIGURE 9.12. Carotid sheath sympathetic neuroma. (A) Coronal T1-weighted image. There is a mass (M) in the parapharyngeal space displacing the carotid artery (C) laterally (arrows). (B) Axial T2-weighted image with markedly increased signal from the lesion (M). Note the loss of surrounding anatomical detail as well as the increased artifact.

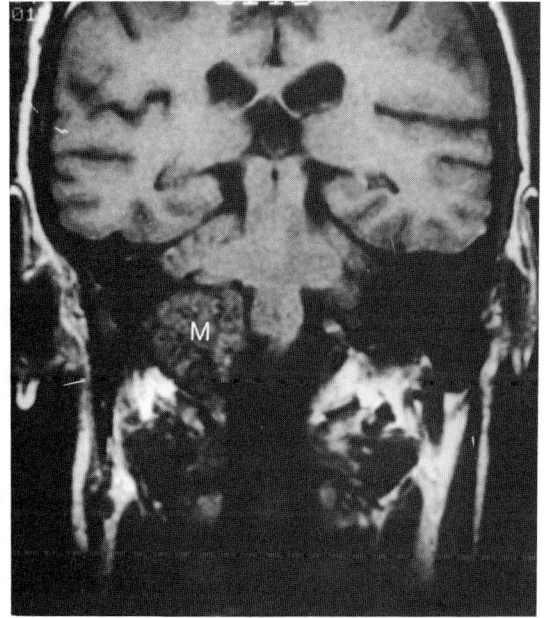
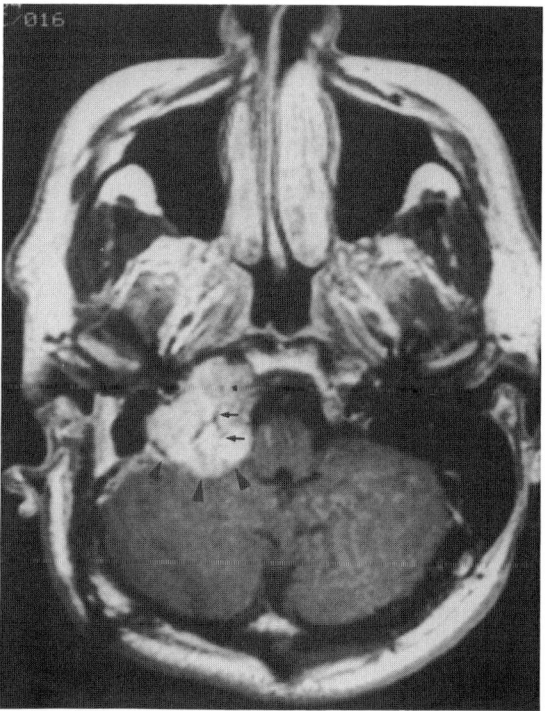

FIGURE 9.13. Glomus jugulare tumor. (A) T1-weighted coronal image demonstrates a heterogeneous speckling of the mass (M), giving a "salt and pepper" appearance. These small areas of signal void (black) correspond to high-flow vessels within the tumor. (B) Axial T1-weighted contrast enhanced image demonstrates the marked enhancement of the mass. Note the small vessels (small arrows) within the lesion. There is erosion of the skull base and a small amount of mass effect on the cerebellum (arrowheads).

Pathology

Masses in the masticator space are relatively asymptomatic until they are of significant size or have invaded adjacent tissues such as the mandible or third division of the fifth cranial nerve. Most malignant tumors in this area are metastatic from adjacent squamous cell carcinoma (Figure 9.14) or minor salivary gland carcinomas or lymphoma (28,35). Primary benign and malignant tumors arising from the muscle, nerve, and bone are less common. Infection of odontogenic or mandibular origin frequently extends into this space, producing facial swelling, pain, and trismus (16). Internal derangements of the temporomandibular joint can cause significant symptomatology referable to this area. In initial evaluation of the temporomandibular joint, MRI is the imaging procedure of choice.

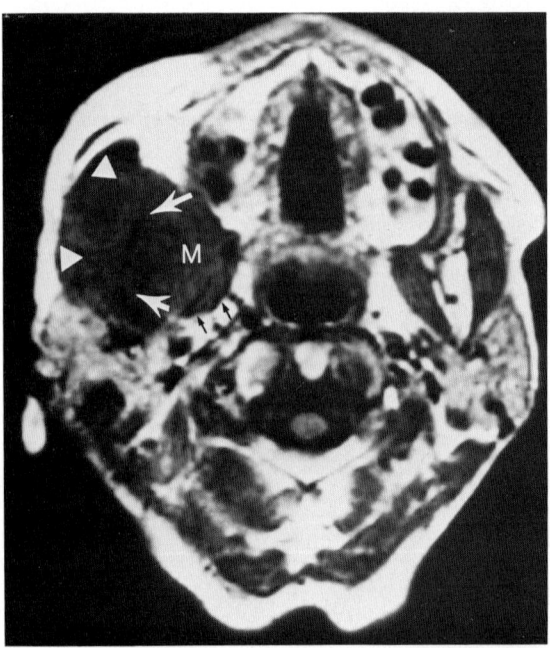

FIGURE 9.14. Metastatic small-cell carcinoma (M) of the mandible. Axial T1-weighted image demonstrates the residual cortical margin of the mandible (white arrows). There is displacement and invasion of the muscles of mastication (arrowheads). Note the posterior displacement of the parapharyngeal fat consistent with a masticator space lesion (small arrows).

Retropharyngeal Space

Anatomy

The retropharyngeal space (a potential rather than a true space) is posterior to the PBF but anterior to the prevertebral musculature. It contains fat and several lymph node groups. The lateral nodes are anterior to the carotid sheath and the longus coli muscle, and the medial nodes are near the midline adjacent to the prevertebral muscles.

Pathology

Malignancy involves the retropharyngeal space either by direct extension or by nodal metastases. Squamous cell carcinoma of the nasopharynx and posterior wall of the oropharynx most commonly extends into this area, although adenopathy from lymphoma is also common. Benign lesions such as hemangiomas are occasionally seen—usually in the pediatric population. Infection may also extend into the retropharyngeal space usually spreading from the peritonsillar region (Figure 9.15).

Paravertebral Space

Anatomy

The paravertebral space, posterior to the retropharyngeal space and anterior to the cervical spine, contains the prevertebral musculature as well as notochord elements. Axial MRI optimally demonstrates the extent of pathological invasion in this area and is invaluable in presurgical planning when a pathological process affects this space.

Pathology

Primary neoplasms are uncommon in the region of the paravertebral space. Common malignant lesions include extensions from vertebral body metastases, lymphoma of the naso- or oropharynx, and direct invasion from squamous cell carcinoma. Benign lesions include schwannoma, chordoma, and degenerative osteophytes.

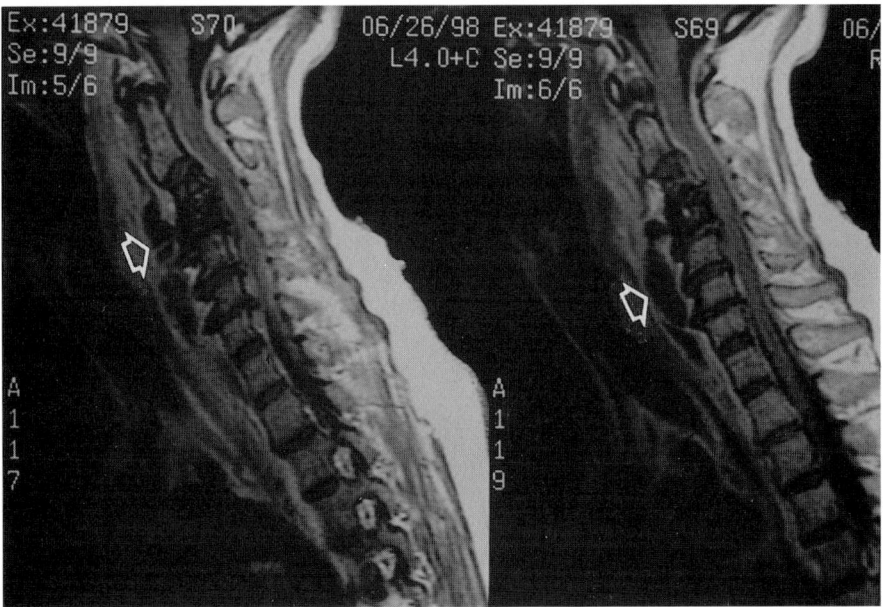

FIGURE 9.15. Retropharyngeal abscess. Sagittal T1-weighted MR image after administration of intravenous contrast material has revealed a retropharyngeal abscess (open arrow).

Lymphatic System

A knowledge of the lymphatic drainage of the cervical region is very important in understanding spread of disease in the lymphatic system. Four main groups can be considered: superficial cervical nodes, deep cervical nodes, junctional nodes, and anterior cervical nodes.

The **superficial cervical nodes** lie external to the deep cervical fascia and are located primarily over the parotid gland and external jugular vein. The more **numerous deep cervical nodes** lie along the course of the carotid sheath and jugular vein; invasion of these nodes is considered to be more ominous than invasion of the superficial nodes. The deep cervical nodes include the jugulodigastric nodes at the level of the digastric tendon, which drain the tonsillar region, and the retropharyngeal nodes, which drain the nasopharyngeal region (12,17).

The **junctional nodes** lie at the junction of the head and neck and receive drainage from the mastoids, parotid gland, submandibular gland, and submental region. The **anterior cervical nodes** lie along the ventral midline and include the infrahyoid nodes, the prelaryngeal nodes near the cricothyroid membrane, and the paratracheal lymph nodes.

Waldeyer's ring is a superficial collection of lymphoid tissue around the pharynx that includes the adenoid tissue superoposteriorly, the faucial tonsils laterally, and the lingual tonsils anteroinferiorly. The ring is an important part of the lymphatic system and can be involved by either primary or secondary disease.

In general, lymphoid tissue is isointense to slightly hyperintense to skeletal muscle on CT and on T1-weighted MR images. Proton density and T2-weighted MR images show this tissue to be quite hyperintense to muscle and slightly brighter than fat. It is not usually possible to differentiate reactive from neoplastic adenopathy on the basis of tissue signal characteristics alone.

Mediastinum

Anatomy

Patients with mediastinal pathology can present with dysphagia, and CT remains the radiological study of choice for the evaluation of the mediastinum (4). The mediastinum is traditionally divided into three anatomical compartments: the anterior mediastinum, the middle mediastinum, and the posterior mediastinum. The anterior mediastinum contains fat, lymphatics, branches of the internal mammary vessels, and the thymus gland. The middle mediastinum contains the heart, major vessels, bronchi, lymph nodes, and phrenic nerve. The posterior mediastinum includes the descending aorta, esophagus, thoracic duct, lymph nodes, nerve, and the paravertebral areas.

Careful evaluation of the esophagus is essential in patients with dysphagia. Both benign and malignant diseases of the esophagus can cause pain or difficulty swallowing. On CT, the esophagus is well visualized owing to the surrounding mediastinal fat. In normal patients the esophagus is usually collapsed, although a small amount of intraluminal air is considered normal (36). A luminal diameter of greater than 10 mm is usually abnormal and may indicate a distal obstruction or esophageal dysmotility. The normal esophageal wall is very thin, usually less than 3 mm when the lumen is well distended (37). The wall may appear thicker (up to 5 mm) when the esophagus is collapsed or at the level of the lower esophageal sphincter. This should not be confused with pathological thickening. If necessary, effervescent granules can be administered and the scan repeated to better distend collapsed segments.

Pathology

Owing to the ability of CT to accurately visualize the esophagus as well as adjacent mediastinal structures, spiral CT is useful in the evaluation of benign and malignant diseases of the esophagus, which can present clinically as dysphagia.

The CT findings of esophagitis usually consist of nonspecific diffuse esophageal wall thickening with inflammatory changes in the periesophageal fat (Figure 9.16) (36,38). Since the CT findings of esophagitis and esophageal cancer can be similar, endoscopy with biopsy may be necessary for definitive diagnosis.

CT in patients with achalasia demonstrates moderate to marked dilatation of the esopha-

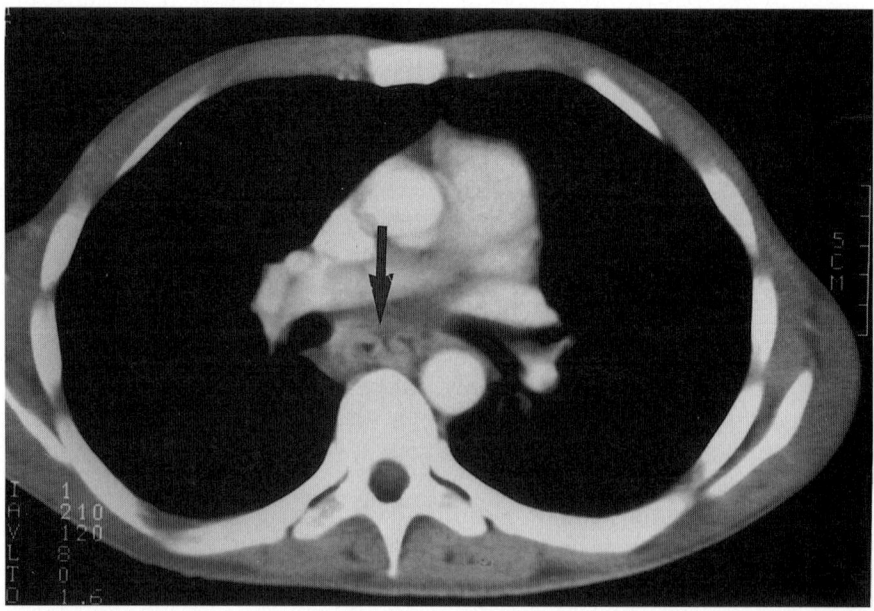

FIGURE 9.16. Esophagitis. Contrast-enhanced spiral CT demonstrates thickening of the esophagus (arrow) and increased density in the adjacent mediastinal fat, compatible with inflammation.

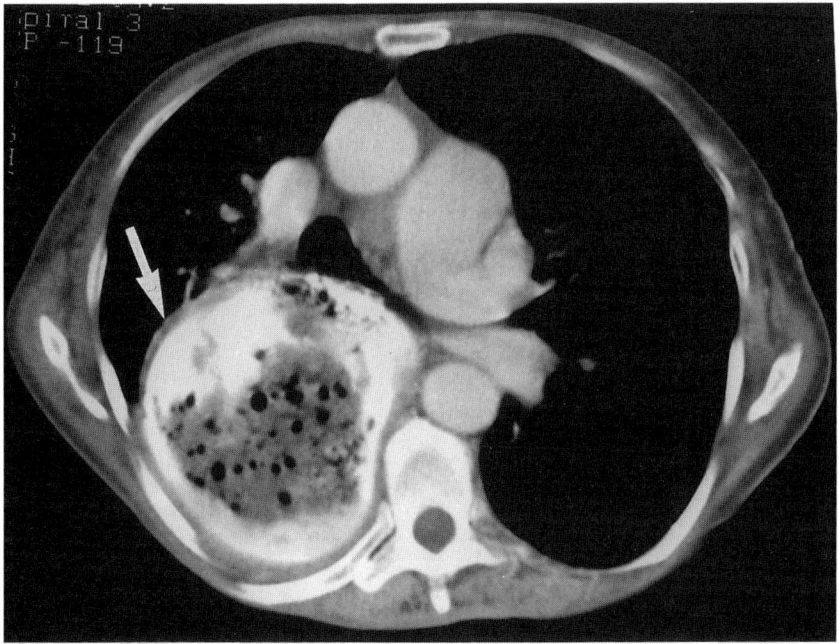

FIGURE 9.17. Achalasia. Contrast-enhanced spiral CT demonstrates marked distension of the esophagus (arrow). The esophagus is filled with contrast and undigested food.

gus (Figure 9.17), with a mean esophageal diameter of 4.5 cm at the level of the carina (39). There is often an abrupt transition from the dilated esophagus to normal at the gastroesophageal junction. Air, fluid, or food particles are often present in the lumen. Since achalasia is associated with the development of esophageal carcinoma, CT can detect and demonstrate the extent of esophageal neoplasms occurring in these patients.

CT is especially valuable in the evaluation and staging of patients with esophageal cancer (40). Although the initial diagnosis of esophageal cancer is typically made with endoscopy or contrast esophagography, CT continues to play a valuable role in surgical and treatment planning as well as a limited role in staging. Preoperative CT can demonstrate tumor size (Figure 9.18), local extension, and invasion of adjacent organs, as well as the presence of distant metastases (Figure 9.19).

Computed tomography is also very useful in detecting involvement of the esophagus by extrinsic structures or mediastinal tumors. For example, congenital anomalies of the thoracic aorta and great vessels can result in compression of the esophagus, producing dysphagia (41,42). Contrast-enhanced spiral CT with 3D reconstruction is an excellent modality for identifying these complex anomalies and demonstrating their effect on the esophagus. With its multiplanar capability and lack of ionizing radiation, MRI is also able to demonstrate these vascular anomalies. The most common congenital anomaly of the aorta is an isolated aberrant right subclavian artery (Figure 9.20). On CT, the aberrant vessel can be identified arising distal to the left subclavian artery and crossing the mediastinum behind the esophagus, resulting in compression and dysphagia. A right aortic arch with an aberrant left subclavian artery is less common, but may also result in esophageal compression. This anomaly can also be reliably detected with contrast-enhanced CT or MR imaging. In addition to vascular anomalies, mediastinal mass or masses invading the mediastinum can compress or invade the esophagus and result in dysphagia.

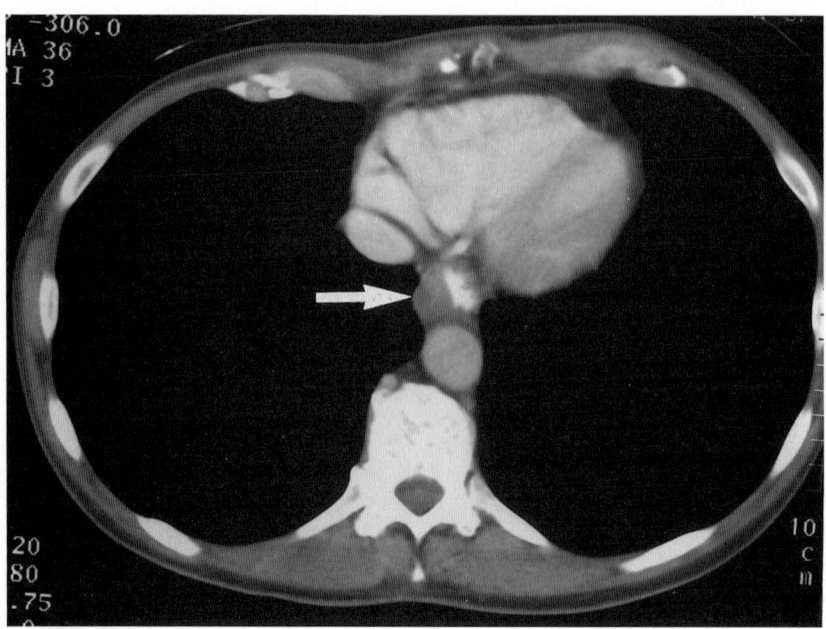

FIGURE 9.18. Esophageal cancer. Contrast-enhanced spiral CT demonstrates a focal mass (arrow) in the esophagus.

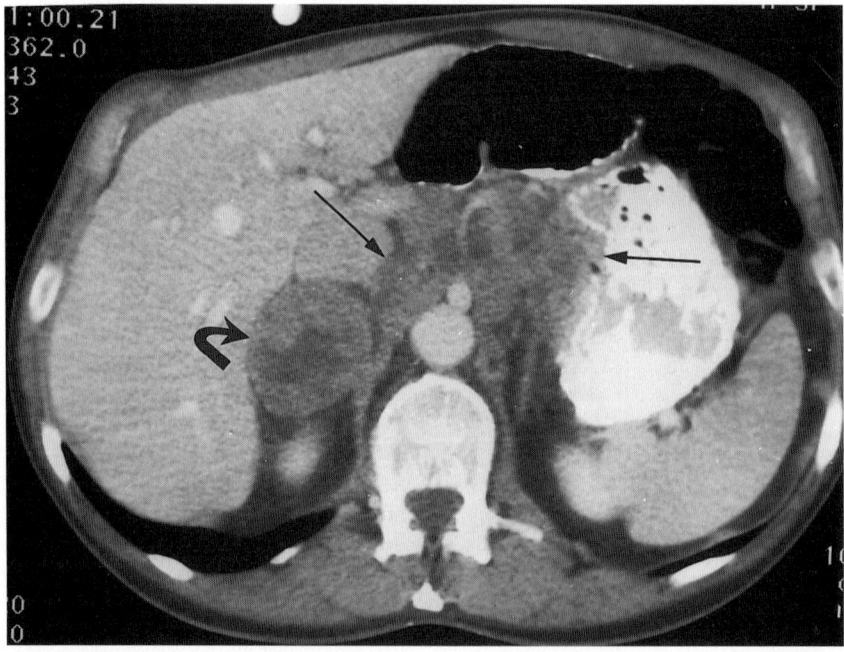

FIGURE 9.19. Metastatic esophageal cancer. Contrast-enhanced spiral CT in a patient with esophageal cancer (not shown) demonstrates adenopathy around the celiac axis (arrows) and metastases to the right adrenal gland (curved arrow).

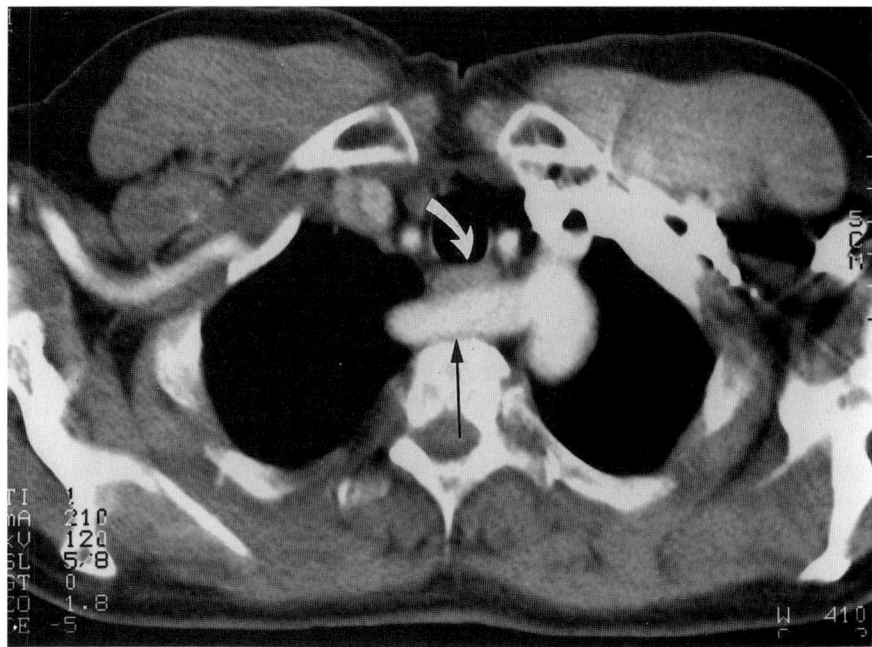

FIGURE 9.20. Aberrant right subclavian artery. Contrast-enhanced spiral CT in a patient with dysphagia demonstrates an aberrant right subclavian artery (arrow) crossing behind and compressing the esophagus (curved arrow).

Neurological Causes of Dysphagia

The second major area in which cross-sectional imaging, predominantly MRI, is proving beneficial in the evaluation of patients with swallowing disorders is that of neurogenic dysphagia. The history and physical examination are often suggestive of the neurological structure most likely responsible for the clinical presentation. Neurological disease usually causes dysphagia by interfering with either the oral or the pharyngeal phase of swallowing (43–45). Esophageal impairment is usually less symptomatic.

An understanding of the relevant neuroanatomy and neurophysiology is necessary for an accurate evaluation of dysphagia with imaging.

Anatomy of Cranial Nerves

A brief review of the nerves involved in the evaluation of deglutition is necessary for accurate assessment of disease in this region.

The **trigeminal nerve (cranial nerve V)**, the largest cranial nerve, is the major sensory nerve for the head and face and the motor nerve for the muscles of mastication. It arises from the lateral pons, coursing anteriorly along the tentorium to the petrous apex in Meckel's cave, where the sensory fibers form the semilunar (Gasserian) ganglion. The upper two divisions are purely sensory, while the lower is both sensory and motor. The third division extends through the foramen ovale to innervate the muscles of mastication as well as the tensor tympani, the anterior belly of the digastric and the mylohyoid muscles.

The **facial nerve (cranial nerve VII)** supplies the motor innervation to the muscles of expression, the platysma and buccinator muscles, the stapedius, and the posterior belly of the digastric and the stylohyoid muscles. The chorda tympani branch supplies taste to the anterior two thirds of the tongue. The facial nerve arises from the upper medulla oblongata, courses within the petrous bone via the internal auditory canal, and exits the skull base from the stylomastoid foramen behind the styloid process.

Small motor fibers exit the nerve to innervate the digastric and stylohyoid muscles prior to entering the parotid gland.

The **glossopharyngeal (cranial nerve IX)** and the **vagus (cranial nerve X) nerves** arise from the upper medulla oblongata. Together, they exit the skull base through the jugular foramen and course inferiorly within the carotid sheath. The glossopharyngeal nerve then courses medially to provide sensory innervation to the pharynx and taste to the posterior third of the tongue. The vagus is both a motor and a sensory nerve, supplying innervation to pharynx, larynx, esophagus, stomach, and heart. Pharyngeal branches exit the carotid sheath to provide motor innervation to the levator veli palatini, the stylopharyngeus, and the constrictor muscles of the pharynx.

The **hypoglossal nerve (cranial nerve XII)** supplies motor innervation to the tongue. Its fibers arise from the medulla in line with the anterior roots of the upper cervical spinal nerves. The nerve then exits the skull through the hypoglossal canal, descending vertically closely associated with the carotid canal. At the level of the angle of the mandible, the nerve follows the course of the digastric muscles and enters the body of the tongue.

Contrast-enhanced MRI with fat suppression is the most accurate means for evaluation of neural or perineural pathology.

Pathological Lesions

Upper Motor Neuron Disease

Diseases affecting the upper motor neurons produce pseudobulbar palsy, primarily associated with difficulty initiating swallowing (46). Each cortical bulbar tract supplies innervation to both sides of the brain stem. For pseudobulbar palsy, bilateral supratentorial disease must be present. Stroke, traumatic injury, tumor, demyelinating disease, or degenerative disease can result in pseudobulbar palsy.

Lower Motor Neuron Disease

Lower motor neuron lesions produce bulbar palsy, characterized by absent or diminished jaw jerk and gag reflex and weakness of the oral and pharyngeal muscles with atrophy and fasciculation. Dysphagia associated with prominent choking or regurgitation of liquids is characteristic. Typical causes of bulbar lesions include stroke, neoplasm, demyelination or degenerative disease, and syrinx.

Cerebrovascular Disease

Cerebrovascular disease is probably the most common neurological cause of dysphagia, and MRI is superior to CT in the detection of cerebral ischemia and infarction in both the acute and the chronic phases. In addition, MRI has been shown to be more sensitive than CT in detection of small lacunar-type infarcts, which are not an uncommon cause of pseudobulbar palsy. Larger areas of infarction may be associated with mass effect in the acute setting; however, over time there is usually encephalomalacia with associated volume loss. Minimal, if any, mass effect is seen in the lacunar-type infarctions.

The CT and MRI findings in ischemic infarction are similar for both supratentorial and posterior fossa infarctions (47). Briefly, hypodensity on CT or increased signal intensity (Figure 9.21) on T2-weighted MR imaging in a vascular distribution are the hallmarks of cerebral infarction (Figure 9.22), which may be associated with edema and mass effect depending on the time course. Because of its sensitivity to soft tissue changes and because of the lack of streak artifacts emanating from the surrounding calvarium, MRI is superior to CT. However, MRI has the disadvantage of requiring greater patient cooperation.

Diffusion-weighted magnetic resonance imaging has the potential to provide unique information regarding the viability of damaged brain tissue. Diffusion-weighted images are very sensitive and specific in the detection of hyperacute and acute infarctions, with a sensitivity of 88 to 100% and specificity of 86 to 100% (48). Lesions with decreased diffusion are strongly suggestive of irreversible infarction (Figure 9.23). Acute neurological defects associated with stroke but without restricted diffusion are typically due to transient ischemic

9. Cross-Sectional Imaging of Dysphagia

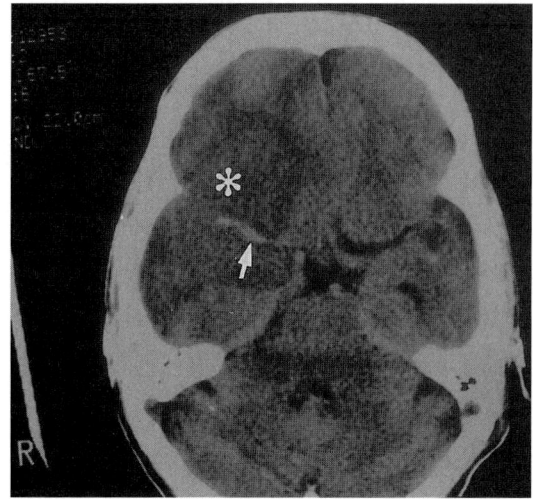

FIGURE 9.21. Acute infarction. Axial CT image obtained without administration of intravenous contrast material reveals a thrombus (arrow) in the right M1 segment of the middle cerebral artery. Note the infarction (asterisk) involving the right middle cerebral artery.

Both diffusion- and perfusion-weighted MR imaging can facilitate the prediction of clinical outcomes relatively quickly after the onset of stroke, thereby allowing the clinician to quickly choose a method of treatment (i.e., thrombolysis or administration of neural protective agents) (49). The combination of these techniques is helpful in the investigation of posterior circulation disorders. Dysphagia is usually caused by posterior rather than anterior circulation disorders, and the 48h treatment window of the former increases the likelihood of success.

Neoplasms

The differential diagnosis of intracranial neoplasm on imaging studies is beyond the scope of this chapter. In general, neoplasms can affect the neural pathways either by intrinsic mass effect and infiltration or by diffuse spread of the tumor in the subarachnoid space via the meninges. Primary or metastatic tumors can involve both hemispheres and cause pseudobulbar palsy, or involve the brain stem and produce bulbar palsy. Metastatic disease is the most common intra-axial neoplasm in the supratentorial and posterior fossa region in adults. These most often result from lung, breast, melanoma, and colon carcinoma, in that

attack, peripheral vertigo, migraine, seizure, intracerebral hemorrhage, functional disorders, amyloid angiopathy, and metabolic disorders. The combination of perfusion-weighted and diffusion-weighted MR imaging may provide more information than either technique alone.

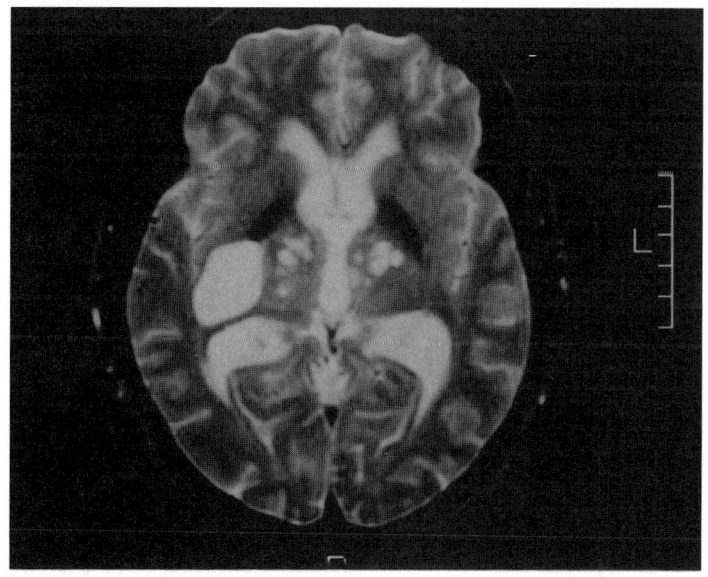

FIGURE 9.22. Stroke: T2-weighted MR image reveals areas of infarction involving the right posterior basal ganglia and the thalamic nuclei bilaterally.

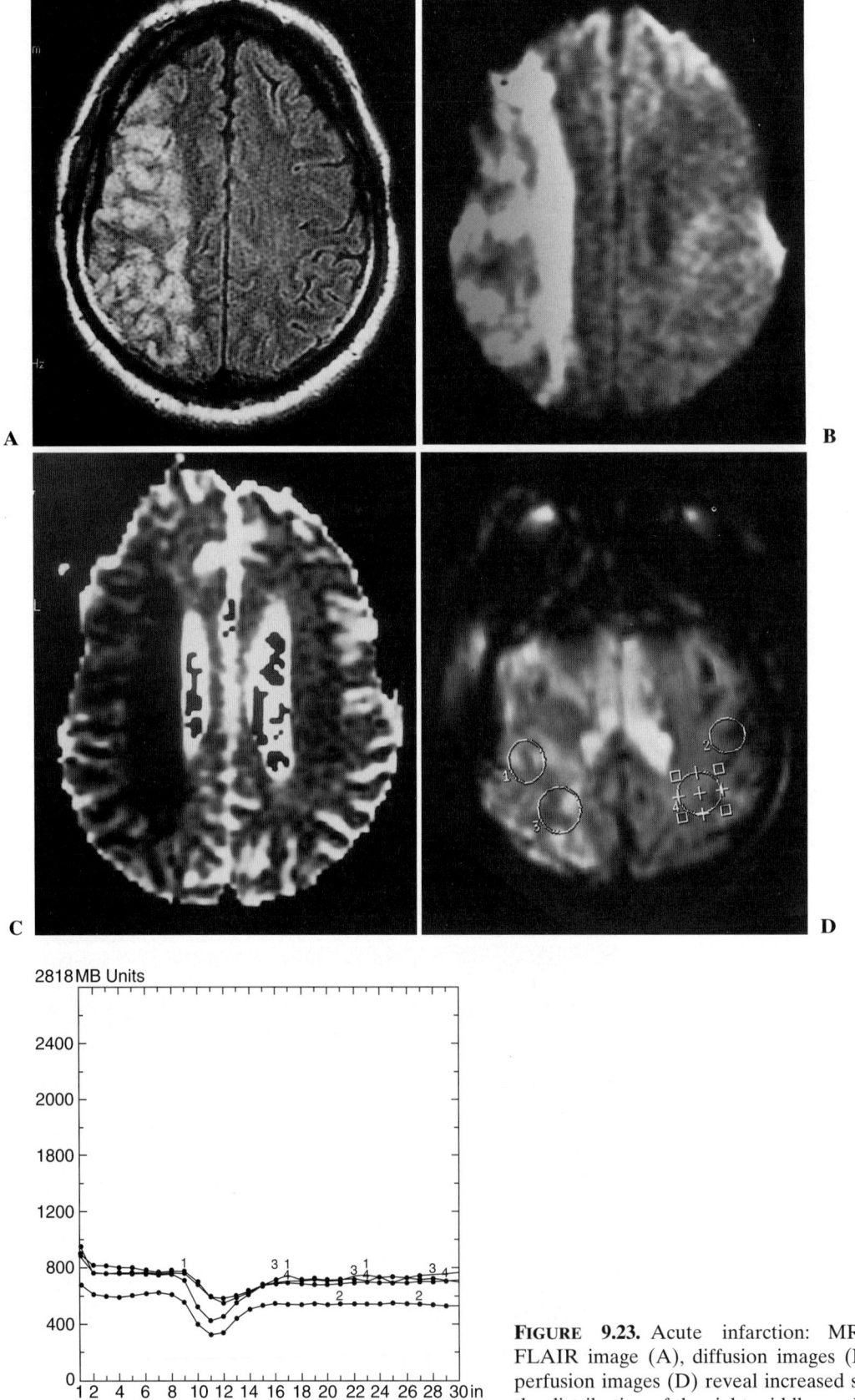

FIGURE 9.23. Acute infarction: MR images. FLAIR image (A), diffusion images (B, C), and perfusion images (D) reveal increased signal with the distribution of the right middle cerebral artery distribution compatible with an acute infarct. (E) Comparative graph.

order of frequency. Metastases are usually associated with significant degrees of surrounding white matter edema (Figure 9.24). Metastases do not commonly cross commissural tracts (the corpus callosum), and this is helpful in differentiating them from primary neoplasms. Sparing of the adjacent gray matter is a helpful differential point in distinguishing tumors from infarction. Extra-axial tumors such as meningiomas, neuromas, or epidermoids can cause significant degrees of brain stem mass compression and produce bulbar palsies.

Skull base lesions such as meningioma, chordoma, primary bone tumors, or metastatic disease may compress and infiltrate cranial nerves as they pass through the foramina, producing significant dysphagia. The multiplanar imaging capabilities of MRI often make this a superior technique in the evaluation of the region. Tissue signal characteristics of neoplasms are not significantly different from those within the head and neck region, generally having intermediate T1 and T2 characteristics. Contrast-enhanced MRI with fat suppression is indicated for accurate evaluation of extracerebral extension.

Demyelinating Disease

Multiple sclerosis is the most common demyelinating process, resulting from immune-mediated damage to the myelin insulating the nerve fibers of the central nervous system. Focal lesions can cause either upper or lower motor neuron deficits. The lesions of MS can be visualized on CT, especially when delayed images are obtained after a double dose of intravenous contrast medium (50). However, MR is more sensitive than CT for the detection of MS plaques (Figure 9.25). Classically, focal areas of hyperintensity are seen within the periventricular white matter on T2-weighted MRI (51–53). The plaques are usually less than 1 cm in diameter, but areas of coalescence can result in a larger homogeneous area of involvement. Magnetic resonance imaging is extremely sensitive in detection of these plaques, with multiecho, T2-weighted, spin-echo images being the most sensitive. Double or triple doses of gadolinium may improve detection of active enhancing lesions in multiple sclerosis (54). A key factor in differentiating multiple sclerosis from other disorders is its deep white matter location, seen in 93% of cases (53).

Degenerative Diseases

Alzheimer's disease, Huntington's disease, and Parkinson's disease, as well as other degenerative diseases, can be associated with symptoms of dysphagia. Nonspecific changes can often be

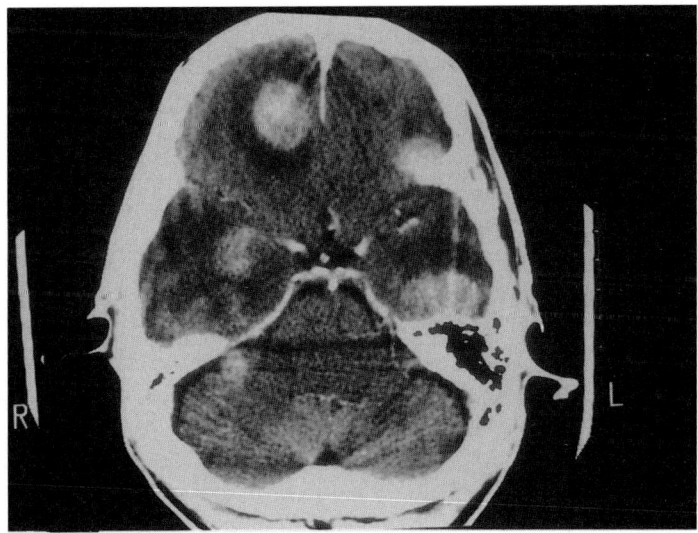

FIGURE 9.24. Intracranial metastasis: axial CT image after administration of intravenous contrast material reveals several enhanced parenchymal lesions compatible with metastasis from pulmonary adenocarcinoma.

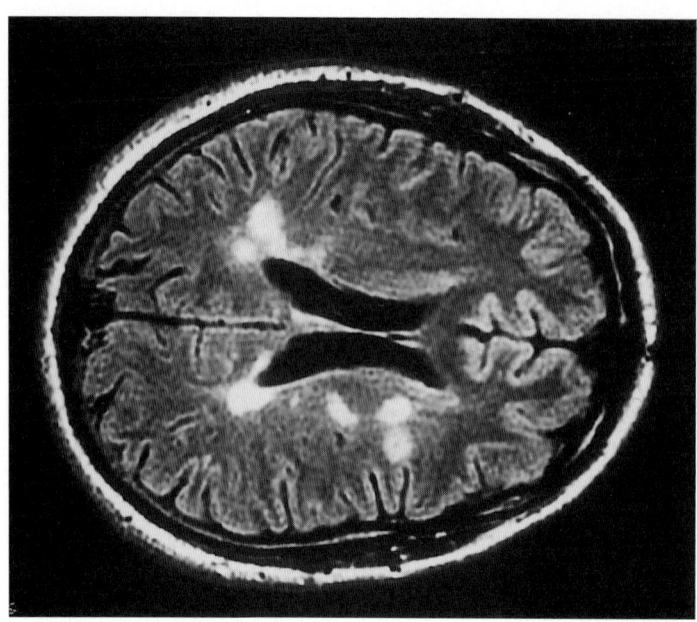

FIGURE 9.25. Multiple sclerosis: FLAIR image reveals the demyelinating disease of multiple sclerosis.

seen in the different entities—a general topic beyond the scope of this chapter.

Inflammatory Processes

Viral or bacterial encephalitis or meningitis can affect the cortical bulbar tracts and the brain stem. Overall, the imaging findings are usually nonspecific, and evaluation with biochemical and laboratory examination is usually necessary for diagnosis. Tuberculous and sarcoid meningitides can involve the basal cisterns and the cranial nerves. Gadolinium-enhanced MRI is the most sensitive imaging test for evaluation of meningeal disease.

Future Directions

Cross-sectional imaging has become a standard and increasingly important diagnostic tool for evaluating the cause of dysphagia. Its main strength is static depiction of gross anatomy in the head and neck region as well as intracranially. In the past, these imaging techniques were very limited in their abilities to evaluate the dynamic physiology of a swallowing disorder. Probably the next major advance in cross-sectional imaging will be "real-time" imaging. This is near reality now with the multidectector and electrom beam CT and echo-planar MRI instruments. As important as fast scan capabilities, is multiplanar flexibility, which would allow cine swallowing studies to be performed in any plane or section and, perhaps, even in three dimensions. Since these examinations are intrinsically digital in nature, temporal and spatial quantitative analysis of swallowing disorders should also be possible. Such advances in imaging allow more precise pathophysiological and anatomical diagnosis to be made, which, it is hoped, will lead to improved patient management.

References

1. Albrecht T, Blomley MY. Spiral computed tomography: principles and clinical use. *Hosp Med* 1998;59:120–125.
2. Brink JA. Technical aspects of helical (spiral) CT. *Radiol Clin North Am* 1995;33:825–841.
3. Brink JA, McFarland EG, Heiken JP. Helical/spiral computed body tomography. *Clin Radiol* 1997;52:489–503.
4. Johnson PT, Fishman EK, Duckwall JR, Calhoun PS, Heath DG. Interactive three-dimensional volume rendering PF spiral CT data: current applications in the thorax. *RadioGraphics* 1998;18:165–187.

5. Zeman RK, Silverman PM, Vieco PT, Costello P. CT angiography. *AJR Am J Roentgenol* 1995; 165:1079–1088.
6. Becker CR, Schoepf UJ, Bruning R, et al. First experiences with multislice CT Somatom Plus 4 Volume Zoom: thoracic combination scan for comprehensive diagnosis of the mediastinum, the thoracic vessels and the lung parenchyma. *Electromedia* 1999;67:47–49.
7. Berland LL, Smith JK. Multidetector-array CT: once again, technology creates new opportunities. *Radiology* 1998;209:327–329.
8. Hu H, Foley WD, Fox SH. Four multidetector-row helical CT: image quality and volume coverage speed. *Radiology* 2000;215:55–62.
9. Horton KM, Fishman EK. 3D CT angiography of the celiac and superior mesenteric arteries with multidetector CT data sets: preliminary observations. *Abdom Imaging* 2000;25:523–525.
10. Kassel E, Keller A, Kuchorczyk W. MRI of the floor of the mouth, tongue and orohypopharynx. *Radiol Clin North Am* 1989;27:331–351.
11. Vogl T, Dresel S, Bilaniuk L, et al. Tumors of the nasopharynx and adjacent areas: MR imaging with GD-DTPA. *Am J Neuroradiol* 1990;154:187–194.
12. Mancuso A, Hanafee W. *Computed Tomography and Magnetic Resonance Imaging of the Head and Neck*. Baltimore: Williams & Wilkins; 1985.
13. Hasso A, Tang T. Magnetic resonance imaging of the pharynx and larynx. *Top Magn Reson Imaging* 1994;6:224–240.
14. Lewine JD, Orrison WW Jr. Magnetic source imaging: basic principles and applications in neuroradiology. *Acad Radiol* 1995;2:436–440.
15. Vogler J III, Murphy W. Bone marrow imaging. *Radiology* 1988:679–693.
16. Yousem DM, Chalian AA. Oral cavity and pharynx. *Radiol Clin North Am* 1998;36:967–981.
17. Mukherji SK, Castillo M. Normal cross-sectional anatomy of the nasopharynx, oropharynx, and oral cavity. *Neuroimaging Clin N Am* 1998;8:211–218.
18. Christianson R, Lufkin R, Vinuela R, et al. Normal magnetic resonance imaging anatomy of the tongue, oropharynx, hypopharynx, and larynx. *Dysphagia* 1987:119–127.
19. Lufkin R, Wortham D, Dietrich R, et al. Tongue and oropharynx findings on MRI. *Radiology* 1986:69–75.
20. Frazell E, Lucas J. Cancer of the tongue: report on the management of 1554 patients. *Cancer* 1962:1085–1099.
21. Laine F, Smoker W. Oral cavity: anatomy and pathology. *Semin Ultrasound Comput Tomogr Magn Reson* 1995;16:527–545.
22. Smoker W. Oral cavity. In: Som PM, ed. *Head and Neck Imaging*. St. Louis, MO: CV Mosby; 1996:61–96.
23. Baker L, Dillon W, Hieshima G, Dowd C, Frieden I. Hemangiomas and vascular malformations of the head and neck: MR characterization. *Am J Neuroradiol* 1993;14:307–314.
24. Yarington C. Pathology of the oral cavity. In: Paparella MM, ed. *Otolaryngology*. Philadelphia: WB Saunders; 1980.
25. Million R, Cassis N. *Management of Head and Neck Cancer*. Philadelphia: JB Lippincott; 1994.
26. Teresi L, Lufkin R, Vinuela F, et al. MR imaging of the nasopharynx and the floor of the middle cranial fossa: II, malignant tumors. *Radiology* 1987:817–821.
27. Halvorsen R. Imaging of the pharynx and esophagus. *Curr Opin Radiol* 1992;418–425.
28. Wertheimer-Hatch L, Hatch III G, Hatch B, et al. Tumors of the oral cavity and pharynx. *World J Surg* 2000;24:395–400.
29. Curtin H. Nasopharynx and paranasopharyngeal space. In: Latchaw R, ed. *Computed Tomography of the Head and Spine*. Chicago: Year Book Medical Publishers; 1985:551–561.
30. Sigal R. Oral cavity, oropharynx, and salivary glands. *Neuroimaging Clin N Am* 1996;6:379–400.
31. Tabor E, Curtin H. MR of the salivary glands. *Radiol Clin North Am* 1989;27:379–392.
32. Weissman J. Imaging of the salivary glands. *Semin Ultrasound Comput Tomogr Magn Reson* 1995;16:546–568.
33. Mancuso A, Dillon W. The neck. *Radiol Clin North Am* 1989;27:407–434.
34. Som P, Braun I, Shapiro M, et al. Tumors of the parapharyngeal space and upper neck: magnetic resonance imaging characteristics. *Radiology* 1987;164.823–829.
35. Batsakis J. *Tumors of the Head and Neck: Clinical and Pathologic Considerations*. Baltimore: Williams & Wilkins; 1979:144–175.
36. Horton KM, Fishman EK. Spiral CT of the esophagus and stomach. In: Fishman EK Jr, ed. *Spiral CT: Principles, Techniques and Practical Applications*. New York: Raven Press; 1998:211–230.
37. Halber MD, Daffner RH. CT of the esophagus: I, normal appearance. *Am J Roentgenol* 1979;133:1047–1050.
38. Noh HM, Fishman EK, Forastiere AA, Bliss DF, Calhoun PS. CT of the esophagus: spectrum of

disease with emphasis on esophageal carcinoma. *RadioGraphics* 1995;15:1113–1134.
39. Rabushka LS, Fishman EK, Kuhlman JE. CT evaluation of achalasia. *J Comput Assist Tomogr* 1991;15:434–439.
40. Van Overhagen H, Lameris JS, Berger MY. CT assessment of resectability prior to transhiatal esophagectomy for esophageal/ gastroesophageal junction carcinoma. *J Comput Assist Tomogr* 1993;17:367–373.
41. McLoughlin MJ, Weisbord G, Wise DH, Yeung HPH. Computed tomography in congenital anomalies of the aortic arch and great vessels. *Radiology* 1981;138:399–403.
42. Proto AV, Cuthbert NW, Raider L. Aberrant right subclavian artery: further observations. *AJR Am J Roentgenol* 1987;148:253–257.
43. Buchholz D. Neurologic causes of dysphagia. *Dysphagia* 1987;1:152–156.
44. Buchholz D. Neurologic evaluation of dysphagia. *Dysphagia* 1987;1:187–192.
45. Buchholz D, Bosma J, Donner M. Adaptation, compensation and decompensation of the pharyngeal swallow. *Gastrointest Radiol* 1985;10:235–239.
46. Kirshner H. Causes of neurogenic dysphagia. *Dysphagia* 1989;3:184–188.
47. Bahn MM, Oser AB, Cross III DT. CT and MRI of stroke. *J Magn Reson Imaging* 1996;6:833–845.
48. Gonzales R, Schaefer P, Buonanno F, et al. Diffusion-weighted MR imaging: diagnostic accuracy in patients imaged within 6 hours of stroke symptom onset. *Radiology* 1999;210:155–162.
49. Schaefer P, Grant P, Gonzalez R. Diffusion-weighted MR imaging of the brain. *Radiology* 2000;217:331–335.
50. Weitze C, Hertel G, Brittner W. Multiple sclerosis: diagnostic value of computerized tomography with delayed scanning after a double dose of contrast medium in comparison with other tests. *Neurosurg Rev* 1988;11:53–58.
51. Miller D. MRI: sensitive and safe in diagnosing multiple sclerosis. *Magn Reson Imaging Decisions* 1988:17–24.
52. Miller D. Multiple sclerosis: use of MRI in evaluating new therapies. *Semin Neurol* 1998;18:317–325.
53. Young I, Randell C, Kaplan P, et al. Nuclear magnetic resonance (NMR) in the white matter disease of the brain using spin-echo sequences. *J Comput Assist Tomogr* 1983:290–294.
54. Gasperini C, Paolillo A, Rovaris M, Yousry T, et al. A comparison of the sensitivity of MRI after double and triple-dose Gd-DTPA for detecting enhancing lesions in multiple sclerosis. *Magn Reson Imaging* 2000;18:761–763.

10
Pharyngography in the Postoperative Patient

STEPHEN E. RUBESIN, DAVID W. EISELE, AND BRONWYN JONES

There are numerous operations involving the oral cavity, oropharynx, larynx, and hypopharynx. This chapter focuses on anatomy and complications in the postoperative patient, including surgery for malignant tumors involving the oral cavity, larynx, and pharynx, or for abnormalities in the pharyngoesophageal segment such as Zenker's diverticulum or "cricopharyngeal achalasia."

General Principles

The Preoperative Videopharyngoesophagogram

Preoperative pharyngography may help delineate the mucosal extent of tumor and fixation of local structures. Pharyngography often visualizes the depths of the valleculae and the pharyngoesophageal segment better than endoscopy. Videofluoroscopy is clearly better than endoscopy for demonstration of baseline motion of structures that may be preserved. If parts of the swallowing tract are proven to be deficient preoperatively, the surgeon may have to alter the intended surgery. Pharyngoesophagography may determine whether there is a second primary tumor, especially in the esophagus, an important consideration because 10 to 20% of patients with head and neck squamous cell carcinomas have a synchronous lesion or will develop a metachronous lesion in the esophagus (1–3). The preoperative examination may demonstrate gastroesophageal reflux or esophageal dysmotility, factors that may alter postoperative healing or lead to aspiration pneumonia.

Unfortunately, the radiologist often sees the patient for the first time after the surgeon has operated. The surgeon has chosen an operation tailored to the tumor's size and location, the depth of tumor invasion, and the presence or size of suspected nodal metastases based on the clinical and endoscopic examinations and cross-sectional imaging. For the reasons stated, however, the authors believe that a baseline videopharyngoesophagram will be of value in most patients.

The Postoperative Videopharyngoesophagogram

Radiologist Preparation

The surgeon should provide to the radiologist a clear description of the surgery that was performed and a request slip stating what information should be demonstrated. A diagram of the surgical procedure is an extremely useful means of transmitting this information to the radiologist. Radiologic request slips that merely state "r/o leak" or "dysphagia" are inadequate directives for this type of radiographic investigation.

Patient Preparation

The remote postoperative patient should not have ingested food or drink after midnight (4).

This results in a pharynx as dry as possible, enabling good double-contrast views for morphology. After many operations, a patient in the immediate postoperative period should not have eaten or ingested fluids before being "cleared" by a negative pharyngogram. Insulin-dependent diabetics should lower or eliminate their morning insulin dose. If a palate or voice prosthesis is being used, initially the patient should have it in place.

Technique

A videopharyngoesophagogram is improved if the patient is studied by a "team approach," with radiology technologist, radiologist, and swallowing therapist present during fluoroscopy. The swallowing therapist is often responsible for a large part of the postoperative care, including retraining in both speech and swallowing.

Pharyngoesophagraphic technique is tailored to the clinical history, the surgical procedure that has been performed, the patient's ability to perform the procedure, and the initial fluoroscopic findings (5). The radiologist tailors the examination depending on whether the larynx has been spared, or partially or entirely removed. The examination is further tailored with respect to whether the patient is in the early or remote postoperative period, because early and late complications are often different (Table 10.1).

Patient Position

The patient is examined in the position used for eating. If the patient can stand without effort, however, the test is done in the standing position, rather than seated, for convenience of positioning. A patient who cannot stand is seated, preferably in a commercially available "swallowing chair." If a chair is not available, the patient can be seated with support upon the footboard of the fluoroscope. If a C-arm fluoroscope or remote control fluoroscope with an overhead tube is available, the patient can be studied while sitting in a wheelchair (6).

TABLE 10.1. Common postoperative complications.[a]

Voice-sparing procedure	Laryngectomy
Early postoperative period	
Wound breakdown	Wound breakdown
Fistula formation	*Fistula formation*
Abscess (wound or fistula)	Abscess (wound or fistula)
Aspiration/pneumonia	*Constrictor dysfunction*
Airway obstruction (edema)	*Tongue dysfunction* (partial resection, immobility, rarely hypoglossal nerve damage)
Hematoma	Hematoma
Mediastinitis	Mediastinitis
Thoracic duct or carotid injury from neck dissection	Thoracic duct or carotid injury from neck dissection
Late postoperative period	
Hoarseness	*Stricture*
Aspiration	*Constrictor dysfunction*
Recurrent tumor	*Recurrent tumor*
Laryngeal stenosis	Stomal stenosis
Velopharyngeal incompetence	Stomal tumor recurrence
Failure of flap graft	Failure of flap graft or jejunal graft
	Hypothyroidism
	Hypoparathyroidism
	Abnormal vocalization

[a] Pharyngography is helpful in evaluation of complications set in italic type.

Because the esophagus is not usually visualized in its entirety when the patient is seated, in all but immediate postoperative patients, the patient must be transferred to the tabletop of the fluoroscope for views of the esophagus. The esophagus need not be studied in the immediate postoperative patient if an esophagogram has been performed prior to surgery or if there is no evidence of esophageal obstruction in the upright views (dilatation, stasis). In rare cases, a patient who cannot sit without support is tested in both the right- and left-side down-decubitus position and in the semierect frontal position. Both right- and left-side down-decubitus positions are necessary because if the pharynx functions asymmetrically, it may appear to be normal while one side is down, but abnormal in the other decubitus position.

Components of the Examination

A "routine" videopharyngoesophagogram includes a dynamic recording (videofluoroscopy) of oral, pharyngeal, and esophageal motility; double-contrast spot films of the pharynx, esophagus, and gastric cardia; and single-column and mucosal relief views of the esophagus (4). When one is evaluating oral and pharyngeal motility, the lateral view best visualizes lip closure, tongue motion, bolus holding at the palatoglossal isthmus, initiation of the pharyngeal phase of swallowing, soft palate elevation, formation of Passavant's cushion, hyoid/laryngeal/pharyngeal elevation, epiglottic tilt, glottic closure, pharyngeal constrictor motion, and opening of the pharyngoesophageal segment. The frontal view lateralizes any abnormality in tongue motion, epiglottic tilt, and constrictor muscle motion. The frontal view should not be ignored (5).

Contrast Media

In the early postoperative period, a water-soluble contrast should be employed first, in case there is contrast extravasation into the soft tissues of the neck (Figure 10.1) or upper mediastinum. Water-soluble contrast is preferred over barium because of the theoretical possibility of mediastinitis made worse by

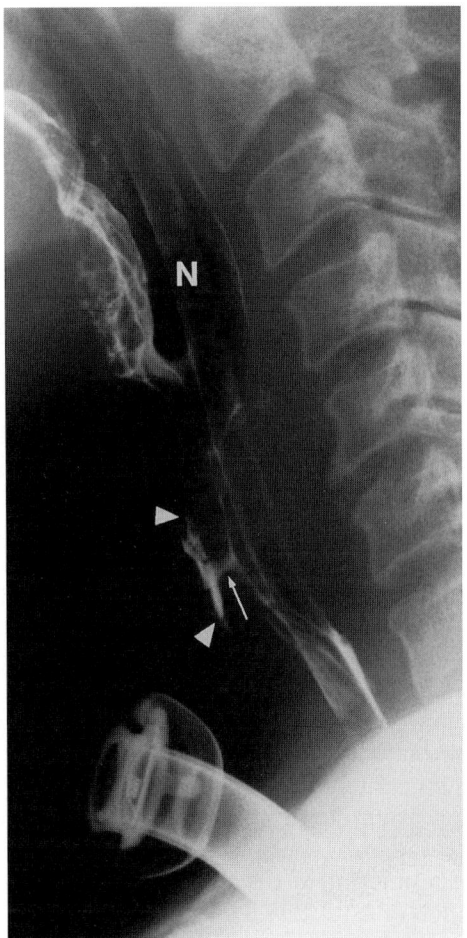

FIGURE 10.1. Postoperative study prior to nasogastric tube removal and feeding. This patient was studied 7 days after total laryngectomy. Lateral view of the pharynx after swallowing water-soluble contrast material shows a 1.5 cm in length contrast-filled track, anterior to the neopharyngeal tube. The track (arrow) rises from the anterior junction line of the neopharyngeal tube. The track is spreading longitudinally in the subcutaneous tissue (arrowheads). A nasogastric tube (N) and tracheostomy tube are in place. (Reproduced with permission from Rubesin SE. Pharynx. In: Levine MS, Laufer I, eds. *Double Contrast Gastrointestinal Radiology.* 2nd ed. Philadelphia: WB Saunders; 1992:74–105; Fig. 4–32.)

combining barium with oral flora. If a patient has a larynx-sparing procedure, nonionic-water-soluble contrast (e.g., Omnipaque) is administered. If a patient has a total laryngectomy, or other procedure that separates the swallowing and respiratory tracts, an ionic-water-soluble contrast (e.g., Gastroview) may be used. Once it has been determined with water-soluble contrast material that there is no gross leak, high-density barium is employed (250% wt/vol, the type used for a double-contrast upper gastrointestinal series).

In the remote postoperative period, the radiologist starts with a small volume of high-density barium unless there is suspicion of a mediastinal perforation. High-density ("thick") barium is preferred over "thin" barium (50–70% wt/vol, the type used for a single-contrast upper gastrointestinal series) for many reasons. First, high-density barium is easier to see than thin barium during both fluoroscopy and reviews of the videotape. Thick barium coats the swallowing tract better than thin barium, enabling the acquisition of spot films showing mucosal detail. Thick barium is probably safer than thin barium because thick barium is manipulated better in the pharynx than thin barium. There is no proof that thin barium demonstrates fistulae better than thick barium. In fact, water-soluble contrast is the "thinnest" contrast of all and has been proven inferior to thin barium in the demonstration of fistulae (7,8).

Order of the Postoperative Examination

The patient is placed in the lateral position: erect, sitting, or decubitus. The entire oral cavity is imaged, from the lips to the cervical spine and from the top of the soft palate to the pharyngoesophageal segment. The videotape and fluoroscope are turned on the moment the bolus approaches the lips, not after the bolus has come to sit in the oral cavity. The videotape and fluoroscope are turned off long after the swallow is over, to demonstrate the physiology of second swallows and to evaluate what happens to barium pooled in the pharynx. One to three swallows of water-soluble contrast are given. A two-in-one spot radiograph of the pharynx is obtained.

Many patients must be turned to a slightly oblique position and the fluoroscope centered on the hypopharynx, if the neck is to be penetrated enough to expose the pharygoesophageal segment. Then the patient is turned to a frontal position and one to three swallows are given to check for contrast extravasation. If no leak is demonstrated, the patient is returned to the lateral position and the study is repeated with high-density barium.

If the esophagus has already been evaluated by a preoperative examination, the oral and pharyngeal phases are the only portions of the swallowing tract that need to be imaged in the immediate postoperative period. If esophageal stasis or dilatation is seen postoperatively, however, the radiologist must also examine the esophagus. After the immediate postoperative period, the entire swallowing tract should be evaluated, including the esophagus: we have found several esophageal cancers within 2 to 6 months of pharyngeal/laryngeal surgery. Therefore, an erect, double-contrast esophagogram and a prone, single-contrast esophagogram will be performed. In some patients, intranasal barium may be instilled into the nares to better visualize the region of the soft palate, Passavant's cushion, and the tonsillar fossa (Figure 10.2).

After viewing the oral and pharyngeal phases in the lateral and frontal positions, the swallowing team decides whether the therapeutic portion of the examination should be started, the esophagus should be imaged, or the examination should be terminated. If moderate aspiration has occurred, the patient's respiratory status is carefully evaluated, and if necessary, suctioning is performed. The examination is aborted if the patient becomes too tired and unable to continue, short of breath, or if aspirated barium reaches the carina.

Surgical Procedures in Which the Larynx Has Been Removed

There is a group of procedures in which the larynx is removed in its entirety, usually for malignant disease. These include total laryngectomy, total laryngectomy with extension (partial pharyngectomy, partial glossectomy), and total pharyngolaryngectomy.

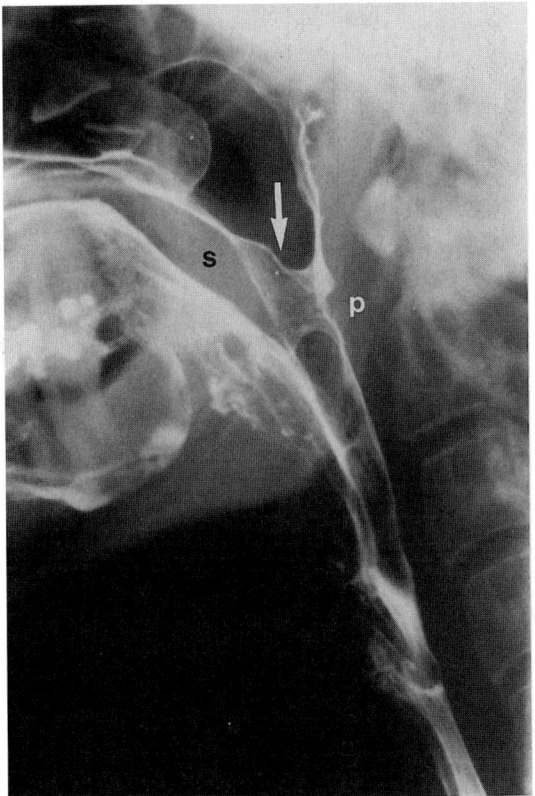

FIGURE 10.2. Use of intranasal barium. In a small percentage of patients, barium is instilled into each naris to outline the superior surface of the soft palate and posterior pharyngeal wall in the region of Passavant's cushion. The tonsillar fossae are better visualized with the use of intranasal barium. This patient had undergone a palatoplasty for cleft palate. A palatal flap (arrow) bridges the soft palate (s) and the posterior pharyngeal wall (p). (From Rubesin SE, et al. Contrast examination of the soft palate with cross-sectional correlation. *RadioGraphics* 1988; 8:641–665; Fig. 16.)

The surgeon carefully selects a procedure based on the clinical history, the physical condition of the patient, the physical examination, the endoscopic findings, and the preoperative radiological studies (CT, MRI, videopharyngoesophagography). This chapter will not review the TNM classification of tumors (9), nor will it discuss the controversial aspects of how to treat tumors of various stages. The reader is referred to several references (10,11) for these discussions. In general, by the time the patient reaches the radiologist, the surgical procedure has already been performed and the radiologist is mainly concerned with the postoperative status of the patient.

Total Laryngectomy

Total laryngectomy is usually reserved for advanced malignancies of the larynx (T3 and T4 tumors, usually squamous cell carcinomas), subglottic cancers, glottic cancers with greater than 1.0 to 1.5 cm subglottic extension, and carcinomas with significant tongue base involvement, or for failed radiation therapy or failed conservation surgery for laryngeal cancer (12–14). Early glottic or supraglottic tumors (T1, T2) can be effectively treated by radiation therapy or endoscopic or partial laryngectomy procedures (13,14). Many hypopharyngeal cancers of the piriform fossae and lateral and posterior pharyngeal walls, as well as postcricoid cancers, are treated by total laryngectomy with partial pharyngectomy or laryngopharyngectomy, depending on the degree of invasion of the retropharyngeal space (14).

During total laryngectomy (Figure 10.3), the larynx is excised, along with its arytenoid, thyroid, and cricoid cartilages. The epiglottis, aryepiglottic folds, and the anterior walls of the piriform fossae are removed. The hyoid bone is usually removed but may be spared. This procedure requires division of the suprahyoid muscles (mylohoid, geniohyoid, hyoglossus, stylohyoid). The infrahyoid muscles (thyrohyoid, sternohyoid, sternothyroid, omohyoid) are also transected. The two parts of the inferior constrictor muscle—the thyropharyngeus and the cricopharyngeus—are detached from their origins on the lateral portions of the thyroid ala and cricoid cartilages, respectively.

The lobe of the thyroid gland on the side of tumor is excised if extralaryngeal spread of disease is suspected. In most cases, however, the thyroid gland and the parathyroid glands are spared. A permanent tracheostoma is required.

The resultant defect in the anterior wall of the pharynx is closed in layers by approximating the residual pharyngeal mucosa. Some surgeons close the constrictor muscles as an

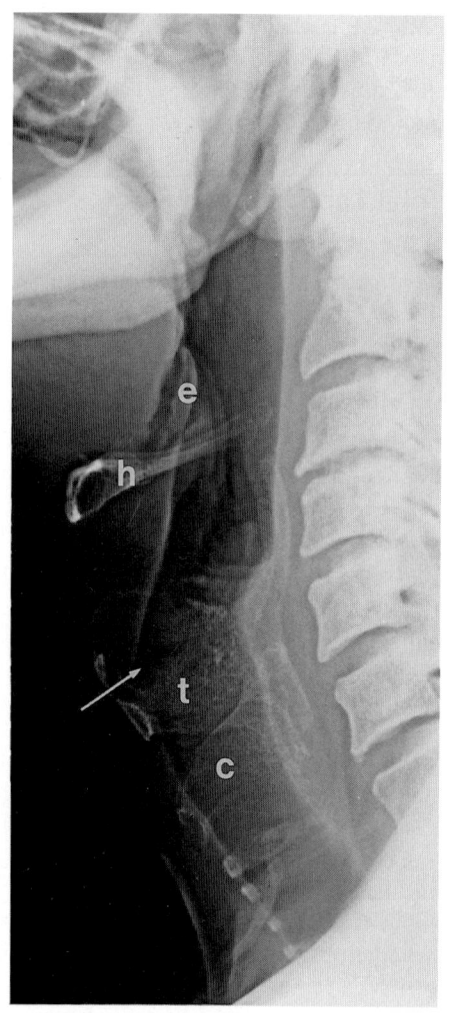 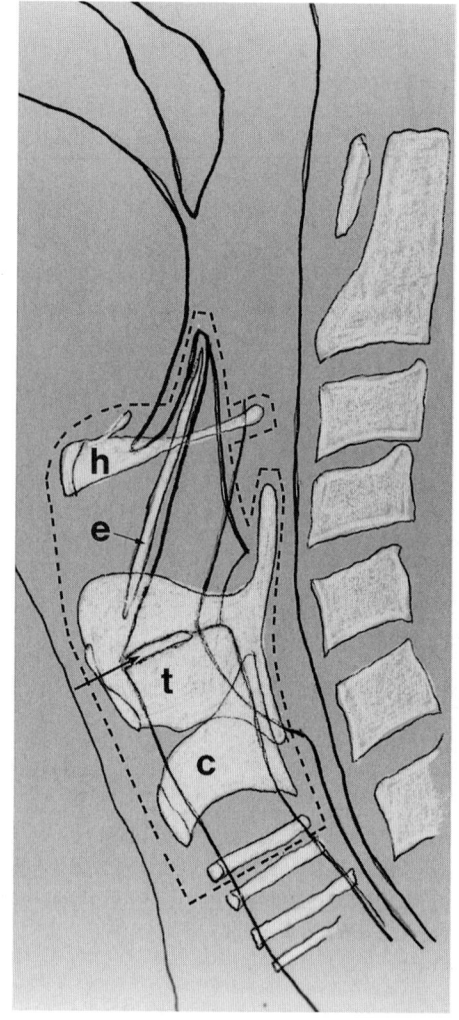

FIGURE 10.3. Structures removed at total laryngectomy. Digital radiograph of the neck with patient in lateral position (A) with corresponding line drawing (B). At total laryngectomy, the hyoid bone (h), thyroid cartilage (t), cricoid cartilage (c), epiglottis (tip, e in A, epiglottic cartilage, arrow, e in B), aryepiglottic folds, and arytenoid cartilages (not shown) are removed. The larynx, including true and false vocal cords, is removed intact with its surrounding thyroid cartilage. A varying number of tracheal rings may be removed. The thyropharyngeus and cricopharyngeus are detached from the thyroid cartilage and cricoid cartilage, respectively. The arrow identifies the air-filled laryngeal ventricle. The dashed line is only a conceptual guide to what the surgeon removes.

additional buttressing layer. If there is insufficient mucosa to form the neopharyngeal tube, a flap (myocutaneous or free flap) may be used to augment the closure. A neck dissection or neck dissections may be performed concomitantly if cervical lymph nodes are clinically or radiographically enlarged or if the tumor arises at sites with a propensity for early nodal spread such as the piriform sinus or supraglottic region (15).

Radiographically, the resultant neopharynx resembles an inverted cone lined by smooth mucosa (Figure 10.4) (12). The hyoid bone may or may not be present. The epiglottis, valleculae, aryepiglottic folds, and the "extrinsic mass" effect of the larynx upon the hypopharynx are absent. The normal neopharyngeal tube has a luminal diameter of 1.0 to 2.5 cm (12). Its posterior wall abuts the vertebral column, and its anterior wall lies closely beneath the skin. A sharp angulation or even sacculation may be present at the closure between the base of the tongue and the anterior neopharyngeal tube. The tube should not be deviated from the midline more than 0.5 cm (12,15). A fold of tissue that courses from the posterolateral wall of the oropharynx to the new base of the tongue–anterolateral neopharyngeal wall may create a filling defect in the barium pool, superficially resembling an epiglottis. This fold of tissue is termed a "pseudoepiglottis" (Figure 10.4B) and resembles and parallels the pharyngoepiglottic fold overlying the stylopharyngeus muscle. The "pseudoepiglottis" is posterior to a space resembling the vallecula, termed the "pseudovallecula."

Common Complications After Total Laryngectomy

Pharyngocutaneous fistula formation is the most common complication in the early

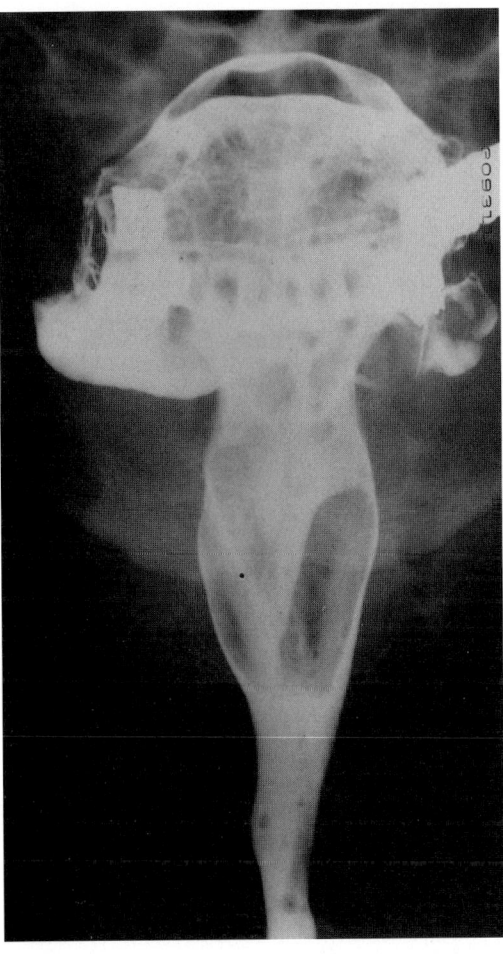
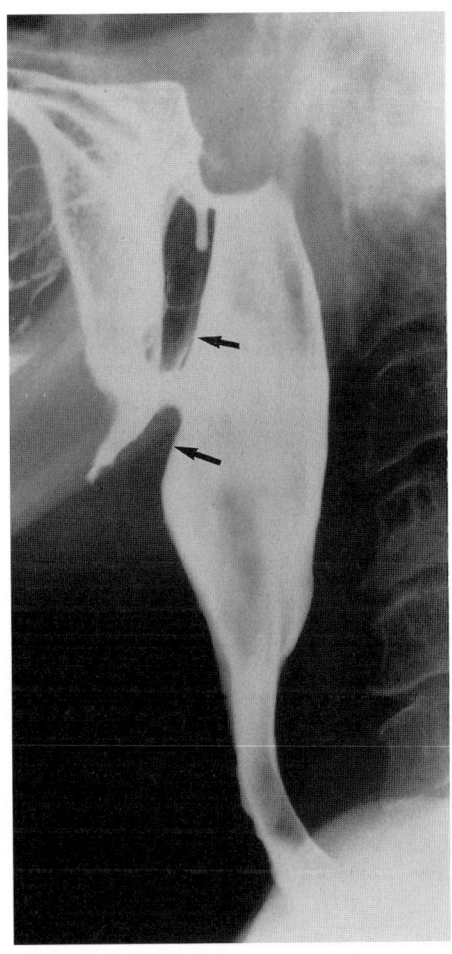

FIGURE 10.4. Normal neopharynx after total laryngectomy. (A) Frontal view obtained during drinking shows a featureless tube that tapers inferiorly. No focal narrowing or nodular mucosa is seen. (B) Lateral view shows a smooth tube tapering inferiorly. Note the "pseudoepiglottis" (arrows), a fold created when the lateral pharyngeal wall is approximated to the tongue base. Note how the fold extends superiorly up the lateral pharyngeal wall.

postoperative period, occurring in 6 to 21% of patients (12,16–19). Most fistulae appear within 10 to 14 days after surgery (12,20). Most patients have signs or symptoms indicating that a fistula is developing, including fever, wound erythema, swelling, and increased drainage from the neck wound (16). Fistulae develop at sites of mucosal approximation: the anterior aspect of the neopharyngeal tube (see Figure 10.1), the junction of the neopharyngeal tube with the base of the tongue (Figure 10.5), along

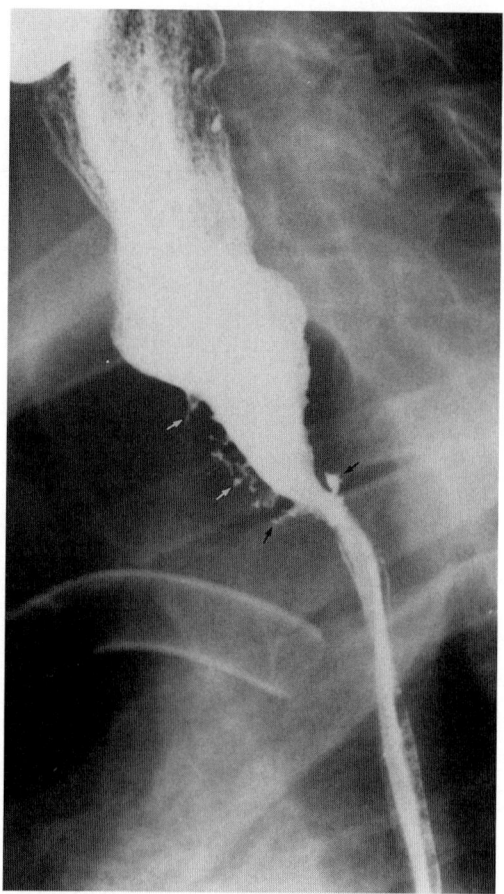

FIGURE 10.6. Flap breakdown and tiny leaks after total laryngectomy. Oblique view of neopharyngeal tube and proximal thoracic esophagus shows numerous contrast-filled tracks that extend into the interstices of the flap (representative fissures identified with arrows).

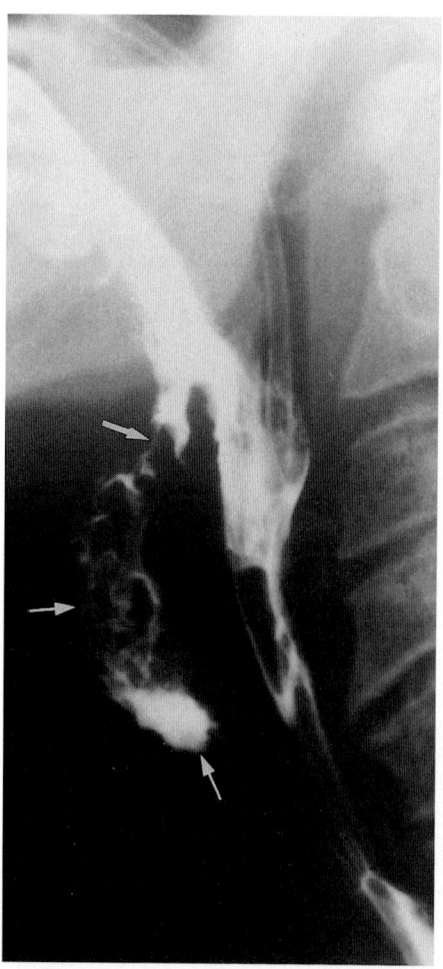

FIGURE 10.5. Leak after total laryngectomy. A contrast-filled track (thick arrow) arises near the base of the tongue and the superior junction line of the nasopharyngeal tube. A $4 \times 1 \times 1 \, cm^3$ collection (thin arrows) is seen in the subcutaneous tissue. (From Rubesin SE. Oral and pharyngeal dysphagia. *Gastrointest Clin North Am* 1995;24:331–352; Fig. 15.)

the margin of a flap (if used) (Figure 10.6), or near the tracheostomy (Figure 10.7). It is controversial whether preoperative irradiation of the neck may (19) or may not (18) increase the risk of fistula formation. Fistulae may extend onto the skin, or end blindly in the soft tissue of the neck or in a subcutaneous abscess. Rarely, fistulae involve the carotid artery or its branches. Most fistulae close spontaneously with delayed feeding and careful nursing (14). Fistulae occurring in the remote postoperative period suggest tumor recurrence.

A subcutaneous hematoma may increase the chance of postoperative wound infection or flap

10. Pharyngography in the Postoperative Patient

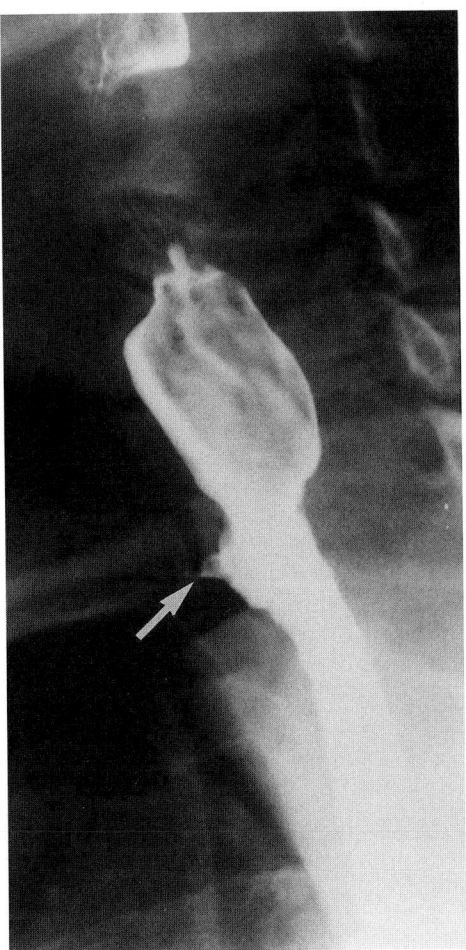

FIGURE 10.7. Leak near tracheostoma. Oblique view of junction neopharynx and cervical esophagus shows a focal outpouching (arrow) of the anterior/distal neopharyngeal wall, just posterior to the tracheostoma.

factors such as ischemia, infection, or fistula healing (12). Radiographically, benign strictures appear as usually short, weblike narrowings less than 5mm long (Figures 10.9 and 10.10), usually forming at the upper or lower end of the closure line, or long, symmetric narrowings greater than 3cm in length involving the majority of the neopharyngeal tube (Figures 10.11 and 10.12) (12). Benign strictures are usually smooth in contour. Weblike strictures are usually the sequelae of infection or fistula formation. Long strictures are usually the sequelae of radiation therapy or insufficient

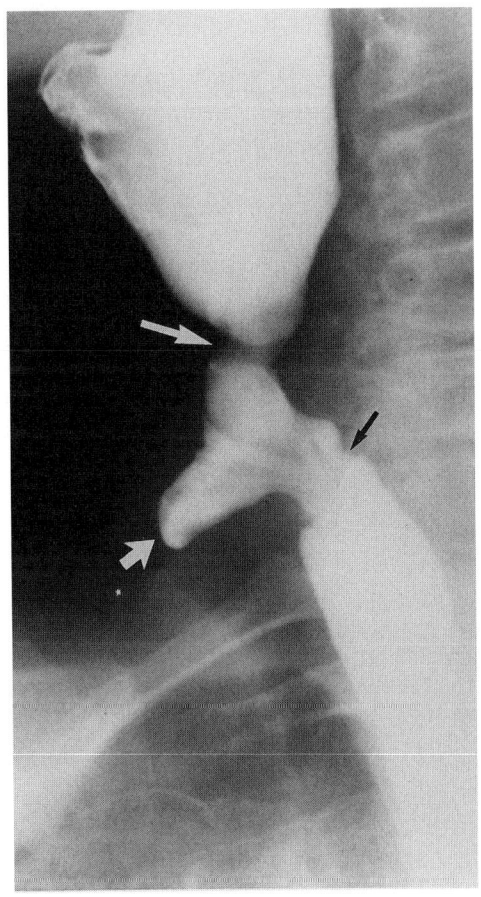

FIGURE 10.8. Stricture and deformity after total laryngectomy. A weblike band (long white arrow) narrows the midneopharyngeal tube. The junction of the neopharyngeal tube and the cervical esophagus is identified (black arrow). The anterior wall of the neopharyngeal tube protrudes anteriorly (short white arrow) near the tracheostoma.

loss. Chylous leakage into the neck may be secondary to thoracic or accessory thoracic duct injury, especially after neck dissection.

In the remote postoperative period, the most common complaint is dysphagia due to benign stricture formation (Figure 10.8) or a retracted thyropharyngeus/cricopharyngeus. Some patients who have strictures will be asymptomatic because they compensate for the luminal narrowing by altering their diet and chewing habits. Benign strictures are usually related to superimposed radiation changes, insufficient mucosa for closure, and local

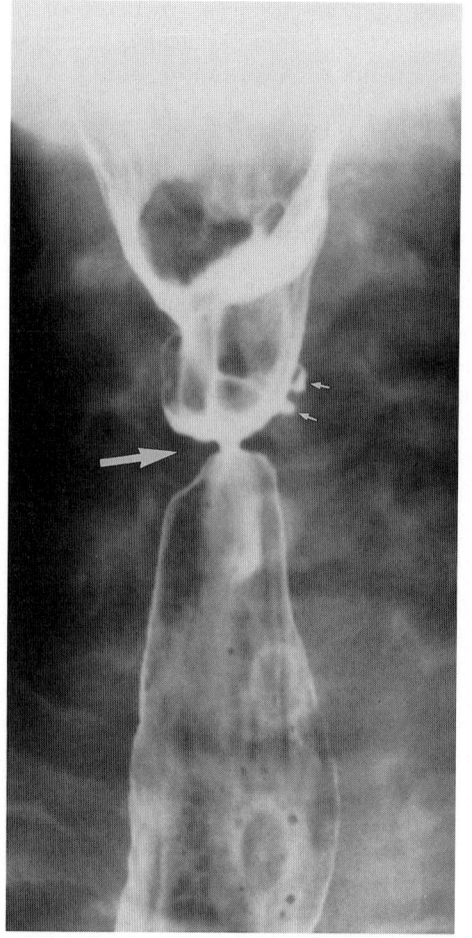 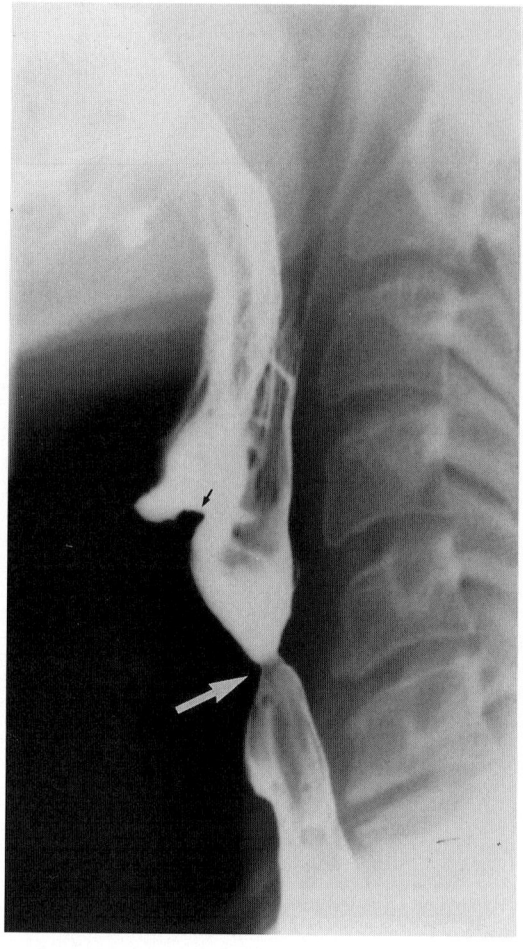

FIGURE 10.9. Weblike stricture after total laryngectomy. (A) Frontal and (B) lateral views show a weblike bar (long white arrow) focally narrowing the neopharyngeal tube to a luminal diameter of 2 to 3 mm. Note the pseudoepiglottis (black arrow) and mild sacculation (short white arrows) due to scarring.

mucosa at time of closure (see Figure 10.12). A luminal narrowing 1 to 3 cm long, with irregular contours and a nodular surface en face, suggests recurrent cancer (Figure 10.13) (12). Although some benign strictures have irregular contours (Figure 10.14), if any portion of the mucosa is nodular or ulcerated, a recurrent cancer must be excluded. Deviation of the neopharyngeal tube from the midline is uncommon and may be due to tumor recurrence or a benign stricture (Figure 10.15) (12). Deviation of the neopharyngeal tube may be investigated by CT/MRI of the neck as well as endoscopy.

After total laryngectomy, the thyropharyngeus and cricopharyngeus have lost their anterior cartilaginous attachments and may be partially or completely denervated. These muscles, especially the retracted cricopharyngeus, may cause dysphagia by not participating in a coordinated contraction wave with the spared superior constrictor muscle and the tongue. Radiologically, there is a smooth, extrinsic impression (mass effect) on the posterior wall of the neopharyngeal tube, which changes size, shape, and position with swallowing (Figure 10.16). Dilatation of the oropharynx or lack of clearance of the barium bolus above the prominent muscles are clues that postoperative dysphagia may be due to a "retracted cricopharyngeus."

hypoglossal nerve damage. The hypoglossal nerves run superficially on the hyoglossus muscle (25). A nerve may be damaged when the suprahyoid muscles are cut to free the hyoid bone. Partial glossectomy or immobility due to wound closure may also cause restriction of tongue motion.

If the thyroid gland is partially or totally removed, or if radiation therapy has been administered, hypothyroidism may ensue. If the

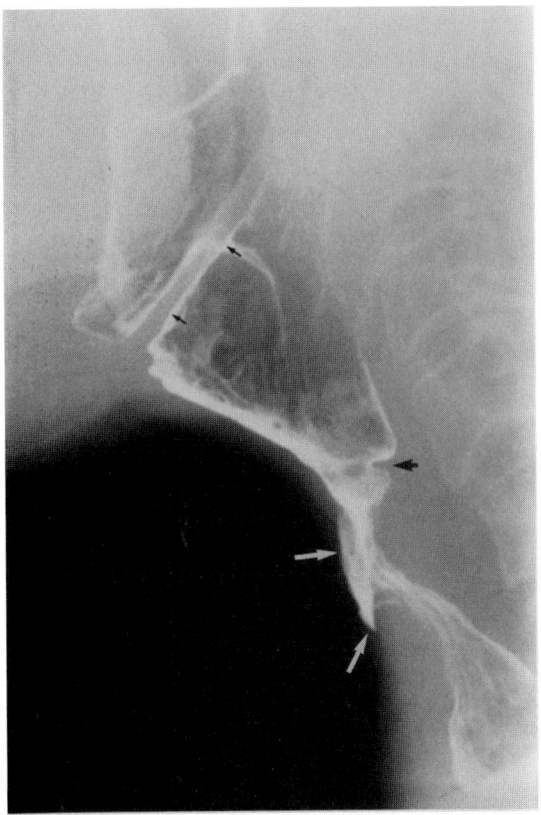

FIGURE 10.10. Deformity, narrowing, and weblike band (large black arrow) after total laryngectomy. The midneopharyngeal tube is pulled and sacculated (white arrows) against the subcutaneous tissue of the anterior neck. Narrowing is seen over a 2 cm length. Note a fold of tissue extending from the junction of the base of the tongue and the oropharynx, the "pseudoepiglottis" (small black arrows).

Tumor recurrence usually develops within the first 2 years after laryngectomy. Radiographically, recurrent tumor is manifested as a mass larger than 1.5 to 2.0 cm, with a coarse, nodular, or ulcerated surface or irregular contour (see Figure 10.13) (21–24). The tumor deviates the pharynx greater than 1 cm from the midline, narrowing the neopharynx at the site of maximal deviation of the tube (23).

Uncommon Complications After Total Laryngectomy

Abnormal tongue motion may result in postoperative dysphagia, especially due to

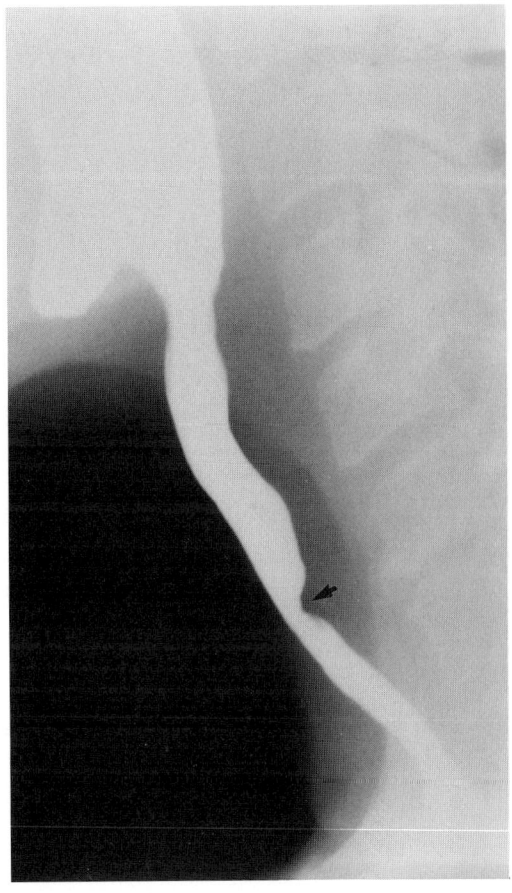

FIGURE 10.11. Long, narrow neopharyngeal tube after total laryngectomy. This patient had dysphagia for solids. The neopharyngeal tube is smooth and not deformed, but is mildly and diffusely narrowed. Only a tiny area of increased focal narrowing is seen (arrow). This diffuse narrowing is presumptively due to the amount of lateral pharyngeal wall left for closure during total laryngectomy. [Balfe et al. (12) define the minimal normal postoperative luminal diameter as 5 mm.]

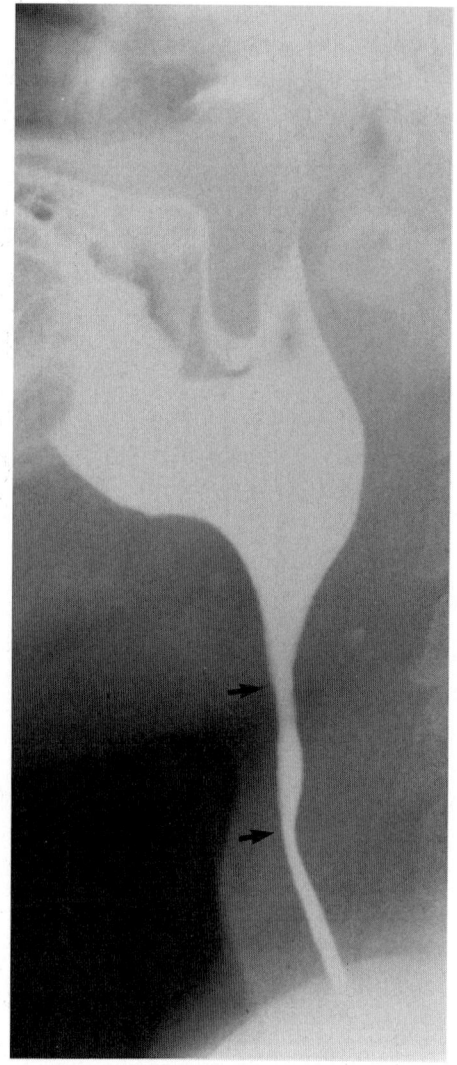 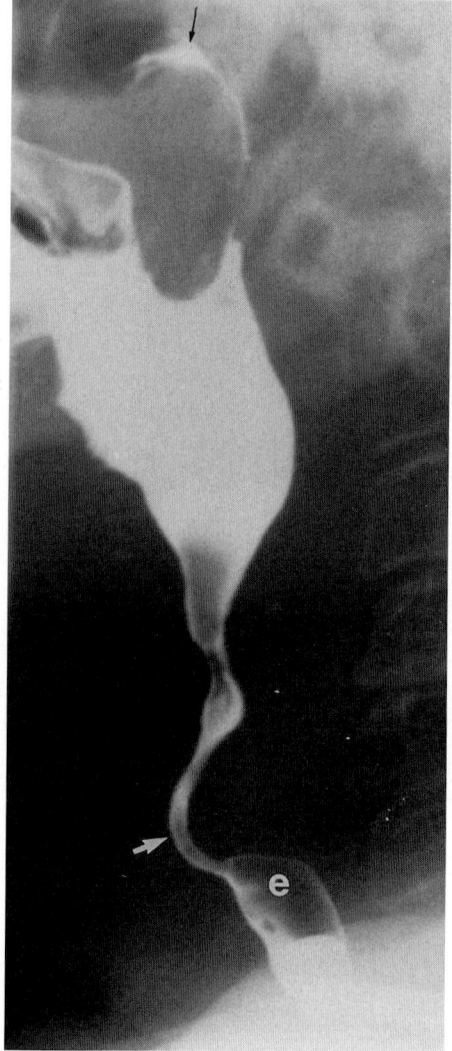

FIGURE 10.12. Diffuse stricture neopharyngeal tube after total laryngectomy. (A) The neopharyngeal tube is diffusely narrowed (arrows) to a luminal diameter of approximately 2 to 3 mm. Note nasal regurgitation. (B) During the early "neopharyngeal" phase of swallowing, the neopharyngeal tube buckles (white arrow) showing that it is not fixed in the soft tissues of the lower neck. Note how the cervical esophagus, e, is now distended. Nasal regurgitation is present (black arrow).

parathyroid glands are not identified and either preserved or reimplanted, hypoparathyroidism may occur.

Chronic complications involving the tracheostoma include stomal stenosis and stomal tumor recurrence.

Voice rehabilitation may be compromised by an inappropriately retracted cricopharyngeus, tracheoesophageal prosthetic device malposition, gastroesophageal reflux, or esophageal motility disorder.

Pharyngolaryngectomy

If a cancer involves the posterior pharyngeal wall, the postcricoid region, or the majority of the piriform sinus, resection of the larynx and the entire hypopharynx may be necessary. The gap between the oropharynx and the cervical esophagus can be bridged by a free jejunal autograft or by bringing the stomach superiorly into the neck to anastomose with the oropharynx (gastric pull-up) (26,27). Jejunal conduits are ideal for pharyngeal replacement because they are lined by mucosa, are similar in caliber to the pharynx, and can withstand radiation therapy (26,27). If tumor extends inferiorly into the thoracic inlet, a transhiatal esophagectomy is performed and the stomach is pulled up into the neck for reconstruction (28). If an extended total laryngectomy has been performed, the defect in the anterolateral pharyngeal wall may be closed a with a myocutaneous flap (e.g., a pectoralis major or platysma myocutaneous flap), or a free flap (e.g., radial forearm (Figure 10.17) or lateral thigh cutaneous flap) (26,29).

Jejunal Free Flap

A proximal jejunal segment with its vascular arcade is harvested from the patient (26). Microvascular revascularization techniques are

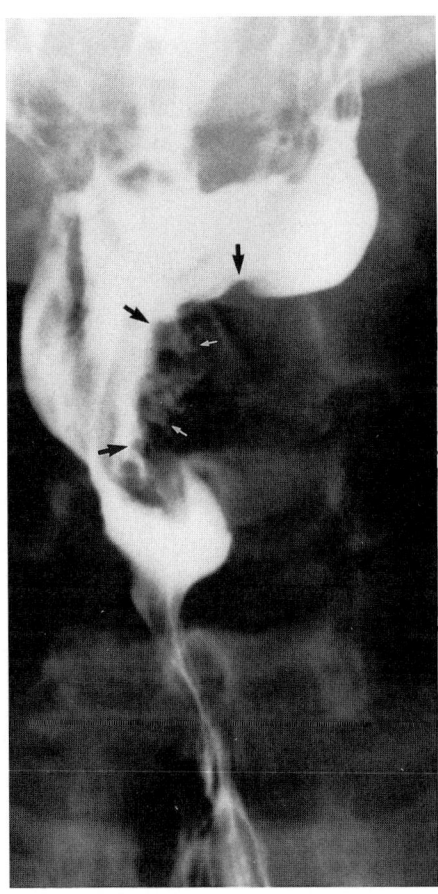
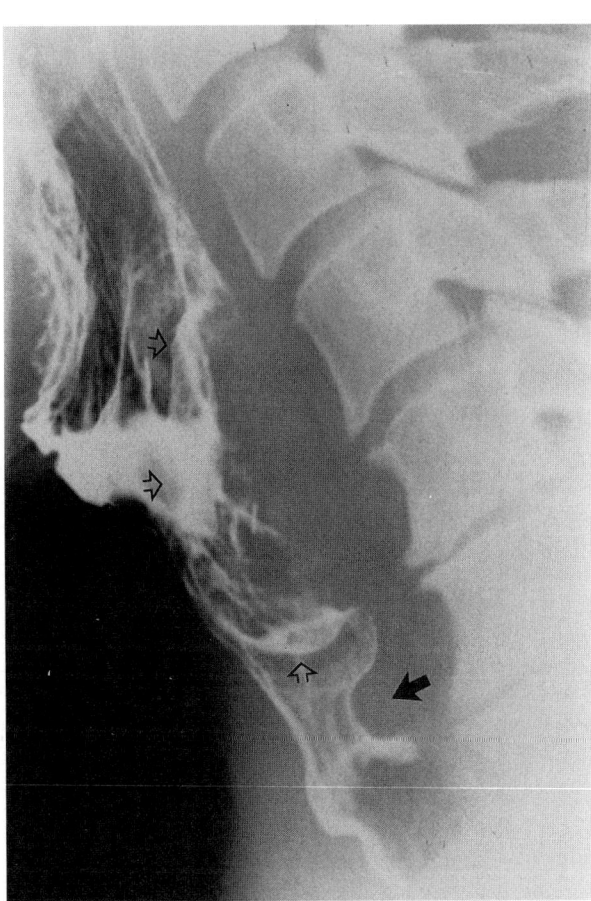

FIGURE 10.13. Recurrent squamous cell carcinoma after total laryngectomy. (A) Frontal view shows loss of the contour of the left lateral wall of the neopharyngeal tube, with a focal mass (black arrows) protruding into the neopharynx. The mucosal surface is nodular. Barium fills the interstices of the tumor (white arrows). (B) Lateral view shows loss of contour of the posterior neopharyngeal wall and barium-etched lines (open arrows) within the expected lumen of the neopharyngeal tube. Compare the irregular surface of the tumor with the smooth surface of a prominent retracted cricopharyngeus (arrow). (Reproduced with permission from Rubesin SE. Pharynx. In: Levine MS, Laufer I, eds. *Double Contrast Gastrointestinal Radiology*. 2nd ed. Philadelphia: WB Saunders; 1992:74–105; Fig. 4–35.)

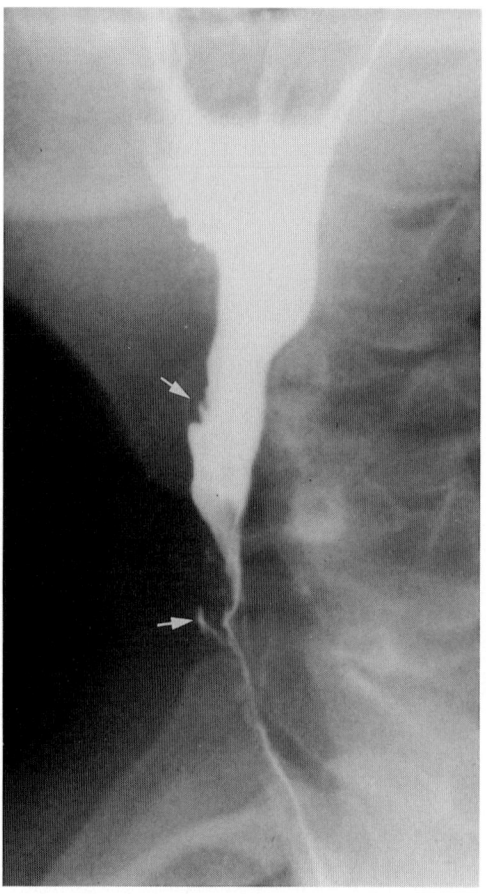

FIGURE 10.14. Scarring of the anterior neopharyngeal wall after total laryngectomy. The anterior wall of the neopharyngeal tube is irregular (arrows). No tumor recurrence was found by endoscopy.

conniventes (Figure 10.18). No acute narrowing or tethering of the tube should be present.

Esophageal Speech After Total Laryngectomy

After total laryngectomy, vocalization may be accomplished by buccal, oropharyngeal, or esophageal speech, or a voice prosthesis may be placed in a surgically created tracheo-

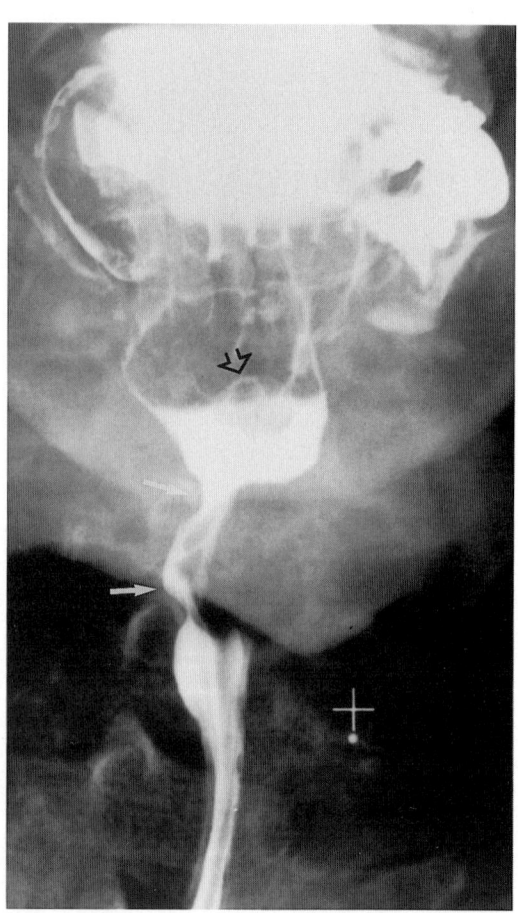

FIGURE 10.15. Stricture with foreign body after laryngectomy. A stricture (white arrow) is seen in the midneopharyngeal tube, which is slightly deviated to the right of midline. (Deviation of the neopharyngeal tube >5 mm suggests tumor recurrence.) A 7 mm foreign body (black open arrow) is seen etched in white on its superior border and as a radiolucent filing defect floating in the barium pool. The patient expectorated a pea immediately after this radiograph was taken.

used to autotransplant the segment into the neck. The jejunal segment is placed in a peristaltic direction. The peristaltic waves, if preserved, occur at a rate of 3 per minute and therefore are not coordinated with swallowing and do not aid in bolus propulsion during swallowing (30). Jejunal free grafts remain open and clear the bolus readily. The clearance of bolus from grafts is indicative of the contribution of gravity and tongue push to pharyngeal clearance (5,28). The visceral graft may become ischemic if its vascular anastomosis or pedicle is compromised. Fistulae are the second major complication of a jejunal free flap. Radiographically, the jejunal free flap should be a tubular segment of bowel with thin valvulae

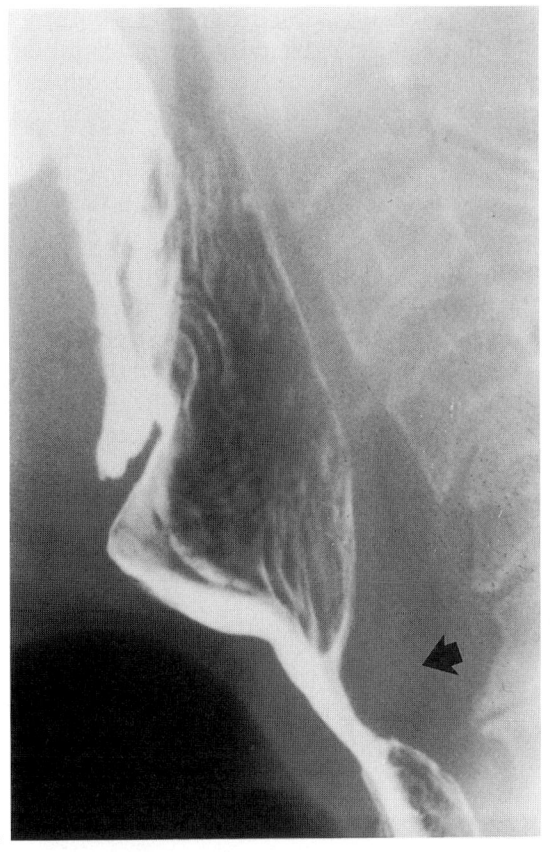 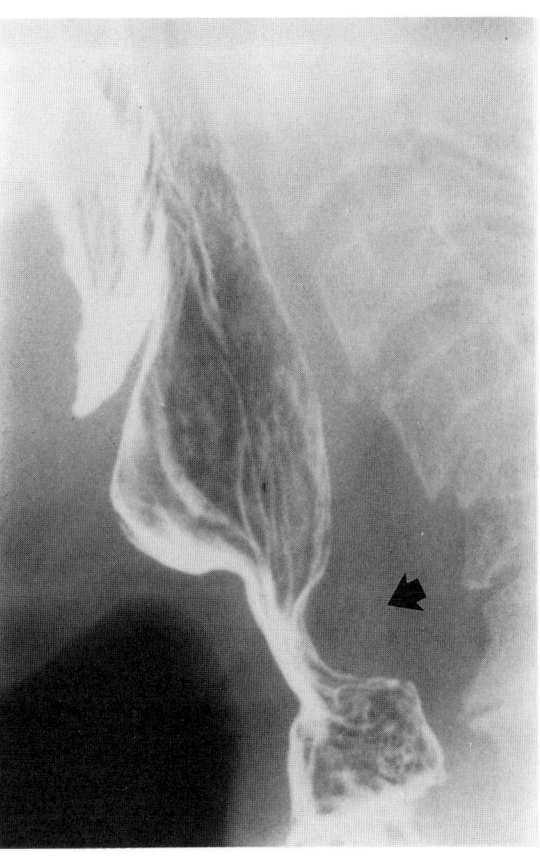

FIGURE 10.16. Prominent "cricopharyngeus" after total laryngectomy. (A) At the end of a swallow as barium passes through the neopharyngoesophageal segment, a mild, smooth indentation of the posterior pharyngeal wall (arrow) is seen. (B) Fractions of a second later, the cricopharyngeus changes its configuration.

esophageal fistula. During esophageal speech, the patient insufflates air into the esophagus, them expels the air through the cricopharyngeus into the neopharynx and oral cavity During esophageal speech, the pharyngoesophageal segment rapidly changes configuration, becoming the vibratory apparatus that replaces the true vocal cords (31). If the pressure gradient crossing the pharyngoesophageal segment is too low, voice will not occur because the air does not create vibration of the pharynx. If the sphincter pressure is too high, air cannot be expelled from the esophagus at a rate high enough to generate a voice.

After total laryngectomy, most patients are unable to use esophageal speech (32). A videopharyngoesophagoram may help determine the cause of this failure to attain esophageal speech. During normal esophageal speech, the pharyngoesophageal segment narrowing varies in length and diameter. In patients who cannot effect esophageal speech, there is relatively fixed and marked narrowing and irregularity of the pharyngoesophageal segment (32). In patients who have adequate speech but of diminished loudness, the barium study will demonstrate either a stricture or flaccid pharyngoesophageal segment.

Neck Dissection

A neck dissection may be performed unilaterally or bilaterally or in conjunction with various head and neck operations. For a discussion of sternocleidomastoid muscle. The surgeon may also select the lymph node groups to be removed or preserved, based on the original site of tumor and its predilection for spread to specific nodal groups (33).

The radiologist must be aware of several complications related to the anatomy of neck dissection. The thoracic duct or the accessory thoracic duct may be disrupted during dissection of the lower neck. Damage to the thoracic duct in the left neck or the accessory thoracic duct in the right neck may result in a collection of chyle. Damage or resection of the hypoglossal nerve may lead to tongue dysfunction. The spinal accessory nerves lie superficially, coursing through the posterior triangle of the neck.

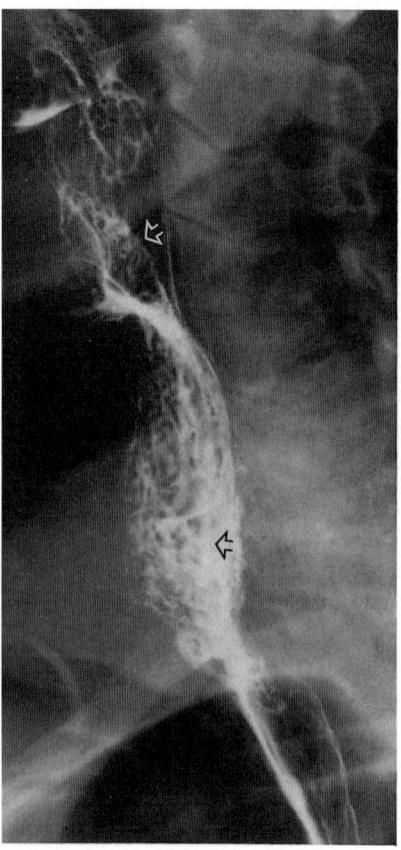

FIGURE 10.17. The "hirsute" neopharynx. After total laryngectomy and radial forearm flap, the mucosa of the neopharyngeal tube is diffusely nodular. The mucosal changes are due to barium coating the skin surface and hair (arrows) of the radial forearm flap, described in the literature as the "hirsute esophagus."

the pattern of lymphatic metastases to various lymph node groups and for the pre- and postoperative radiographic evaluation for nodal metastases, the reader is referred to References 33 to 35.

The nodal dissection performed depends upon the initial location and size of the primary tumor; the size, location, and fixation of clinically or radiologically suspected nodal masses; and whether prior radiation or surgery has been performed. The surgeon has the option to preserve or resect the submandibular gland, internal jugular vein, spinal accessory nerve, hypoglossal nerve, external carotid artery, and

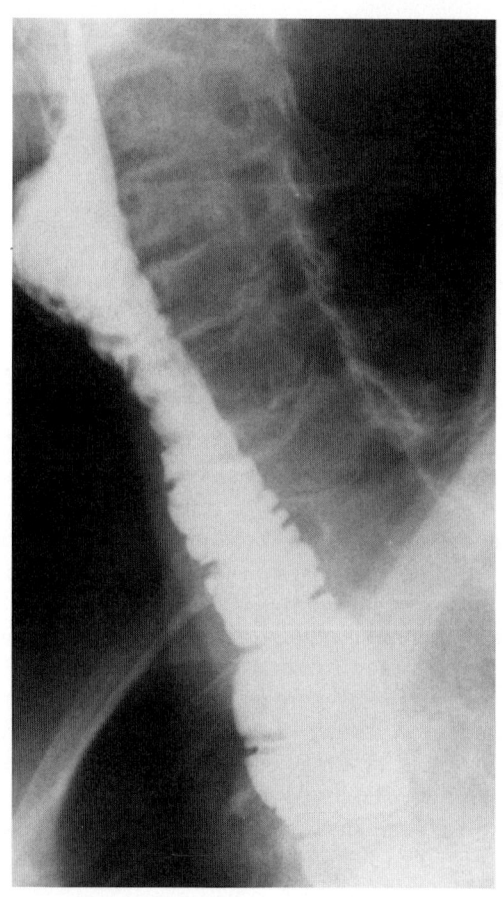

FIGURE 10.18. Jejunal free flap. A tube with valvulae conniventes spans the region from the base of the tongue to the proximal thoracic esophagus.

Damage or resection of a spinal accessory nerve may lead to shoulder dysfunction due to interruption of the neural supply to the trapezius muscle (34).

Voice-Preserving Surgical Procedures

Horizontal (Supraglottic) Laryngectomy

Patients with tumors above the plane of the laryngeal ventricle may be candidates for horizontal (supraglottic) laryngectomy, a procedure designed to preserve voice. Lesions amenable to this type of operation are T1 and T2 supraglottic cancers (36,37). Some T3 and T4 tumors, such as those invading the pre-epiglottic space, the low base of tongue, and upper piriform sinus may also be treated by supraglottic laryngectomy (37).

While the true vocal cords have a paucity of lymphatics, the supraglottic region has rich lymphatic drainage. Therefore, supraglottic cancers spread earlier to lymph nodes than glottic cancers. Furthermore, in the supraglottic region, lymph drains to both sides of the neck. Therefore, unilateral or bilateral lymph node dissections are often performed concurrently with supraglottic laryngectomy.

During supraglottic laryngectomy, the surgeon removes the entire epiglottis, aryepiglottic folds, false vocal cords, and upper one third to one half of the thyroid cartilage (Figure 10.19). Thus, while the supraglottic region is removed, the true vocal cords and arytenoid cartilages remain. In some patients, one arytenoid cartilage or a small portion of the medial wall of the piriform sinus on the side of the tumor is resected (38). The surgeon transects the thyroid cartilage at the level of the laryngeal ventricle (38). In some patients, the lateral portion of the thyroid cartilage is preserved on the side contralateral to the tumor (36). The hyoid bone is usually removed if there is tumor invasion of the pre-epiglottic space. In some patients the hyoid bone may be preserved, or the hyoid bone lateral to the lesser horn on the side contralateral to the tumor may

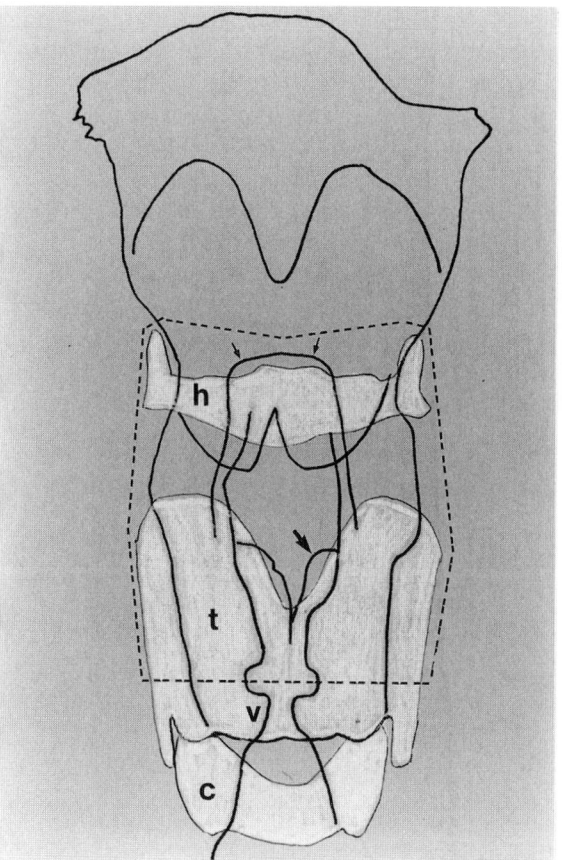

FIGURE 10.19. Supraglottic laryngectomy. Line drawing of the pharynx and larynx in the frontal view shows the contours of the pharynx and larynx with a thick black line and the cartilages in white. A total supraglottic laryngectomy is illustrated by the dashed line, with removal of the entire upper thyroid cartilage and supraglottis. The epiglottis (tip of epiglottis identified by small arrows), majority or all of the upper thyroid cartilage (t), and false vocal cords are removed. The hyoid bone (h) is frequently removed. At least one arytenoid cartilage is preserved. The arytenoids (left arytenoid identified by large arrow) are spared; c, cricoid cartilage; v, right true vocal cord.

be preserved. Hyoid or partial hyoid preservation helps in reconstruction and postoperative swallowing (37). A cricopharyngeal myotomy may be performed (36).

The remaining larynx is suspended underneath the shelf of the tongue base. The thyroid perichondrium is approximated to the tongue base (36). If the hyoid bone has been preserved, the remaining lower half of the thyroid cartilage is approximated to the hyoid bone. The mucosa of the piriform sinuses is also pulled up to the tongue base. The free anterior margin of the piriform sinus is pulled anteromedially to the mucosal margin of the laryngeal ventricle, creating a fold superior to the true vocal cord.

During postoperative pharyngography, the epiglottis and aryepiglottic folds are missing (Figure 10.20). The remaining true vocal cords are usually visible because some barium usually penetrates the remaining portion of the larynx. In the lateral view, the true vocal cords are pulled up underneath the shelf of the tongue (see Figure 10.20A). Barium coats the mucosa overlying the arytenoid cartilages. The folds of piriform sinuses pulled anteromedially to form "pseudofalse cords" may be seen (38). There may be slight prominence and irregularity of the mucosa at the junction line between the tongue base and the true vocal cords (38).

In the frontal view, one sees the smooth mucosa overlying the muscular processes of the arytenoids and the true vocal cords. If part of an arytenoid cartilage or piriform sinus has been removed, the mucosa appears asymmetric. If a neck dissection has been performed, the

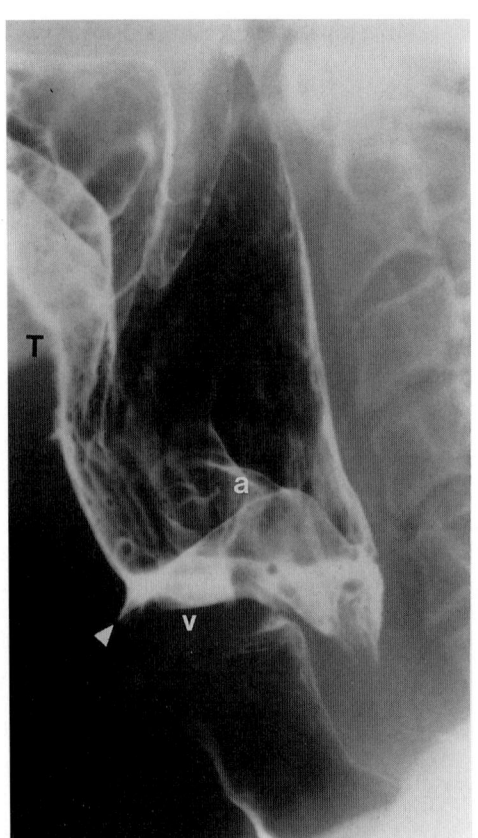
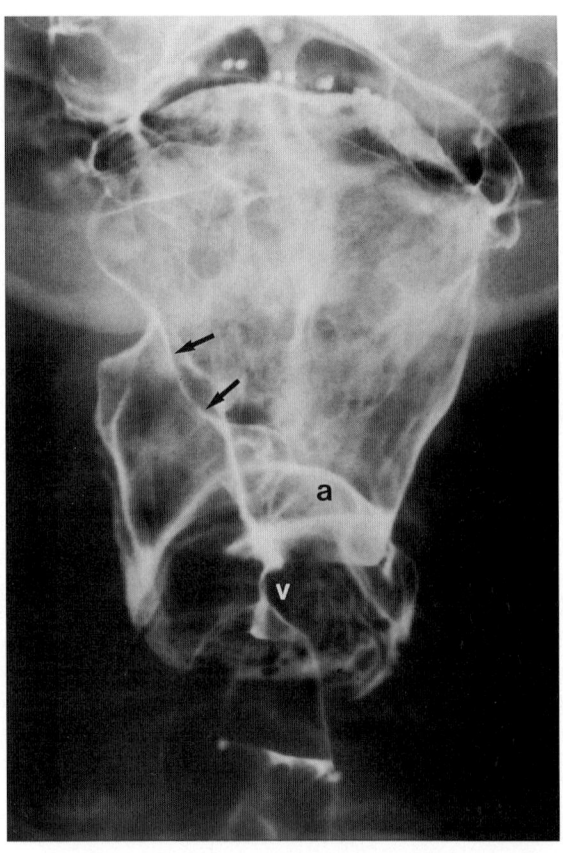

FIGURE 10.20. Supraglottic laryngectomy. (A) Lateral view shows a smooth line between the tongue base (T) and the elevated anterior commissure (arrowhead). The true vocal cords (v) are coated by aspirated barium. The arytenoids (a) are slightly asymmetric. The epiglottis and the valleculae are missing. (B) Frontal view demonstrates the barium-coated true vocal cords (left vocal cord, v). A mucosal fold (black arrows) courses medially from the lateral pharynx. This fold is created when the anterior margin of the piriform sinus is pulled medially to create a fold above the ipsilateral vocal cord. The arytenoids (left arytenoid, a) are asymmetric. The epiglottis, valleculae, and aryepiglottic folds are missing.

manifested as an asymmetric mass lesion with mucosal irregularity. Smooth asymmetry should be interpreted with caution, to ensure that a mucosal recurrence is not missed (38). Cross-sectional imaging may help detect recurrent cancer as a soft tissue recurrence or nodal metastasis (38).

The Family of Vertical Partial Laryngectomy Procedures

Treatment of early glottic carcinoma includes endoscopic removal, radiotherapy, and open surgical procedures. Cancer involving the anterior commissure has a high local recurrence rate after endoscopic removal. The surgeon can perform one of a family of open procedures for relatively large T1 cancers of the true vocal cord, depending on the extent of local disease. These procedures are especially aimed at treatment of cancers involving the anterior portion of the true vocal cord and the anterior commissure. The family of procedures, grouped as "vertical partial laryngectomy" includes cordectomy, vertical partial laryngectomy, and vertical hemilaryngectomy, as well as other variants (41–45).

Laryngofissure and Cordectomy

In the simplest of the family of vertical procedures, laryngofissure and cordectomy, the surgeon removes the involved vocal cord and internal perichondrium of the thyroid cartilage via a midline vertical opening of the thyroid cartilage. This procedure is indicated for cancer limited to the true vocal cord with or without limited extension to the contralateral anterior true vocal cord (43,44).

Vertical Partial Laryngectomy

Glottic cancers with extension to the vocal process of the arytenoid, vocal cord cancers with involvement of the floor of the laryngeal ventricle, transglottic cancers without vocal cord fixation, or recurrent cancers after radiation therapy may be treated by vertical partial laryngectomy. The surgeon removes a varying amount of the ala of the thyroid cartilage on the

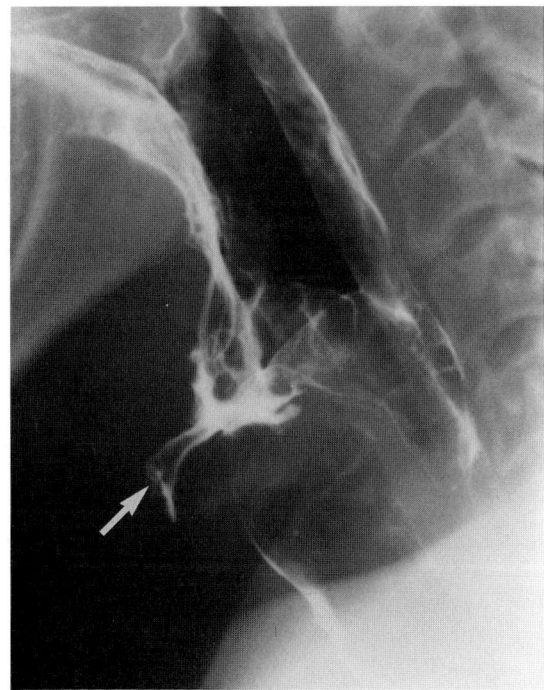

FIGURE 10.21. Leak after supraglottic laryngectomy. A contrast-filled track (arrow) protrudes into the subcutaneous tissue at the level of the anterior commissure. Note the absence of valleculae, epiglottis, and aryepiglottic folds. The distance between the base of the tongue and the vocal cords is short. A nasogastric tube is in place.

lateral pharyngeal wall is flattened on the side of the neck dissection (38).

In the immediate postoperative period, common complications include aspiration pneumonia, fistula formation (Figure 10.22), postoperative edema, and airway obstruction. Edema and fibrosis will be radiographically manifested as smooth symmetric or asymmetric enlargement of the mucosa overlying the muscular processes of the arytenoid cartilages. Fistula formation occurs in about 16% of patients (39).

In the remote postoperative period, the major complications are aspiration (Figure 10.22), in over 40% of patients (40), and recurrent cancer, in 19 to 33% of patients (38). Removal of one arytenoid leaves an open space in the glottis and increases the risk of aspiration (28). Recurrent cancer is radiographically

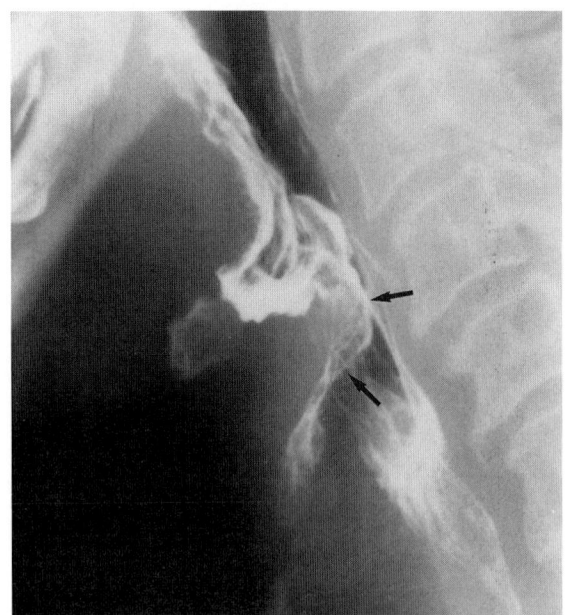
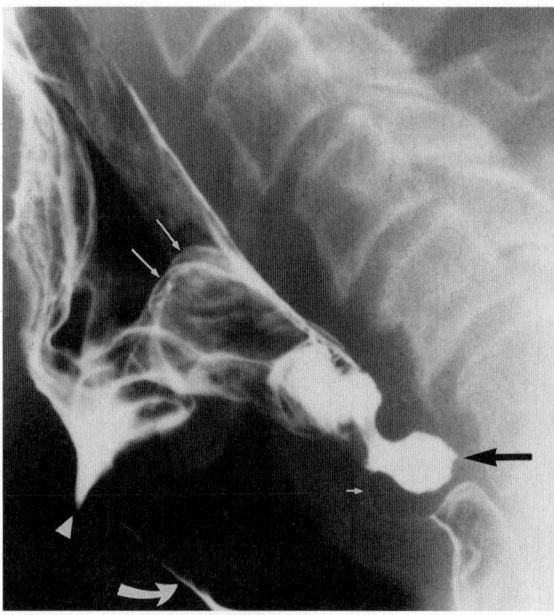
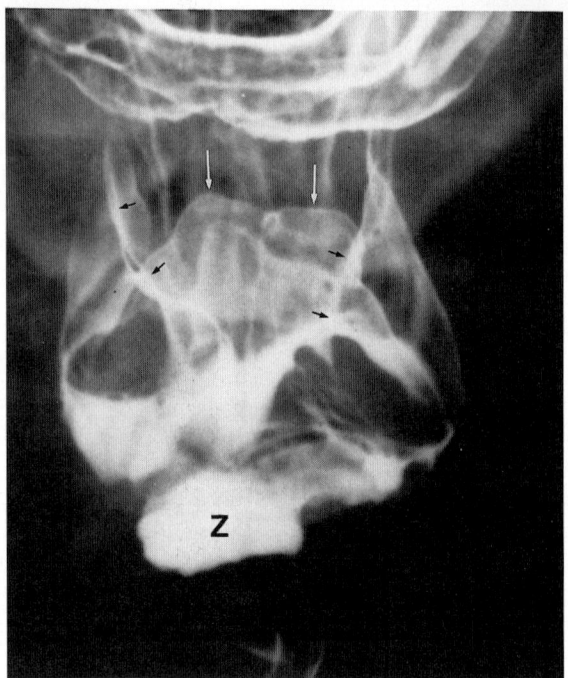

FIGURE 10.22. Pre- and postoperative supraglottic laryngectomy. (A) Preoperative lateral view of the pharynx shows an epiglottic carcinoma. The midepiglottis is enlarged, with an irregular contour (arrows). The proximal part of the pharyngoesophageal segment is at the edge of the (bottom) radiograph. (B) Lateral view of the same patient after supraglottic laryngectomy. The hyoid bone, epiglottis, valleculae, and aryepiglottic folds are missing. The larynx is pulled superiorly. The arytenoids (long white arrows) are elevated. The anterior commissure (arrowhead) is in a straight line with the tongue base. The pharyngoesophageal segment and the upper cervical esophagus are now elevated to the level of the anterior commissure. Aspirated barium coats the anterior wall of the trachea (curved white arrow). A small Zenker's diverticulum (black arrow) has developed postoperatively. The cricopharyngeus (short white arrow) is now prominent. (C) Frontal view shows prominent and elevated arytenoids (white arrows). Folds of mucosa (black arrows) have been pulled anteriorly to cover the true vocal cords. The Zenker's diverticulum (Z) is seen as a midline, ovoid barium collection.

side of the true vocal cord cancer, depending on the extent of tumor. This often amounts to about one third of the ala of the thyroid cartilage on the side ipsilateral to the tumor. The cartilaginous defect is closed with various techniques, including use of the residual perichondrium from the excised thyroid cartilage and the strap muscles (45). The epiglottis is preserved to help prevent aspiration. The base of the epiglottis is reattached. A "neocord" may be created by attaching the false vocal cord to the remaining ipsilateral thyroid cartilage.

Vertical Hemilaryngectomy

The true vocal cord, the false vocal cord, the arytenoid cartilage, and the thyroid cartilage on the side of the tumor are removed (Figure 10.23). Complete vertical hemilaryngectomy may be complicated by poor voice, laryngeal incompetence, stenosis, and aspiration.

Pharyngography

The radiographic findings vary with the extent of surgery. Since the epiglottis and lateral and posterior walls of the hypopharynx are preserved, if no laryngeal penetration occurs, the pharynx may appear relatively normal during pharyngography (46). If a complete vertical hemilaryngectomy has been performed, including removal of the ipsilateral arytenoid cartilage (as well as the true and false vocal cords and the ipsilateral thyroid cartilage), the aryepiglottic fold on the operated side will be missing. Barium will coat the preserved contralateral false and true vocal cords (Figure 10.24).

Recurrent cancer is radiographically manifested as narrowing and irregularity of the residual laryngeal vestibule or subglottic airway (46). An irregular mass may indent the airway. Postoperative deformity, edema, and granulation tissue mimic tumor recurrence. Diagnosis of recurrent cancer may require a combination of endoscopy, barium studies, and cross-sectional imaging (47).

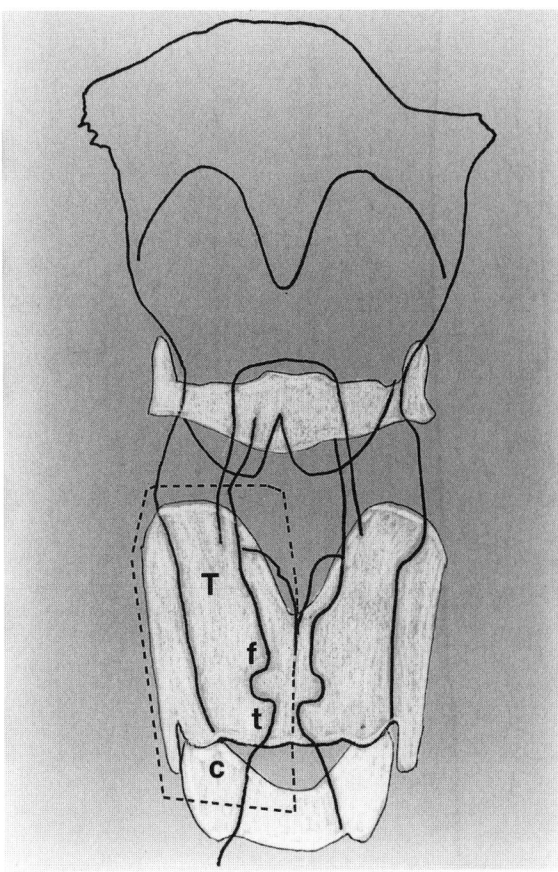

FIGURE 10.23. Vertical hemilaryngectomy. Line drawing of pharynx in frontal view shows approximate resection for a vertical hemilaryngectomy. The surgeon removes a variable amount of the ipsilateral thyroid cartilage (T) and the true (t) and false (f) vocal cords. During some operations portions of the thyrohyoid and cricothyroid ligaments and a variable portion of the cricoid cartilage (c) are removed. If the base of the epiglottis is spared, the risk of aspiration is less.

Other Procedures

There are myriad subtle variations of partial laryngectomies. A surgeon may tailor a laryngeal operation in a way the radiologist is not familiar with. Communication between radiologist and surgeon will help radiological interpretation of images (Figure 10.25).

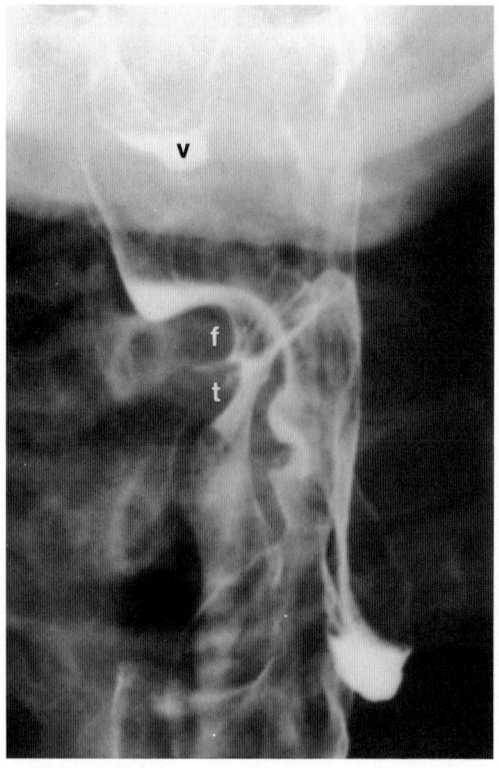 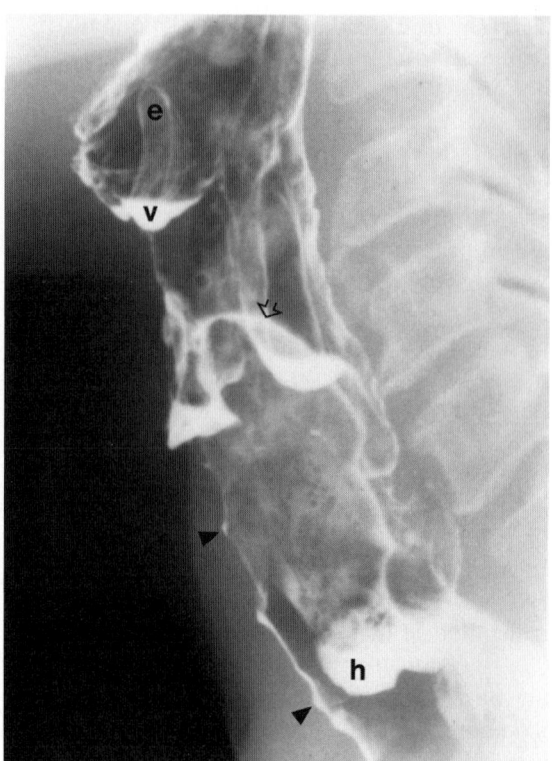

FIGURE 10.24. Vertical hemilaryngectomy. (A) Frontal view shows the right true (t) and false (f) vocal cords coated with aspirated barium. The right vallecula (v) is seen, indicating that part of the epiglottis remains, even though it is not visible on this radiograph. The left side of the epiglottis, left aryepiglottic fold, and left true and false vocal cords have been resected. (B) Lateral view shows residual right vallecula (v), epiglottic tip (e), and right arytenoid (arrow). Note barium coating the trachea (arrowheads) and the dilated hypopharynx/pharyngoesophageal segment (h).

Surgery for Tongue or Oropharyngeal Cancers

Glossectomy

There are numerous surgical approaches to the tongue, depending on the size, location, and spread of tumor (48,49). A *transoral approach* may be used for small anterior lesions less than 2 cm in size. A *mandibulotomy* may be performed for lesions that do not involve the mandible, but a *segmental mandibulectomy* may be necessary for lesions involving the mandible. A *transhyoid approach* may be used for small lesions of the posterior tongue. The transhyoid approach may alter pharyngeal and laryngeal elevation in the postoperative patient if there is damage to the suprahyoid muscles. Postoperative tongue motion may be abnormal in the presence of damage to the hypoglossal nerve, adhesions, or loss of the majority of the tongue volume. Damage to the superior laryngeal nerve may also occur during this approach (48).

A near total or *total glossectomy* may be performed for large tumors of the posterior tongue. Tissue from the adjacent floor of the mouth, retromolar trigone, or lateral pharyngeal wall may also be removed. The soft tissue defect may be filled with a skin graft, tissue flap (Figure 10.26), or microvascular free flap (28). A cricopharyngeal myotomy may be performed. Occasionally, a total laryngectomy is performed concurrently with total glossectomy (Figure 10.27).

Radiographically, the oral phase of swallowing is carefully evaluated for bolus collection (if some tongue tissue remains), stasis in the oral cavity (Figure 10.28), and premature spill into the hypopharynx, which may result in poor timing between oral and pharyngeal phases, in turn causing laryngeal penetration. Approximately one third to one half of the tongue can be removed without significant swallowing disability (50). If bolus collection and transfer is abnormal, patients may tilt the head superiorly to decant the bolus into the oropharynx. A large proportion of the bolus may remain in the oral cavity, especially if a barium-impregnated solid bolus is tested. The defect in the tongue may be apparent. Irregularity of the contour of the postoperative defect may reflect postoperative change or recurrent cancer. Therefore, demonstration of recurrent cancer requires direct visualization or cross-sectional imaging.

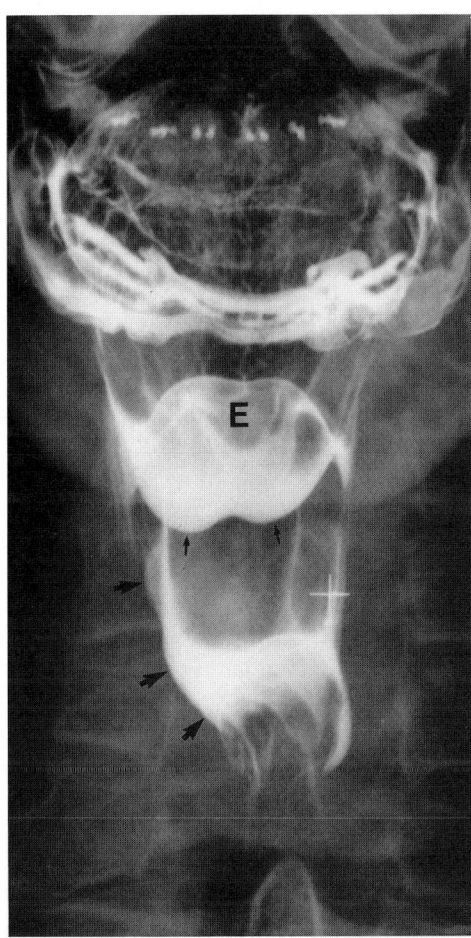
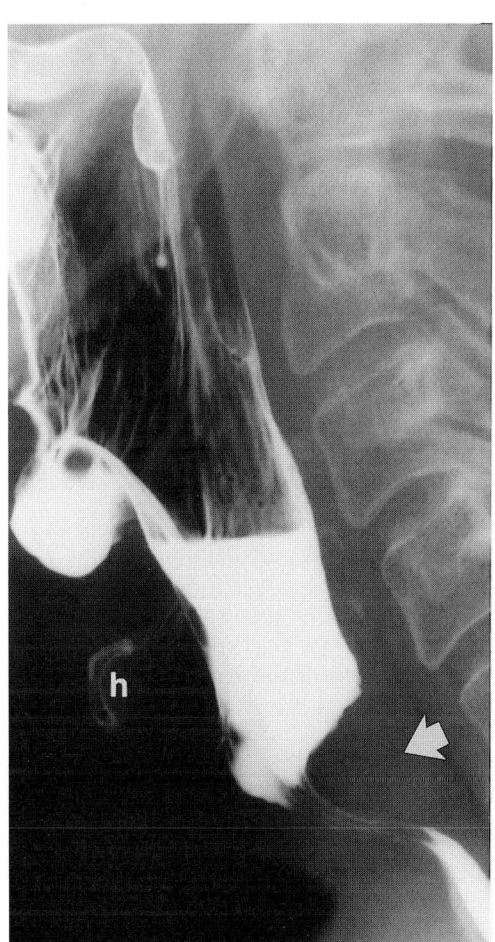

FIGURE 10.25. Partial pharyngectomy, subtotal laryngectomy, and radiation changes. (A) Frontal view shows an enlarged bulbous epiglottis (E) and flattened valleculae (short arrows). The right hypopharynx (arrows) is small. The tip of the piriform sinus is missing, reflecting local resection. The normal mass effect of the larynx is not demonstrated. (B) Lateral view shows residual hyoid (h), valleculae, and epiglottis. The cricopharyngeus is prominent (arrow). Air within the larynx is not seen, reflecting partial laryngectomy. A tracheostoma is present. (Reproduced with permission from Rubesin SE. Pharynx. In: Levine MS, Laufer I, eds. *Double Contrast Gastrointestinal Radiology*. 2nd ed. Philadelphia: WB Saunders; 1992:74–105; Fig. 4–34.)

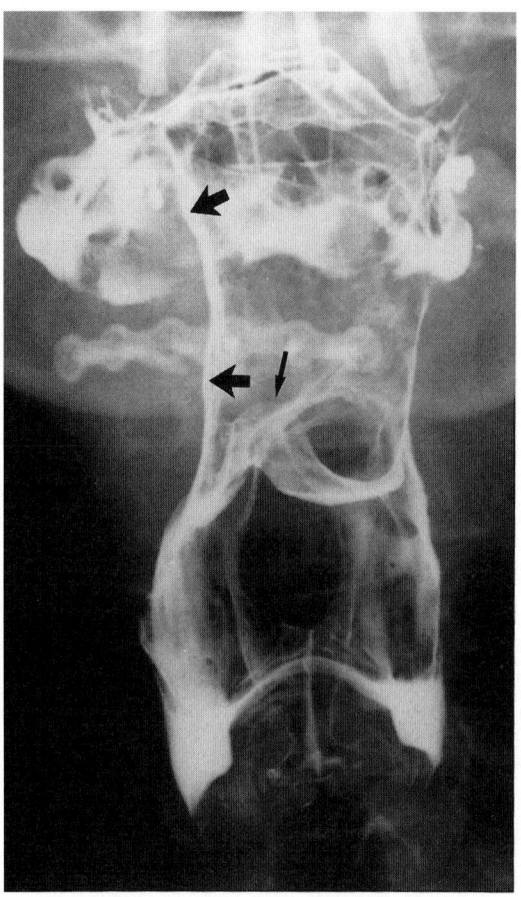

FIGURE 10.26. Base of tongue surgery and flap. The flap bulges (large arrows) into the right lateral oropharyngeal wall. There is volume loss of the right side of the tongue. A mandibular fixation device is seen. Radiation therapy changes include a smooth, enlarged epiglottis (small arrow) and flattening of the valleculae.

The role of pharyngography in most postglossectomy patients is to assess dysphagia and aspiration. The radiologist needs to carefully evaluate pharyngeal and laryngeal elevation, since the suprahyoid muscles may be damaged.

Postoperative complications include dysphagia, coughing or aspiration due to poor bolus manipulation, and premature spill of oral contents (Figure 10.28). Aspiration occurs in 10 to 33% of patients after total glossectomy (51). A large changeable space may appear in the oral cavity, in the space previously occupied by the tongue (see Figure 10.27). Irregular mucosa may be due to recurrent tumor (Figure 10.29) or to postoperative changes. Orocutaneous fistulae may form (Figure 10.30). Also, flap necrosis may occur, leading to fistula formation.

Malignant Oropharyngeal Lesions

The surgeon has many options for malignant lesions of the oropharynx based on the subsite or spread of tumors of the palatine tonsil, soft palate, posterior oropharyngeal wall, or tongue base. Many tumors often involve more than one subsite (52). Surgical approaches include transoral, lip splitting with or without mandibulotomy, mandibulotomy or subsegmental mandibulectomy, or transcervical. A neck dissection is often performed in conjunction with primary tumor resection. Reconstruction options may include a skin graft, myocutaneous flap (Figure 10.31) (e.g., pectoralis major or latissimus dorsi), or free flap (52).

Portions of the palate may be removed for primary squamous cell carcinoma or minor salivary gland cancers. A portion of the soft palate may be removed if a tumor in the tonsil or retromolar trigone has spread to the palate. If more than one third to one half of the soft palate is resected, the patient may complain of hypernasal speech or nasal regurgitation (Figure 10.32). If a portion of the hard palate is removed, an oronasal or sinonasal fistula may occur. Difficulty in swallowing or chewing may occur if the tongue base is tethered or partially removed.

The radiologist should remember to examine the patient. If an anterior mandibulectomy has been performed, the muscular attachments of the genioglossus are detached, which may lead to drooling (53). Loss of the inferior alveolar nerve with partial mandibulectomy results in anesthesia of the ipsilateral mandibular teeth, alveolar ridge, lower lip, and skin of chin.

The radiologist looks for orocutaneous and pharyngocutaneous fistula (Figure 10.33) and flap or graft breakdown, so the oral cavity should be included in radiographs. When surgery involving the tongue base or soft palate results in premature leak from the oral cavity into the oropharynx, laryngeal penetration may occur as a result of abnormal timing between oral and pharyngeal phases. Tonsillar resection may result in nasopharyngeal reflux and nasal speech due to adjacent soft palate resection or functional damage. Nasal regurgitation may be tested for with the patient in a decubitus position on the side down where palate damage is suspected. Placing the patient in the decubitus position pools contrast at the site of the surgical defect.

Tracheostomy

A tracheostomy may be permanent (e.g., for total laryngectomy and pharyngolaryngectomy) or temporary, to assist breathing during complicated larynx-sparing procedures. Tracheostomy alone can cause dysphagia and chronic aspiration (28). Laryngeal elevation is diminished with tracheostomy owing to tracheal tethering and postoperative neck changes. Desensitization of the cough reflex

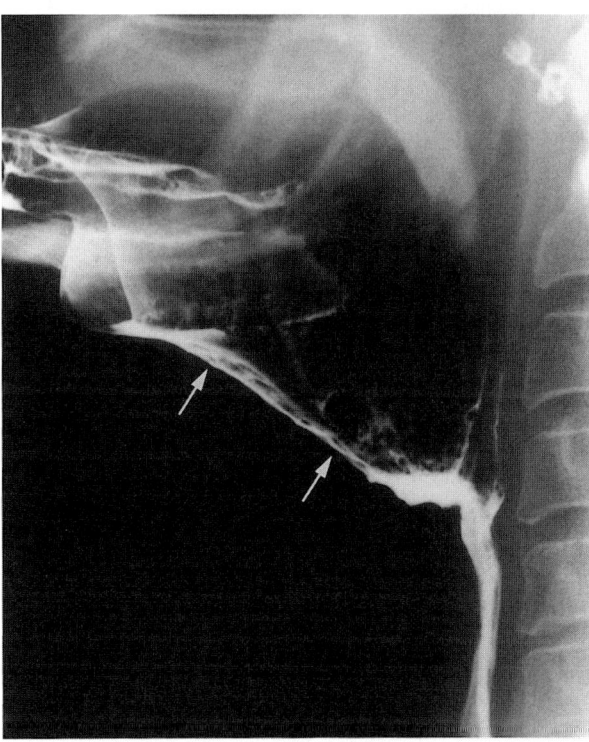

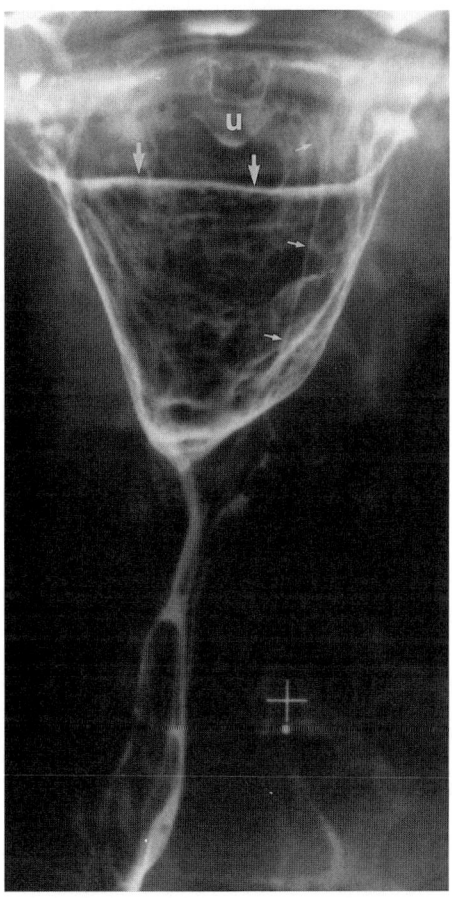

FIGURE 10.27. Total glossectomy and laryngectomy. (A) Lateral view shows barium outlining a triangular, air-filled space in an area normally occupied by the soft tissue density of the tongue and structures of the upper anterior neck. The barium-coated base of this space (arrows) is a flap. The nasopharyngeal tube is mildly narrowed. The patient is edentulous. (B) Frontal view shows the superior/anterior edge of the flap as a straight line (large arrows). The surface of the flap is nodular. The entire left palatopharyngeal fold (small arrows) is seen; the distal portion of the palatopharyngeal fold is normally obscured by the tongue in the frontal view; u, uvula.

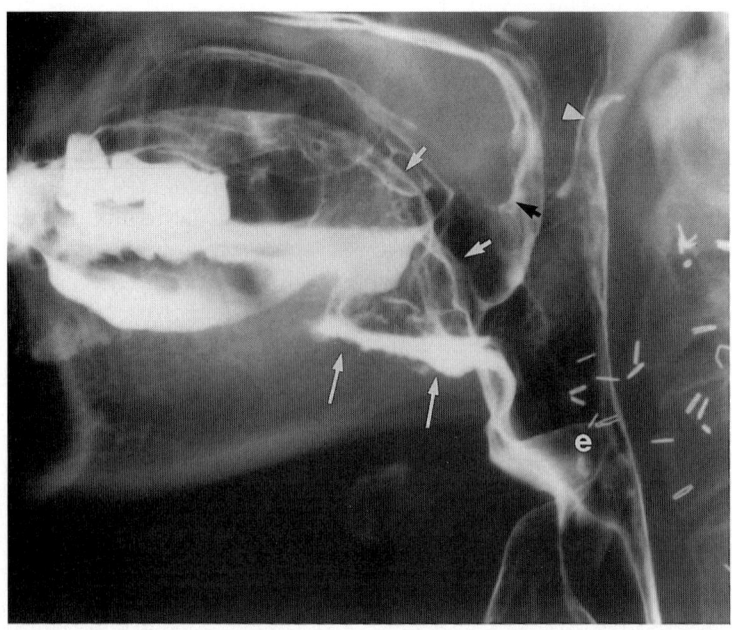

FIGURE 10.28. Partial glossectomy, stasis in the glossectomy defect, partial soft palate resection, neck dissection, and radiation therapy changes. A large, barium-filled defect (long white arrows) is in the base of the tongue. Barium outlines the normal curve of the unresected contralateral portion of the base of the tongue (small white arrows). The soft palate is asymmetric, with loss of volume of half the soft palate (black arrow). The velopharyngeal portal is open, despite phonation. Passavant's cushion (arrowhead) is seen. The epiglottis (e) is smoothly enlarged as a result of radiation therapy. Laryngeal penetration was due to poor bolus control and poor timing between the oral and pharyngeal phases of swallowing. The tongue defect results in both premature spillage of bolus into the oropharynx and stasis, with overflow of bolus into the oropharynx after a swallow.

may occur. Loss of coordination of laryngeal closure may also result in aspiration (54).

Surgery for Zenker's Diverticulum and Lateral Pharyngeal Pouches

Some patients with Zenker's diverticulum are asymptomatic. Many patients complain about food sticking in their throat requiring repeated swallows, or regurgitation of food. Other patients have halitosis, hoarseness, weight loss due to inability to eat, or pneumonia or lung abscess as the sequelae of aspiration (55). Some patients complain only of symptoms related to gastroesophageal reflux, as over 94% of patients with Zenker's diverticulum have a hiatal hernia and gastroesophageal reflux disease (56,57). Some patients with Zenker's diverticulum do not complain of symptoms until after the pharyngeal function has been secondarily compromised by coexistent neural or neuromuscular disease (e.g., stroke) (57).

Several endoscopic and surgical procedures have been devised for the treatment of patients with symptomatic Zenker's diverticulum (58,59), and these are described next.

1. **Endoscopic dilatation** of the prominent pharyngoesophageal segment frequently fails because the pouch is left in place and the upper esophageal sphincter is not disrupted enough to allow drainage of pharyngeal contents.

2. **Dohlman's operation** is the endoscopic procedure in which a special endoscope is placed so that the anterior lip of the instrument

10. Pharyngography in the Postoperative Patient

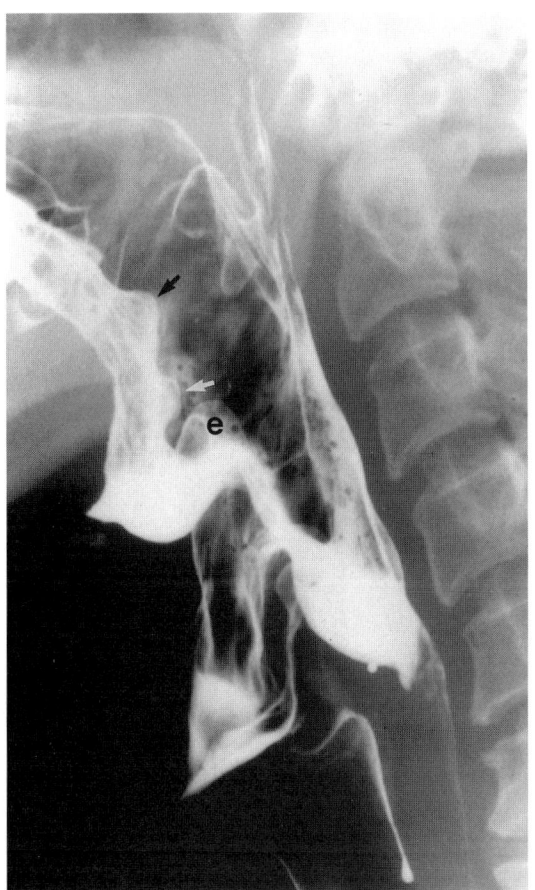

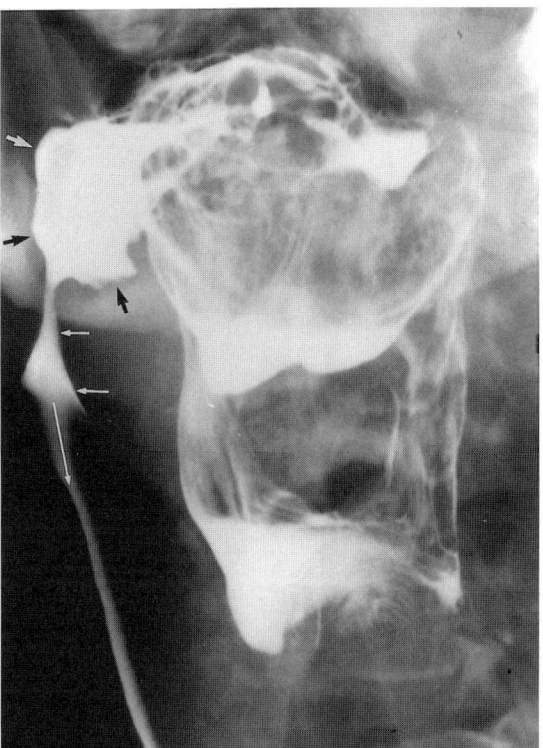

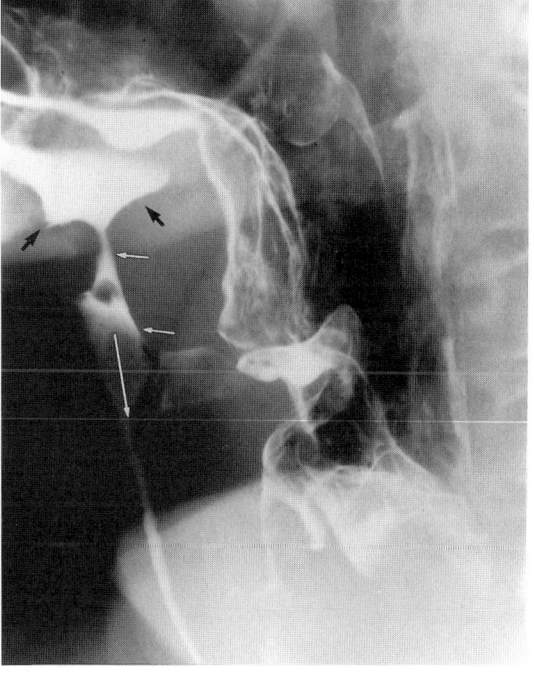

FIGURE 10.29. Recurrent squamous cell carcinoma after base of tongue and retromolar trigone surgery. Loss of volume of the base of the tongue is due to previous surgery. The surface of the base of the tongue is lobulated (arrows) in this patient, owing to recurrent tumor. Radiation therapy changes include soft palate atrophy and an enlarged, bulbous epiglottic tip (e). Laryngeal penetration was due to a combination of poor bolus control and diminished epiglottic tilt. Radiological demonstration of lobulation and nodularity of the postoperative tongue is not specific for recurrent cancer nor postoperative deformity. Direct visual examination and biopsy are needed.

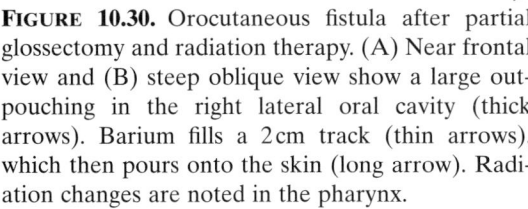

FIGURE 10.30. Orocutaneous fistula after partial glossectomy and radiation therapy. (A) Near frontal view and (B) steep oblique view show a large outpouching in the right lateral oral cavity (thick arrows). Barium fills a 2 cm track (thin arrows), which then pours onto the skin (long arrow). Radiation changes are noted in the pharynx.

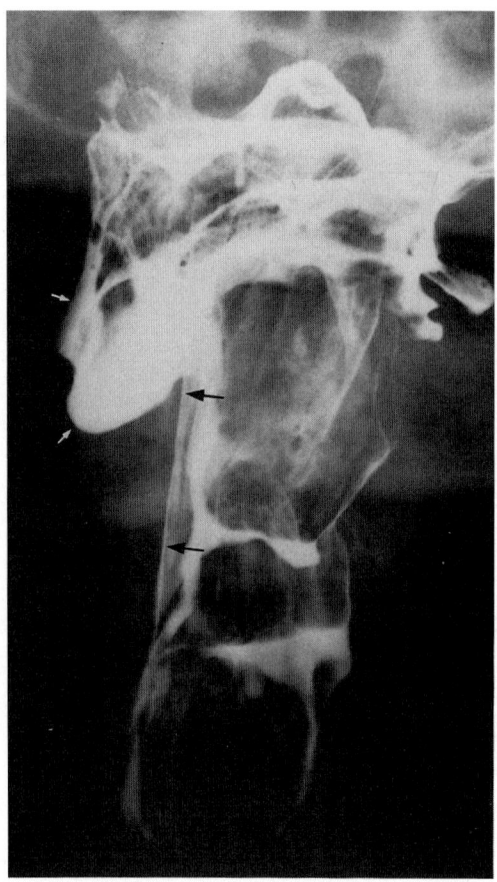

FIGURE 10.31. Right tonsillar fossa and base-of-tongue surgery with myocutaneous flap. A large, barium-filled defect (white arrows) is seen in the right oral cavity. A flap is seen as a straight line (black arrows) indenting the right neo-oropharyngeal wall.

4. A small Zenker's diverticulum may be inverted into the lumen (64).

5. **Diverticulopexy**, which may be performed in high-risk patients, avoids opening the pharynx. The surgeon sutures the apex of the diverticulum superiorly to the prevertebral fascia (64,65). A cricopharyngeal myotomy is usually part of this procedure. Although the sac may partially fill during swallowing, it drains early through the pharyngoesophageal segment, diminishing the risk of aspiration.

6. **Diverticulectomy combined with cricopharyngeal myotomy** is the most successful approach for the treatment of Zenker's divertic-

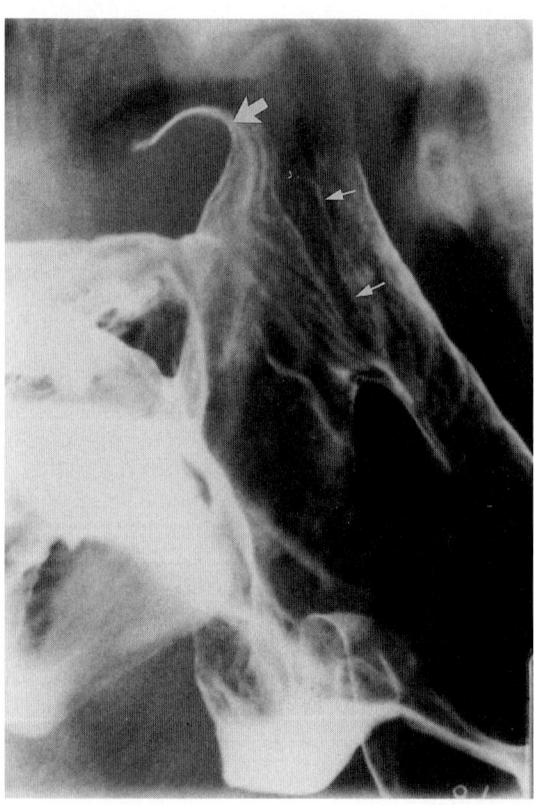

FIGURE 10.32. Partial soft palatectomy. The soft palate is truncated (large arrow), having a round posterior margin rather than the long tapered uvula. Mild nasal regurgitation of barium coats one of the paired salpingopharyngeal folds (small arrows) overlying the salpingopharyngeal muscle on the lateral nasopharyngeal wall. These folds are visualized only by nasal regurgitation or intranasal instillation of barium.

lies in the pharyngoesophageal segment and the posterior lip inserts into the diverticulum (60,61). The endoscopist then divides the septum between the sac and the pharyngoesophageal segment/upper cervical esophagus with a laser or endoscopic stapler (58,61). The Zenker's diverticulum is left in situ. This procedure is usually reserved for debilitated and elderly patients who are poor operative risks (62).

3. **Cricopharyngeal myotomy** alone has been used to treat Zenker's diverticulum, but its success rate is poor (63).

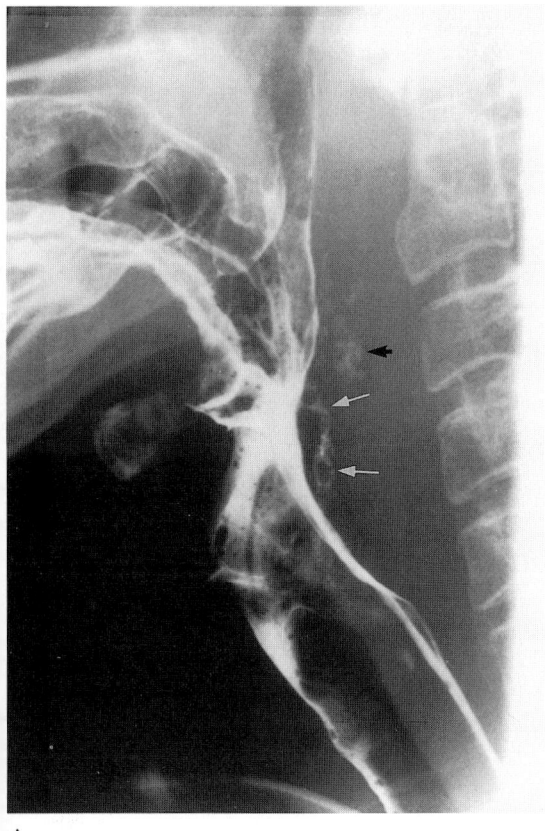 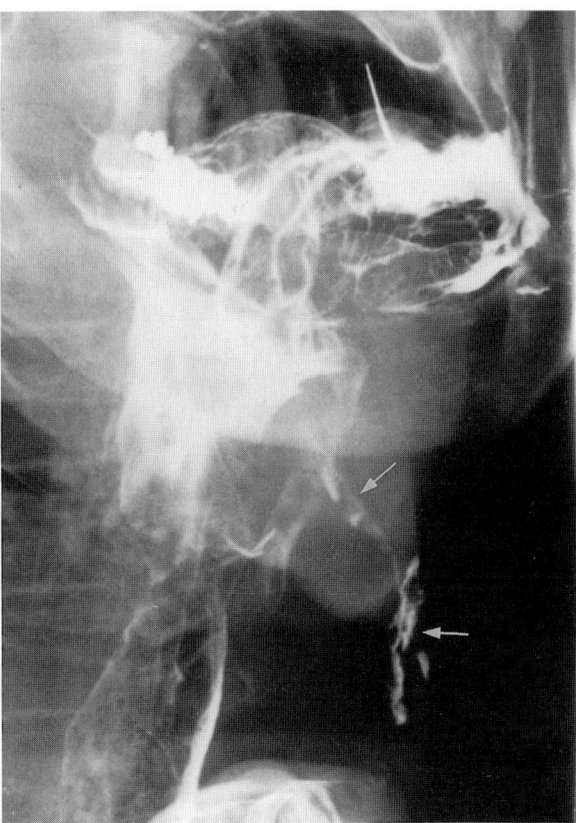

FIGURE 10.33. Fistula to carotid sheath. (A) Lateral and (B) oblique views of the pharynx show deformity of the left side of the oropharynx. The soft palate is asymmetric. The retropharyngeal space is widened. Barium enters the laryngeal vestibule and extends into the trachea. A track of barium (white arrows) extends posteriorly and laterally. On the lateral view, the barium lies just below calcification in the carotid artery (black arrow in A). This patient was expectorating blood. At surgery, a fistula to the carotid sheath was found.

ulum. An extended cricopharyngeal myotomy is performed, including division of the inferior fibers of the thyropharyngeus. The sac is then carefully excised, without removing mucosa of the pharyngoesophageal segment (66).

When the sac is not excised during a procedure (diverticulopexy, Dohlman's procedure, isolated myotomy), part or all of the diverticulum remains radiographically visible. To assess the success of the procedure, the radiologist must evaluate opening of the pharyngoesophageal segment, clearance of the bolus from the hypopharynx, and presence or absence of overflow aspiration. A preoperative video-pharyngoesophagogram is necessary to compare the preoperative and post–sac sparing procedure state.

In evaluating Dohlman's procedure, success is defined as diminished height of wall between the cervical esophagus and the pouch, free flow of bolus into the esophagus, and diminished height of barium in the residual pouch (62). In assessing myotomy with or without diverticulopexy, there should be limited filling of the pouch and easy bolus passage into the esophagus.

Postoperative complications include pharyngocutaneous fistula formation or mediastinitis due to a leak along the line of cricopharyngeal myotomy or at the site of sac excision. A fistula will usually close spontaneously with conservative treatment.

The recurrent laryngeal nerve lies in the tracheoesophageal groove just anterior to the esophagus and passes behind the inferior cornu of the thyroid cartilage. Transient vocal cord paralysis can be seen in up to 19% of patients (55). Permanent injury to the recurrent laryngeal nerve results in unilateral vocal cord paralysis (58).

If the myotomy is incomplete, dysphagia may persist. If normal mucosa is pulled out of Killian's dehiscence and excised along with the sac, a stricture may develop owing to excessive pharyngeal mucosal resection (58).

Cricopharyngeal Myotomy for Neuromuscular Disorders

The indications for cricopharyngeal myotomy as an isolated surgical procedure are controversial. Cricopharyngeal myotomy has been used as a "drainage" procedure in patients with dysphagia or aspiration due to an abnormally functioning pharyngoesophageal segment, a global pharyngeal motor disorder, or a Zenker's diverticulum (66–68). The principle of surgically dividing the cricopharyngeus to allow drainage from a neuromuscularly compromised pharynx is similar to performance of a pyloroplasty in patients who will develop abnormal gastric emptying due to vagotomy. Cricopharyngeal myotomy is probably not indicated in patients with globus symptoms, defined as long-standing, near-constant sensations of a lump in the throat, sensations that do not disappear between swallows (66).

The major risks of isolated cricopharyngeal myotomy are postoperative leak and the surgical destruction of one protective mechanism (upper esophageal sphincter function) that prevents reflux of esophageal contents into the pharynx and subsequently into the lungs. Thus, the surgeon has to balance the risk of aspiration from a neuromuscularly compromised pharynx with the risk of aspiration of esophageal contents. Another risk, although low, is injury to the recurrent laryngeal nerve with resultant vocal cord paralysis.

Radiographically, following a cricopharyngeal myotomy, there should be diminished stasis of barium in the hypopharynx, especially in the apices of the piriform sinuses. During swallowing, the cricopharyngeal bar should be absent or diminished in its compromise of the luminal diameter of the pharyngoesophageal segment in comparison to a preoperative videopharyngoesophagogram. The complications detected by videopharyngoesophagography are leak, with fistula or abscess formation, and incomplete myotomy, manifested as a persistent cricopharyngeal bar.

Radiation Therapy

Radiation therapy is utilized either as primary treatment for squamous cell carcinoma of the head and neck or as adjuvant postoperative therapy. Radiation therapy causes acute mucositis and edema, which usually subside 6 to 8 weeks after treatment (69,70). Biopsy samples taken 2 to 12 days after radiation therapy reveal acute necrosis, hemorrhage, leukocyte infiltration, and accumulation of histiocytes in irradiated tissue (71,72). Endothelial cell damage leads to acute interstitial edema. Within 1 to 4 months after therapy, obliterative endothelial cell proliferation occurs in small arteries, veins, and lymphatics, and collagen is deposited in connective tissue. Muscles can undergo necrosis, fibrosis, and fatty replacement. Lymph tissue in nodes and Waldeyer's ring atrophies in about one third of patients (73). Re-formation of capillary and lymphatic channels occurs after about 8 months, leading to diminished interstitial fluid. Accelerated atherosclerosis also occurs.

Pharyngography is helpful in the approximately 10% of patients who have persistent dysphagia after the cessation of radiation treatments and in patients in the remote posttreatment period who present with new symptoms such as dysphagia, odynophagia, hoarseness, and aspiration. If radiation therapy is combined with a surgical procedure, there is probably an increased risk of a postsurgical complication,

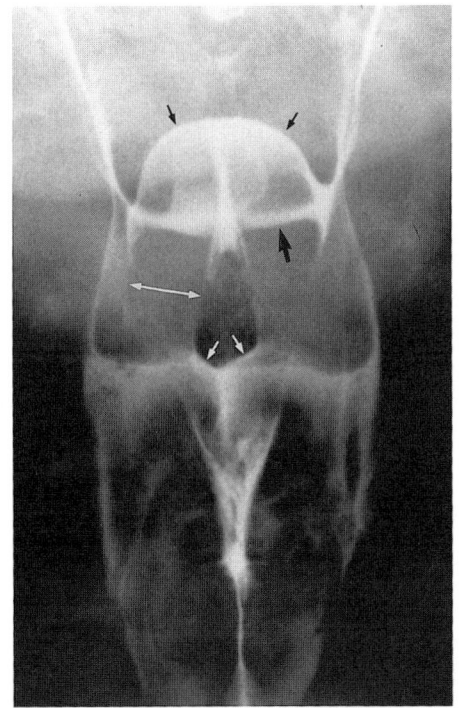

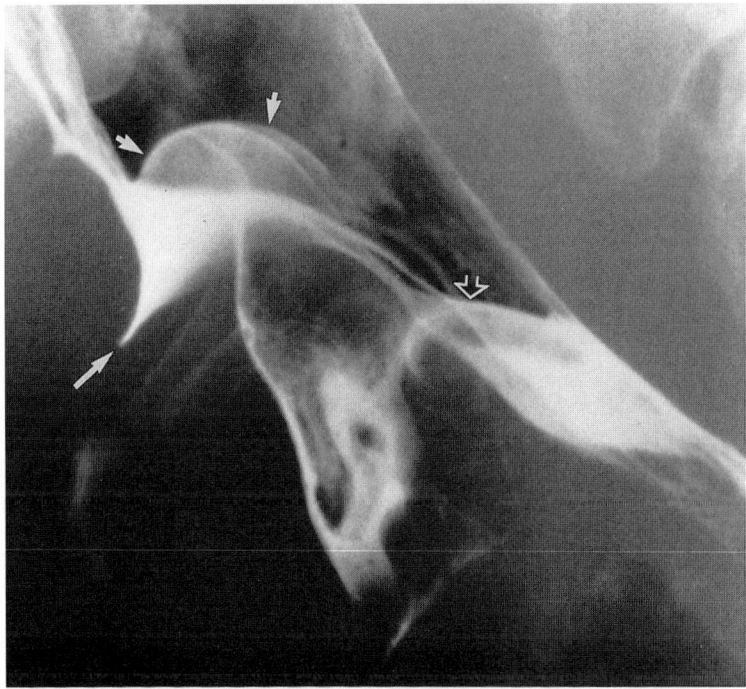

FIGURE 10.34. Radiation therapy changes. (A) Frontal view of the pharynx shows a smooth, enlarged, bulbous epiglottic tip (small black arrows), marked widening of the aryepiglottic folds (right fold identified with double white arrow), flattening of the valleculae (left vallecula, long black arrow), and elevation of the mucosa overlying the muscular process of the arytenoid cartilages (small white arrows). The resultant mucosal swelling results in marked narrowing of the laryngeal aditus. Note barium coating the false and true vocal cords. (B) Lateral view of the pharynx shows beaklike valleculae (long arrow), an enlarged, bulbous epiglottic tip (short arrows), and elevation of the mucosa overlying the arytenoid cartilages (open arrow). Also note moderate barium in the laryngeal vestibule. (From Rubesin SE, Yousem D. Structural abnormalities. In: Gore RM, Levine MS, Laufer I, eds. *Textbook of Gastrointestinal Radiology*. Philadelphia: WB Saunders; 1994:244–276; Fig. 17–38A,B.)

such as wound infection, pharyngocutaneous fistula, or flap necrosis (69). Pharyngography in the postoperative period will help distinguish persistent radiation changes from a surgical complication. Late complications of radiation therapy can include chronic aspiration, chondronecrosis, osteonecrosis, fistula formation, hypothyroidism, and neck fibrosis (74,75).

Radiographically, radiation-induced edema and early fibrosis appear as diffuse, symmetric enlargement of pharyngeal structures lying within the radiation portal (Figure 10.34) (22,23,76). The epiglottis is smoothly enlarged.

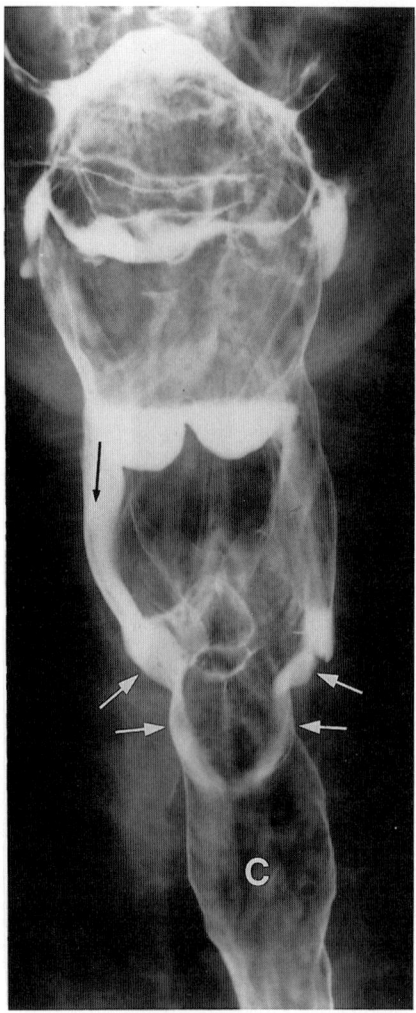

FIGURE 10.35. Pharyngeal paresis after radiation therapy. In this static image, paresis is manifested by visibility of portions of the hypopharynx that are not usually visible. The lower hypopharynx remains open, seen as a tubular structure (white arrows) in an area that is normally closed by intrinsic muscular contractility and the normal mass effect of the larynx. The normal arcuate line, seen as the "bottom" of the hypopharynx on static images, has disappeared. The cervical esophagus (c) is also atonic and is open when it should not be open. Moderate stasis in the valleculae reflects diminished epiglottic tilt. Note the barium overflowing (black arrow) from the valleculae into the right piriform sinus.

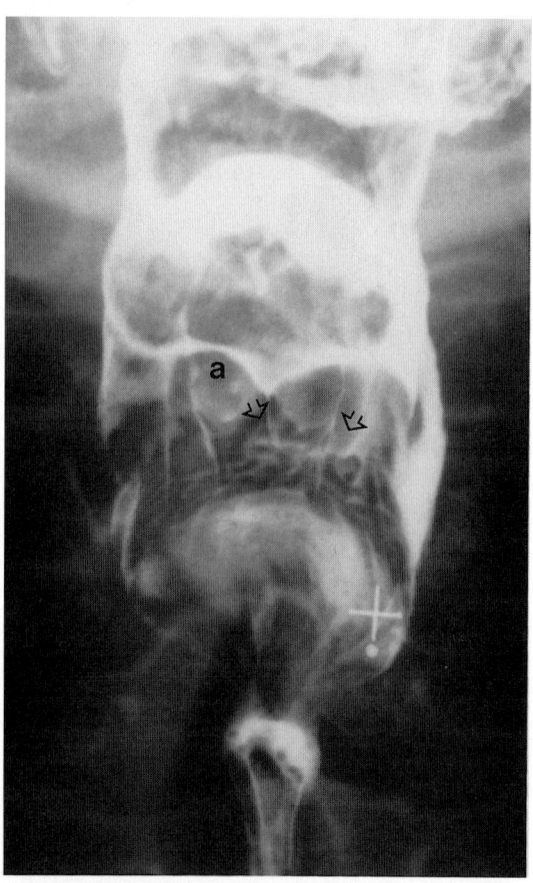

FIGURE 10.36. Recurrent squamous cell carcinoma after radiation therapy. A focal area of mucosal nodularity (arrows) in the hypopharynx was due to recurrent cancer after radiation therapy. The arytenoids are slightly enlarged and asymmetric (right arytenoid, a). (Reproduced with permission from Rubesin SE, et al. Lines of the pharynx. *Radio-Graphics* 1987;7:217–237; Fig. 15.)

the laryngeal vestibule is narrowed by the swollen epiglottic tip, aryepiglottic folds, and arytenoids.

The most common abnormality seen with dynamic imaging is that the swollen epiglottis is immobile or shows diminished tilt, leading to aspiration (76). Aspiration of barium is seen in about 90% of patients referred for pharyngography after radiation therapy (22). Dynamic imaging also demonstrates late closure of the laryngeal vestibule, paresis of the constrictor muscles (Figure 10.35), and in one quarter of patients, delayed opening of the pharyngoesophageal segment (76). Elevation of the larynx and pharynx is relatively preserved. Closure of the true vocal cords is also relatively preserved (76).

Persistence of edema 6 to 8 weeks after radiation therapy suggests infection, voice abuse, or

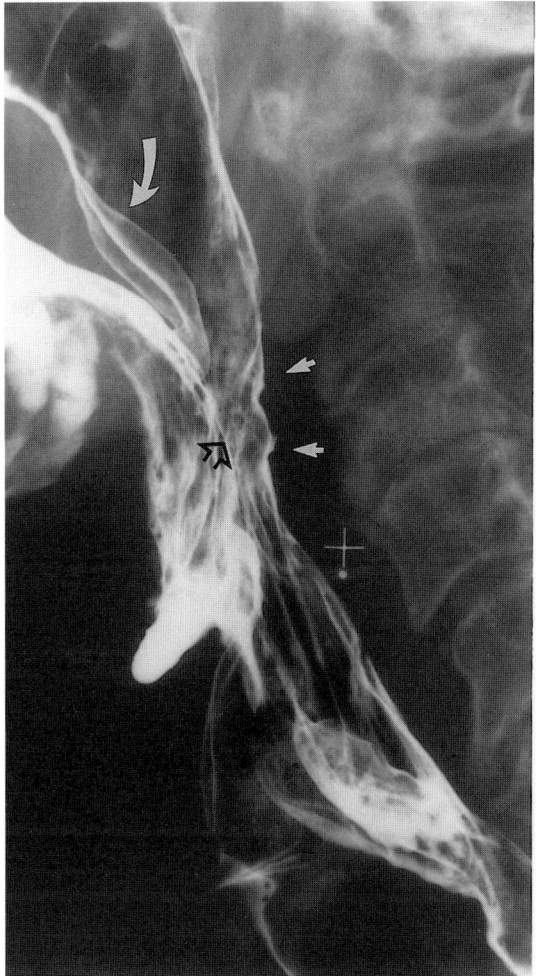

FIGURE 10.37. Recurrent squamous cell carcinoma posterior pharyngeal wall. Focal irregularity of the contour (short white arrows) and focal nodularity of the mucosa (open arrow) of the posterior pharyngeal wall indicate the site of recurrent squamous cell carcinoma. The soft palate is compensating (curved arrow) to hold the bolus in the oral cavity.

The valleculae are flattened, and there is broadening of the median glossoepiglottic fold. If aspirated barium outlines both sides of the aryepiglottic folds, these folds appear smoothly widened. Smooth, symmetric elevation of the mucosa overlying the muscular processes of the arytenoids is seen. Asymmetric swelling of the mucosa overlying the muscular process of the arytenoid cartilage may be seen on the side ipsilateral to the original tumor. The lumen of

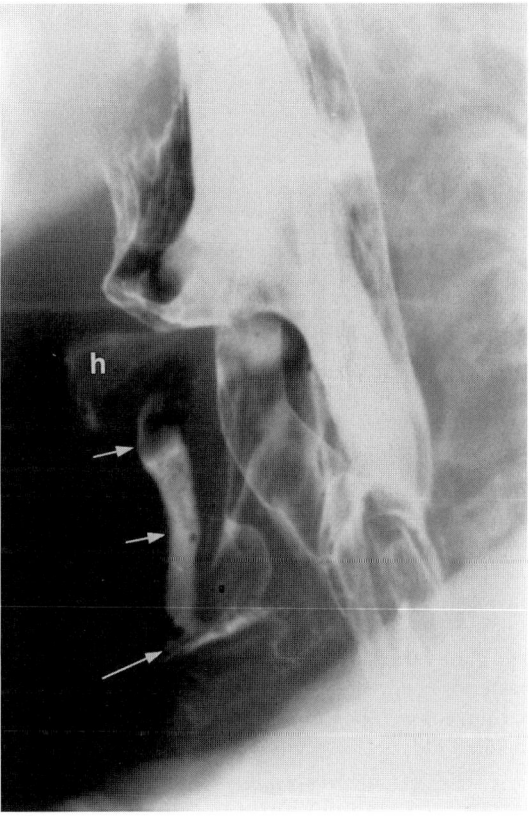

FIGURE 10.38. Fistula formation after radiation therapy for laryngeal carcinoma. A barium-filled track (short arrows) rises from the larynx just above the anterior commissure (long arrow). The fistula extends superiorly to the level of the hyoid bone (h).

residual tumor (22). Endoscopy and biopsy do not always lead to a diagnosis of recurrent tumor because persistent tumor may be hidden within or behind swollen structures. During pharyngography, mucosal irregularity, ulceration, nodularity, or a focal mass suggests tumor recurrence (Figures 10.36 and 10.37) (22). Other complications demonstrated by pharyngography include fistula formation (Figure 10.38) and atrophy of structures leading to dysfunction such as laryngeal penetration (see Figure 10.34) or nasal regurgitation (Figure 10.39).

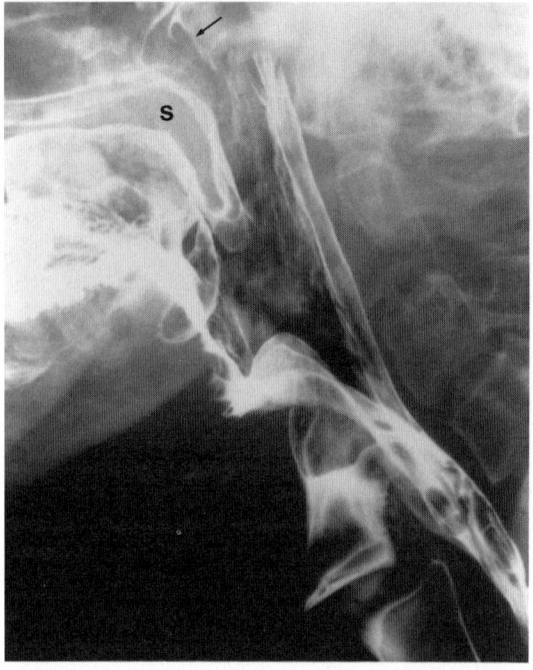

FIGURE 10.39. Soft palate atrophy long after radiation therapy. The soft palate (s) is small, resulting in moderate nasal regurgitation. Barium coats portions of the nasopharynx, including the salpingopharyngeal fold (arrow). Loss of soft tissue in the upper posterior pharyngeal wall is manifested as the barium-coated posterior pharyngeal wall overlapping the anterior cortex of the C2 vertebral body. Note the flat valleculae, bulbous epiglottis, and elevated aryepiglottic folds, all signs of radiation change. Barium coats the laryngeal vestibule and proximal trachea. (Reproduced with permission from Rubesin SE, et al. Contrast examination of the soft palate with cross-sectional correlation. *RadioGraphics* 1988;4:641–665; Fig. 23.)

References

1. Goldstein HM, Zornoza J. Association of squamous cell carcinoma of the head and neck with cancer of the esophagus. *AJR Am J Roentgenol* 1978;131:791–794.
2. Thompson WM, Oddson TA, Kelvin F, et al. Synchronous and metachronous squamous cell carcinoma of the head, neck, and esophagus. *Gastrointest Radiol* 1978;3:123–127.
3. Wagonfeld DJH, Harwood AR, Bryce EP, et al. Second primary respiratory tract malignant neoplasms in supraglottic carcinoma. *Arch Otolaryngol* 1981;107:135–137.
4. Rubesin SE, Yousem DM. Pharynx: normal anatomy and techniques. In: Gore RM, Levine MS, Laufer I, eds. *Textbook of Gastrointestinal Radiology*. Philadelphia: WB Saunders; 1994:202–225.
5. Rubesin SE, Stiles TD. Principles of performing a "modified barium swallow" examination. In: Balfe DM, Levine MS, eds. *Categorical Course in Diagnostic Radiology: Gastrointestinal*. Oak Brook, IL: RSNA Publications; 1997:7–20.
6. Davis M, Palmer P, Kelsey C. Use of the C-arm fluoroscope to examine patients with swallowing disorders. *AJR Am J Roentgenol* 1990;1655:986–988.
7. Ott DJ, Gelfand DW. Gastrointestinal contrast agents: indications, uses, risks. *JAMA* 1984;249:2380–2384.
8. Buecker A, Wein BB, Neuerberg JM, Guenther RW. Esophageal perforation: comparison of use of aqueous and barium-containing contrast media. *Radiology* 1997;202:683–686.
9. Fleming ID, Cooper JS, Henson DE, et al., eds. *AJCC Cancer Staging Manual*. 5th ed. Philadelphia: Lippincott-Raven; 1997:21–46.
10. Bailey BJ, Calhoun KH, Coffee AR, Neely JG, eds. *Atlas of Head and Neck Surgery—Otolaryngology*. Philadelphia: Lippincott-Raven; 1996:66–118,138–217,770–786.
11. Bleach N, Milford C, Van Hasselt A, eds. *Operative Otorhinolaryngology*. Oxford: Blackwell Science; 1997:295–396.
12. Balfe DM, Koehler RE, Setzen M, et al. Barium examination of the esophagus after total laryngectomy. *Radiology* 1982;143:501–508.
13. Wong F. Total laryngectomy. In: Bailey BJ, Calhoun KH, Coffee AR, Neely JG, eds. *Atlas of Head and Neck Surgery—Otolaryngology*. Philadelphia: Lippincott-Raven; 1996:200–203.
14. Gregor RT. Total laryngectomy. In: Bleach N, Milford C, Van Hasselt A, eds. *Operative Otorhi-

nolaryngology. Oxford: Blackwell Science; 1997: 365–372.
15. Balfe DM. Imaging of the pharynx after surgical therapy. In: Jones B, Donner MW, eds. *Normal and Abnormal Swallowing.* New York: Springer-Verlag; 1991:147–171.
16. Moses BL, Eisele DW, Jones B. Radiologic assessment of the early postoperative total-laryngectomy patient. *Laryngoscope* 1993;103: 1157–1160.
17. Muller-Miny H, Eisele DW, Jones B. Dynamic radiographic imaging following total laryngectomy. *Head Neck* 1993;15:342–347.
18. Fradis M, Podoshin L, Ben David J. Postlaryngectomy pharyngocutaneous fistula—a still unresolved problem. *J Laryngol and Otol* 1955;109: 221–224.
19. Hier M, Black MJ, Lafond G. Pharyngocutaneous fistulas after total laryngectomy: incidence, etiology and outcome analysis. *J Otolaryngol* 1993;22:164–166.
20. DiSantis DJ, Balfe DM, Hayden RE, et al. The neck after total laryngectomy: CT study. *Radiology* 1984;153:713–717.
21. Wippold FJ II, Balfe D. Imaging of the postoperative neck In: Gore RM, Levine MS, Laufer I, eds. *Textbook of Gastrointestinal Radiology.* Philadelphia: WB Saunders; 1994:277–290.
22. Quillen SP, Balfe DM, Glick SN. Pharyngography after head and neck irradiation: differentiation of postirradiation edema from recurrent tumor. *AJR Am J Roentgenol* 1993;161:1205–1208.
23. Balfe DM, Heiken JP. Contrast evaluation of structural lesions of the pharynx. *Curr Probl Diagn Radiol* 1986;15:77–160.
24. Rubesin SE, Jessurun J, Robertson D, et al. Lines of the pharynx. *RadioGraphics* 1987;7:217–237.
25. Pernkof E. *Atlas of Topographical Applied Human Anatomy,* Vol I. *Head and Neck.* Baltimore: Urban & Schwarzenberg; 1980:231–339.
26. Stepnick DW, Hayden RE. Options for reconstruction of the pharyngoesophageal defect. *Otolaryngol Clin North Am* 1994;27:1151–1158.
27. Haughey BH. The jejunal free flap in oral cavity and pharyngeal reconstruction. *Otolaryngol Clin N Am* 1994;27:1159–1170.
28. Kronenberger MB, Meyers AD. Dysphagia following head and neck cancer surgery. *Dysphagia* 1994;9:236–244.
29. Wong F. Total pharyngolaryngectomy. In: Bailey BJ, Calhoun KH, Coffee AR, Neely JG, eds. *Atlas of Head and Neck Surgery—Otolaryngology.* Philadelphia: Lippincott-Raven; 1996:206–209.
30. Wilson JA, Maran AG, Pyrde A, Walker WS, Heading RC. The function of free jejunal autografts in the pharyngoesophageal segment. *J R Coll Surg Edinburgh* 1995;40:363–366.
31. Sloane PM, Griffin JM, O'Dwyer TP. Esophageal insufflation and videofluoroscopy for evaluation of esophageal speech in laryngectomy patients: clinical implications. *Radiology* 1991;181:433–437.
32. Gatenby RA, Rosenblum JS, Leonard CM, et al. Esophageal speech: double contrast evaluation of the pharyngo-esophageal segment. *Radiology* 1985;157:127–131.
33. Som PM, Urken ML, Biller H, Lidov M. Imaging the postoperative neck. *Radiology* 1993;187:593–603.
34. Medina JE. Radical neck dissection. In: Bailey BJ, Calhoun KH, Coffee AR, Neely JG, eds. *Atlas of Head and Neck Surgery—Otolaryngology.* Philadelphia: Lippincott-Raven; 1996:140–143.
35. Urquhart AC. Radical and conservative neck dissections. In: Bleach N, Milford C, Van Hasselt A, eds. *Operative Otorhinolaryngology.* Oxford: Blackwell Science; 1997:444–453.
36. Wong F. Supraglottic laryngectomy (horizontal hemilaryngectomy). In: Bailey BJ, Calhoun KH, Coffee AR, Neely JG, eds. *Atlas of Head and Neck Surgery—Otolaryngology.* Philadelphia: Lippincott-Raven; 1996:190–193.
37. Gregor RT. Horizontal (supraglottic) Laryngectomy. In: Bleach N, Milford C, Van Hasselt A, eds. *Operative Otorhinolaryngology.* Oxford: Blackwell Science; 1997:383ff.
38. Niemeyer JH, Balfe DM, Hayden RE. Neck evaluation with barium-enhanced radiographs and CT scans after supraglottic subtotal laryngectomy. *Radiology* 1987;162:493–498.
39. Tabb HG, Druck NS, Thorton RS, Gibbert WP. Supraglottic laryngectomy. *South Med J* 1978;71: 114–117.
40. Gregor RT, Oei SS, Baris G, et al. Supraglottic laryngectomy with neck dissection and postoperative radiation in the management of supraglottic laryngeal cancer. *Am J Otolaryngol* 1996; 17:316–321.
41. Roberson JB Jr, Fee WE Jr. Conservation surgery for laryngeal carcinoma. *Ann Acad Med* 1991;20:656–664.
42. Olsen KD. Vertical partial laryngectomy. In: Bleach N, Milford C, Van Hasselt A, eds. *Operative Otorhinolaryngology.* Oxford: Blackwell Science; 1997:373–382.
43. Rassekh CH. Laryngofissure and cordectomy. In: Bailey BJ, Calhoun KH, Coffee AR, Neely

JG, eds. *Atlas of Head and Neck Surgery—Otolaryngology*. Philadelphia: Lippincott-Raven; 1996:174–176.
44. Bailey BJ: Vertical partial laryngectomy. In: Bailey BJ, Calhoun KH, Coffee AR, Neely JG, eds. *Atlas of Head and Neck Surgery—Otolaryngology*. Philadelphia: Lippincott-Raven; 1996:184–187.
45. Gopal HV, Fried MP. Vertical partial laryngectomy including the thyroid cartilage. In: Bailey BJ, Calhoun KH, Coffee AR, Neely JG, eds. *Atlas of Head and Neck Surgery—Otolaryngology*. Philadelphia: Lippincott-Raven; 1996:176–179.
46. DiSantis DJ, Balfe DM, Koehler RE, et al. Barium examination of the pharynx after vertical hemilaryngectomy. *AJR Am J Roentgenol* 1983;141:335–339.
47. DiSantis DJ, Balfe DM, Hayden R. The neck after vertical hemilaryngectomy: computed tomographic study. *Radiology* 1984;151:683–687.
48. Cannon CR. Surgical approaches. In: Bailey BJ, Calhoun KH, Coffee AR, Neely JG, eds. *Atlas of Head and Neck Surgery—Otolaryngology*. Philadelphia: Lippincott-Raven; 1996:66–69.
49. Johnson RC. Near total glossectomy. Total glossectomy. In: Bailey BJ, Calhoun KH, Coffee AR, Neely JG, eds. *Atlas of Head and Neck Surgery—Otolaryngology*. Philadelphia: Lippincott-Raven; 1996:78–83.
50. Hirano M, Kuroiwa Y, Tanaka S, et al. Dysphagia following various degrees of surgical resection for oral cancer. *Ann Otol Rhinol Laryngol* 1992;101:138–142.
51. Weber RS, Ohlms L, Bowman J, et al. Functional results after total or near-total glossectomy with laryngeal preservation. *Arch Otolaryngol Head Neck Surg* 1991;117:512–516.
52. Waldron J. Surgery for malignant lesions of the oropharynx. In: Bleach N, Milford C, Van Hasselt A, eds. *Operative Otorhinolaryngology*. Oxford: Blackwell Science; 1997:357–362.
53. Logemann JA, Bytell DE. Swallowing disorders in three types of head and neck surgical patients. *Cancer* 1979;44:1095–1105.
54. Nash M. Swallowing problems in the tracheotomized patient. *Otolaryngol Clin North Am* 1988;21:701–709.
55. Bonafede JP, Lavertu P, Wood BG, Eliachar I. Surgical outcome in 87 patients with Zenker's diverticulum. *Laryngoscope* 1997;107:720–725.
56. Delahunty JE, Margulies SE, Alonso UA, et al. The relationship of reflux esophagitis to pharyngeal pouch (Zenker's diverticulum). *Laryngoscope* 1971;81:570–577.
57. Rubesin SE. Pharynx: structural abnormalities. In: Gore RM, Levine MS, eds. *Textbook of Gastrointestinal Radiology*. 2nd ed. Philadelphia: WB Saunders; 2000:227–255.
58. Vilantis AC. Surgery of hypopharyngeal diverticula. In: Bleach N, Milford C, Van Hasselt A, eds. *Operative Otorhinolaryngology*. Oxford: Blackwell Science; 1997:343–348.
59. Cassisi NJ. Pharyngeal pouches (Zenker's diverticulum). In: Bailey BJ, Calhoun KH, Coffee AR, Neely JG, eds. *Atlas of Head and Neck Surgery—Otolaryngology*. Philadelphia: Lippincott-Raven; 1996:256–257.
60. Dohlman G, Mattsson O. The endoscopic operation for hypopharyngeal diverticula. A roentgencinematographic study. *Arch Otolaryngol* 1960;71:744–752.
61. Collard JM, Otte JB, Kastens PJ. Endoscopic stapling technique of esophagodiverticulostomy for Zenker's diverticulum. *Ann Thoracic Surg* 1993;56:573–576.
62. Hadley JM, Ridley N, Djazaeri B, Glover G. The radiological appearances after endoscopic cricopharyngeal myotomy: Dohlman's procedure. *Clin Radiol* 1997;52:613–615.
63. Schmit PJ, Zuckerbraun L. Treatment of Zenker's diverticula by cricopharyngeus myotomy under local anesthesia. *Am Surg* 1992;18:710–716.
64. Bowdler DA, Stell PM. Surgical management of posterior pharyngeal pulsion diverticula: inversion versus one-stage excision. *Br J Surg* 1987;74:988–990.
65. Konowitz PM, Biller HF. Diverticulopexy and cricopharyngeal myotomy: treatment for the high risk patient with a pharyngoesophageal (Zenker's) diverticulum. *Otolaryngol Head Neck Surg* 1989;100:146–153.
66. McKenna A, Dedo HH. Cricopharyngeal myotomy: indications and technique. *Ann Otol Rhinol Laryngol* 1992;101:216–221.
67. Overbeek JJM. Upper esophageal sphincterotomy in dysphagic patients with and without a diverticulum. *Dysphagia* 1991;6:228–234.
68. Schechter GL. Cricopharyngeal myotomy and myectomy. In: Bailey BJ, Calhoun KH, Coffee AR, Neely JG, eds. *Atlas of Head and Neck Surgery—Otolaryngology*. Philadelphia: Lippincott-Raven; 1996:262–263.
69. Tartaglino LM, Rao VM, Markiewicz DA. Imaging of radiation changes in the head and neck. *Semin Roentgenol* 1994;29:81–91.
70. Fu KK, Woodhouse RJ, Quincy JM, et al. The significance of laryngeal edema following

radiotherapy of carcinoma of the vocal cord. *Cancer* 1982;49:655–658.
71. Goldman JL, Cheren RJ, Zak FG, et al. Histopathology of larynges and radical neck specimens in combined radiation and surgery for advanced carcinoma of the larynx and hypopharynx. *Ann Otol* 1966;75:313–321.
72. Mukherji SK, Mancuso AA, Kotzur IM, et al. Radiologic appearance of the irradiated larynx, I: expected changes. *Radiology* 1994;193:141–148.
73. Mukherji SK, Mancuso AA, Kotzur IM, et al. Radiologic appearance of the irradiated larynx, II: primary site response. *Radiology* 1994;193:149–154.
74. Larson DL, Lindberg RD, Lane E, et al. Major complications of radiotherapy in cancer of the oral cavity and oropharynx. A 10-year retrospective study. *Am J Surg* 1983;146:431–436.
75. McCombe AW, Jones AS. Radiotherapy and complications of laryngectomy. *J Laryngol Otol* 1993;107:130–132.
76. Ekberg O, Nylander G. Pharyngeal dysfunction after treatment for pharyngeal cancer with surgery and radiotherapy. *Gastrointest Radiol* 1983;8:97–104.

11
Swallowing in Children

SANDRA S. KRAMER AND PEGGY S. EICHER

Swallowing difficulty may occur in children as an isolated problem, but it is more commonly seen as one of a constellation of issues in patients with multiple abnormalities (1). Pediatric feeding problems are often complex because systems are already stressed by the demands of growth and development, nutritional needs are usually greater than those of adults, anatomic structures grow and their relationships change, and the central nervous system is maturing.

Although there may be similarities, dysfunctional feeding in children is very likely to be different from that of adults. For example, children with congenital problems must learn feeding skills without a foundation of existing skills and in the presence of neurological impairment and/or anatomic anomalies. Such a situation is often further complicated by the child's inability to communicate clinical information or to fully comprehend instructions. Children with neurological and myopathic impairments, congenital malformations of the head and neck, and syndromes (2–4) (Table 11.1) are especially at risk. Central nervous system injuries (from infection, anoxia, trauma, or vascular accident), hydrocephalus, mental retardation, and cerebral palsy are the most common problems encountered in this patient population.

A multidisciplinary approach is particularly appropriate for pediatric feeding problems. Most feeding difficulties are complicated and necessitate a coordinated approach by specialists from different disciplines to correctly diagnose the contributing factors, appreciate the problem's effect on the patient's daily life, and construct a successful treatment plan.

Clinical Assessment

Symptoms of dysfunctional feeding (2,3,5,6) include gagging or vomiting during feeding, nasopharyngeal reflux with leak from the nostrils, malnutrition and failure to thrive, food refusal, choking or coughing while eating, and respiratory problems including recurrent pneumonias, upper respiratory tract infections, bronchospasm, and apnea. Because of the significant influence of medical, motor, and developmental factors on the swallowing process, the evaluation of a child with dysphagia should reflect a multidisciplinary approach. For effective assessment and coordinated treatment, team expertise should include pediatric medicine, nutrition, development, psychology and family function, positioning, oral motor skills, and radiology.

The diagnostic evaluation (7) of a child with dysphagia should emphasize problem presentation, medical and feeding history, physical exam, and observation of feeding performance. The summation of this information aids in the development of a working impression or hypothesis. Diagnostic exams then serve to clarify the hypothesis. The goal is to understand the underlying pathophysiology and expected developmental progression, so that an optimal treatment strategy can be designed and monitored.

TABLE 11.1. Causes of clinical swallowing difficulties in children.

> Local anatomical abnormality
>   Choanal atresia
>   Cleft lip and palate
>   Micrognathia (Pierre-Robin syndrome)
>   Macroglossia, ankyloglossia
>   Pharyngeal tumors, cysts
>   Laryngeal cleft, tracheoesophageal fistula
>   Pharyngeal diverticulum: congenital, posttraumatic
>   Trauma, caustic burns to mouth and pharynx
>   Inflammation, infection of mouth and pharynx
>   Foreign bodies
>   Esophageal lesions: congenital anomalies (e.g., esophageal atresia/tracheoesophageal fistula), vascular rings, duplication cysts, reflux esophagitis, caustic burns, esophageal dysmotility, infection, strictures, achalasia, postoperative complications
> Neuromuscular abnormality
>   Delayed maturation, prematurity
>   Brain damage due to infection, anoxia, trauma, metabolic disease, hydrocephalus, vascular accident
>   Mental retardation
>   Cerebral palsy
>   Cranial nerve palsy: V, VII, IX, X, XI, XII
>   Bulbar and pseudobulbar palsy, Moebius syndrome, poliomyelitis
>   Werdnig-Hoffman disease
>   Familial dysautonomia (Riley-Day syndrome)
>   Huntington's chorea
>   Syndromes: Cornelia DeLange, Prader-Willi, chromosomal defects, etc.
>   Muscular disorders: myotonic dystrophy, myasthenia gravis, dermatomyositis
>   Local anesthesia of the pharynx

Source: Reprinted with permission from Kramer SS. Special swallowing problems in children. *Gastrointest Radiol* 1985;10:241–250.

History

A thorough medical history should include information on all organ systems and the child's pattern of growth. Any medical problem, from otitis media to constipation, may have an adverse effect on feeding. It is helpful to organize the medical information into abnormalities of structure and function. For example, cleft palate and tracheoesophageal fistula are structural problems that can be successfully treated by surgery, whereas motor incoordination in cerebral palsy and gastroesophageal reflux are dynamic functional problems whose influence on feeding may change over time with growth and development.

The developmental history should document the child's developmental progression, current developmental level, and any qualitative difficulties with attention, tolerance, or transitions. The developmental history will facilitate accurate interpretation of the child's response to past events and future interventions.

The feeding history should review the child's current feeding regimen, including associated problems that occur with eating such as coughing, gagging, vomiting, or wheezing. The child's progress through each transition phase of oral feeding (introduction of bottle, spoon, and cup) and through the introduction of advancing textures (purées, junior foods, and table foods) (8) should be documented. If difficulty is encountered at any step, it can be correlated temporally with medical and developmental events. A description of a typical mealtime elucidates the mealtime social environment and the caretaker's response to the feeding problem. From the history, hypotheses are developed about the components contributing to the feeding problem.

Exam and Observation

The general physical exam should include growth parameters as well as assessment of the structure and function of the head and neck, oral cavity, chest, and abdomen. Dysmorphic findings should prompt investigation into associated syndromes or genetic disorders. The neurodevelopmental examination highlights neurological dysfunction and its effect on gross motor, fine motor, and language skills (9).

The oral motor exam looks at anatomy of the oral pharyngeal cavity, the relationship of the individual structures to each other, and their coordinated function (10,11). The mealtime observation gives information on the level of competency of demonstrated oral skills, coordination, and fatigue. Cervical auscultation of a swallow with different textures gives insight into pharyngeal function and the coordination of the oral transport phase with the pharyngeal phase and respiration. If the child behaves typically, the evaluator can see firsthand the antecedents to any associated problems. The caretaker's response can also be observed.

Original hypotheses are reviewed in light of information obtained from the exam and feeding observation, and those that do not fit are discarded. The remaining hypotheses focus the direction of radiological and laboratory investigation. These tests can then substantiate the working hypotheses and document the impact of a potential intervention.

Radiological Examination (5,12)

Technique

The radiological examination provides the best demonstration of the swallowing mechanism and, therefore, plays a central role in the diagnostic evaluation of any child with a swallowing impairment (3,5). It helps the clinical staff design the most appropriate treatment plan for the child, and in follow-up it gives helpful information about changing function resulting from that treatment. Thus, the effort put into careful examination technique and radiological interpretation of a swallowing study may have a significant effect on a child's care.

The best diagnostic studies are obtained when one is able both to formulate questions based on the patient's clinical assessment and to design an examination that will answer those questions as clearly as possible. All pertinent clinical information should be available to the radiologist and the examination goals clarified before the study is performed.

The events in a swallowing sequence happen in fractions of a second; no fluoroscopic observer could follow everything as it occurs. Therefore, dynamic recording of swallowing with videotape is imperative to allow the examiner to carefully analyze at a later time the swallowing events with slow motion, backup, and stop-frame viewing.

Scout films of the chest and sometimes also of the neck may be made prior to the examination. They will show the anatomical structures involved in swallowing and related areas where complications may arise (e.g., the airway and the lung parenchyma). The swallowing act itself must be recorded dynamically in lateral and, if possible, posteroanterior projections and should include evaluation of the oral cavity, pharynx, and esophagus.

The swallowing study of an infant or child poses special challenges to the examiner. Infants are frequently difficult to examine, as are children with mental retardation and severe neurological impairment; yet these are the very children who will benefit the most from good-quality examinations. Patience and planning are necessary components of these pediatric studies. Efforts should be made to keep radiation exposure, a special concern when dealing with children, to a diagnostic minimum.

The success of the examination, to a large extent, depends on the cooperation of the patient. Preparations made prior to the study may have a big impact on this. We have found that withholding the meal prior to the exam encourages infants and small children to drink barium more readily. Once in the examination room, every attempt is made to put the child at ease. If the child is old enough to understand, the procedure is explained in appropriate terms. Whenever possible, the feeding technique is practiced with the patient before filming. Involvement of the parents and caretakers helps in allaying the child's anxiety and frequently elicits additional information about problems and aid in feeding the child.

Special personnel may be invaluable in planning and conducting the examination of significantly impaired patients. Key people include the occupational therapist or speech and language pathologist involved in the patient's care and feeding program and an experienced nurse who can remain in the radiographic room to provide oxygen and suction for patients likely to aspirate.

Whenever possible, one should examine children in the position in which they commonly eat. Infants are usually studied in the supine or semiupright position and children in the sitting position. Special immobilization devices and radiolucent car seats and chairs may be especially useful (Figure 11.1). Cooperative older patients may be examined standing.

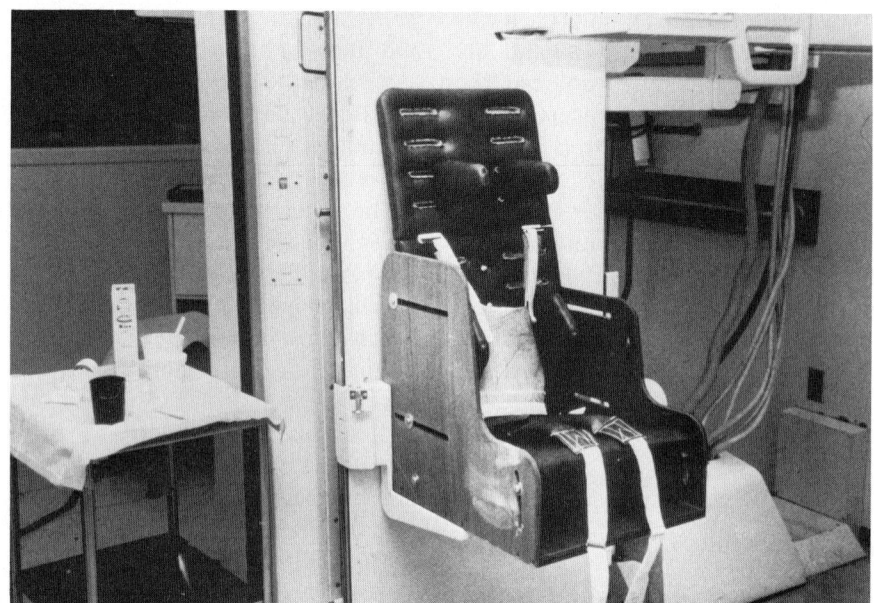
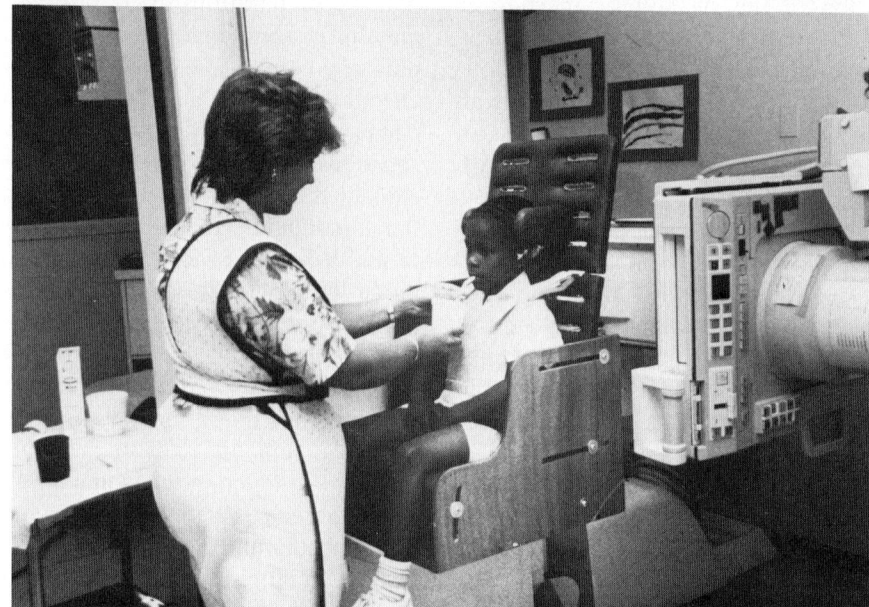

FIGURE 11.1. A custom-constructed chair is attached to an upright fluoroscopic table for examinations in sitting position. It is radiolucent, fully adjustable, and can be rotated 90° so that filming can be performed in posteroanterior and lateral projections. (Reprinted with permission from Kramer SS. Radiologic examination of the swallowing impaired child. *Dysphagia* 1989;3:117–125.)

The examination should try to mimic the feeding pattern appropriate for the patient's age and development. The examiner should attempt to reproduce circumstances that cause feeding difficulty within the limits of safety and good judgment. Barium mixtures of various consistencies from thin liquid to purées to solids may be used, depending on the patient's symptoms or on the question to be answered. Thin or thick liquid barium is often used initially, employing a nipple and bottle for infants and a cup or straw for older children. Liquid barium is relatively safe if aspirated and easily removed with suctioning. Specialized feeding methods and devices may be employed for patients with specific handicaps.

If oral feeding proves difficult because of either oral-motor dysfunction or lack of patient cooperation, other approaches can be taken to gain important information. Small amounts of barium can be injected under fluoroscopic control through a small feeding tube placed in the buccal pouch or oral cavity, or transnasally into the nasopharynx. It is usually possible with this technique to evaluate at least the pharyngeal phase of swallowing and esophageal function in problem cases.

One must keep in mind that the child's span of attention and cooperation may be short. Complete studies may require more than one visit, especially when a detailed evaluation of the esophagus is needed.

Normal Age-Related Anatomy and Swallowing Function (3,5,10,11,13–20)

The radiologist interpreting children's swallowing studies must understand normal growth and age-related change in anatomical structures and relationships (3,8,10,13–16) and normal maturation in neuromuscular function (8,10,11,15–20) pertinent to swallowing; usually these parallel each other in child development. It should also be remembered that, in the broader context, feeding is interrelated with the maintenance of a patent airway, breathing, speech, and posture, and the pharynx plays a central role in all of these functions.

The Infant

The tongue, which apposes the hard and soft palates (Figure 11.2), occupies most of the oral cavity in the infant. The pharynx is relatively small, and the hyoid bone and larynx lie at a higher level than in the adult (Figure 11.3). These anatomical relationships are in many ways ideal for the normal feeding pattern in infancy, suckle feeding from a nipple (Figures 11.4 and 11.5).

Suckle feeding, a reflex feeding behavior regulated at a subcortical level, probably in the medulla or pons, is mature in the full-term newborn but may not be fully developed in premature infants. In established suckle feeding, suckling, swallowing, and breathing between swallows recur in a stable pattern characteristic for each infant.

Suckling is accomplished by the rhythmic compression of the nipple by the lower jaw and tongue against the upper jaw and palate. The tongue moves in a rhythmic and peristaltic motion, expressing liquid from the nipple. A repetitive negative pressure is developed, alternating with compression. During suckling, the soft palate is apposed to the posterior tongue, and, at times, may even bow forward, closing off the oral cavity posteriorly (Figure 11.4). Accumulated liquid bolus fills the posterior reservoir between the soft palate and the tongue, and, in some instances, the valleculae between the soft palate and the epiglottis.

When one or more suckling motions have collected enough liquid posteriorly, the pharynx is filled and a normal pharyngeal swallow is initiated. Breathing stops momentarily, the soft palate elevates and angulates to close off the nasopharynx, the laryngeal airway closes, and a pharyngeal contraction wave strips the lumen from top to bottom, propelling the bolus past the reflexly relaxed cricopharyngeal sphincter into the esophagus (Figure 11.5). This pharyngeal phase of swallowing is similar to that in the adult, but the posterior wall may move forward more markedly to appose the tongue, causing a prominent posterior pharyngeal wave. Sometimes the mobility of the posterior wall is quite striking (Figure 11.6). The "laryngeal sphincter" appears to play an important role in laryngeal protection in infants. During suckle feeding, the pharyngeal swallow occurs more frequently and with greater speed than in the adult.

At the end of the pharyngeal swallow, the cricopharyngeal sphincter contracts again, and is often more readily seen in the infant, outlined by barium. The nasal, pharyngeal, and laryngeal airway usually opens immediately after the swallow.

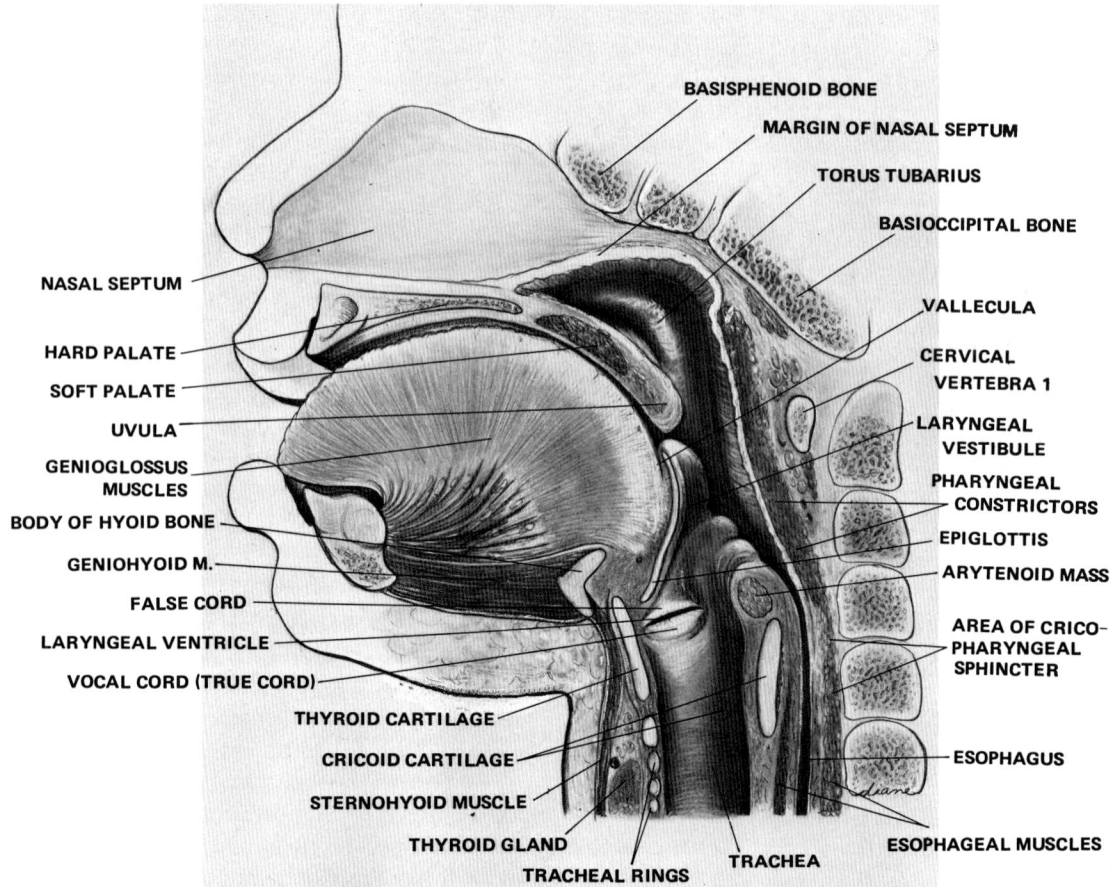

FIGURE 11.2. Normal infant anatomy in midsagittal plane. (Reprinted with permission from Kramer SS. Special swallowing problems in children. *Gastrointest Radiol* 1985;10:241–250.)

Some infants are such vigorous suckle feeders that they may take several swallows rapidly in a row without reopening the airway or taking a breath until the end of the sequence. It is easy to see why in this group of infants the last swallow in the sequence might either be incomplete or abnormal, lead to aspiration, or be associated with a drop in arterial oxygen saturation.

With rapid swallowing, peristaltic waves in the esophagus tend to summate, so that the esophagus remains "filled" in appearance (3) (Figure 11.7). The last pharyngeal swallow in the sequence triggers an esophageal peristaltic wave that results in complete esophageal stripping. In most instances, oral suckling, pharyngeal filling and contraction, and esophageal peristalsis occur in a smooth continuum or sequence of events.

The Older Child

As higher centers of central nervous system (CNS) feeding function evolve in the thalamus and then in the cerebral cortex, more and more voluntary control over the oral phase of deglutition is possible. It is at the oral stage that the greatest change occurs in feeding behavior with the growth and development of the child. Transitional feeding (19,20) develops with maturation of the CNS between the ages of 6 and 36 months. Midline mashing of purées by the tongue gives way to better manipulation of the bolus and lateralized processing of textured materials by vertical biting and chewing, a process that is accompanied by the eruption of teeth. This is followed by the development of more mature, adultlike feeding behavior. The evolution of neural function is accompanied by an anatomical evolution: development of dentition, enlargement of the oral cavity (growth of the face and base of the skull), enlargement of the pharynx, and descent of the hyoid bone and larynx (Figure 11.3). For all the change toward voluntary control in oral function, the pharyngeal and esophageal phases of swallowing remain under involuntary control, with only minor differences from the infant or child to the adult.

A number of mechanisms play a role in protecting the laryngeal airway during deglutition (Table 11.2). Their relative merits are controversial and may depend in each case on the individual patient and his or her age. However, among the more important mechanisms are the temporary cessation of respiration, the closure of the laryngeal aditus and the vocal cords, the elevation of the larynx, and an intact cough reflex.

Abnormal Swallowing Function (3,5,21–27)

A swallowing disorder may present as an isolated problem or in combination with multiple abnormalities. Only one or any number of the components of swallowing may be affected. It is important to remember that many different causes may result in the same radiographic finding. For example, deficient suckling activity in a small infant may be the consequence of anoxic brain damage, extreme prematurity, general debility, sedating medication, or respiratory decompensation. The finding must be

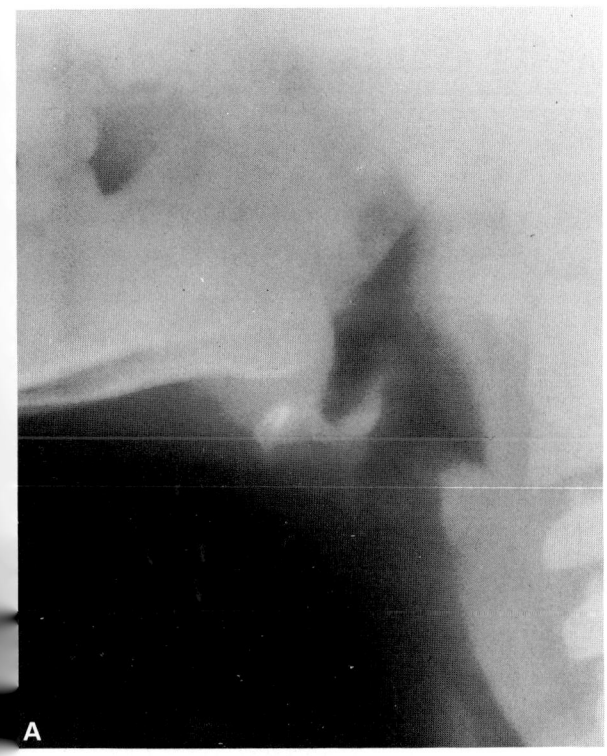
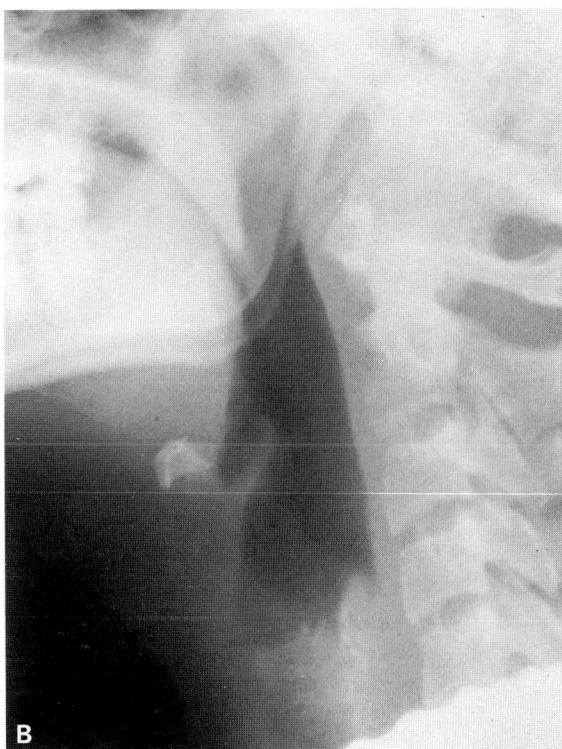

FIGURE 11.3. Comparison of (A) infant and (B) adult anatomical relationships of the pharynx and larynx to adjacent bony structures as seen on lateral radiographs. (Reprinted with permission from Kramer SS. Special swallowing problems in children. *Gastrointest Radiol* 1985;10:241–250.)

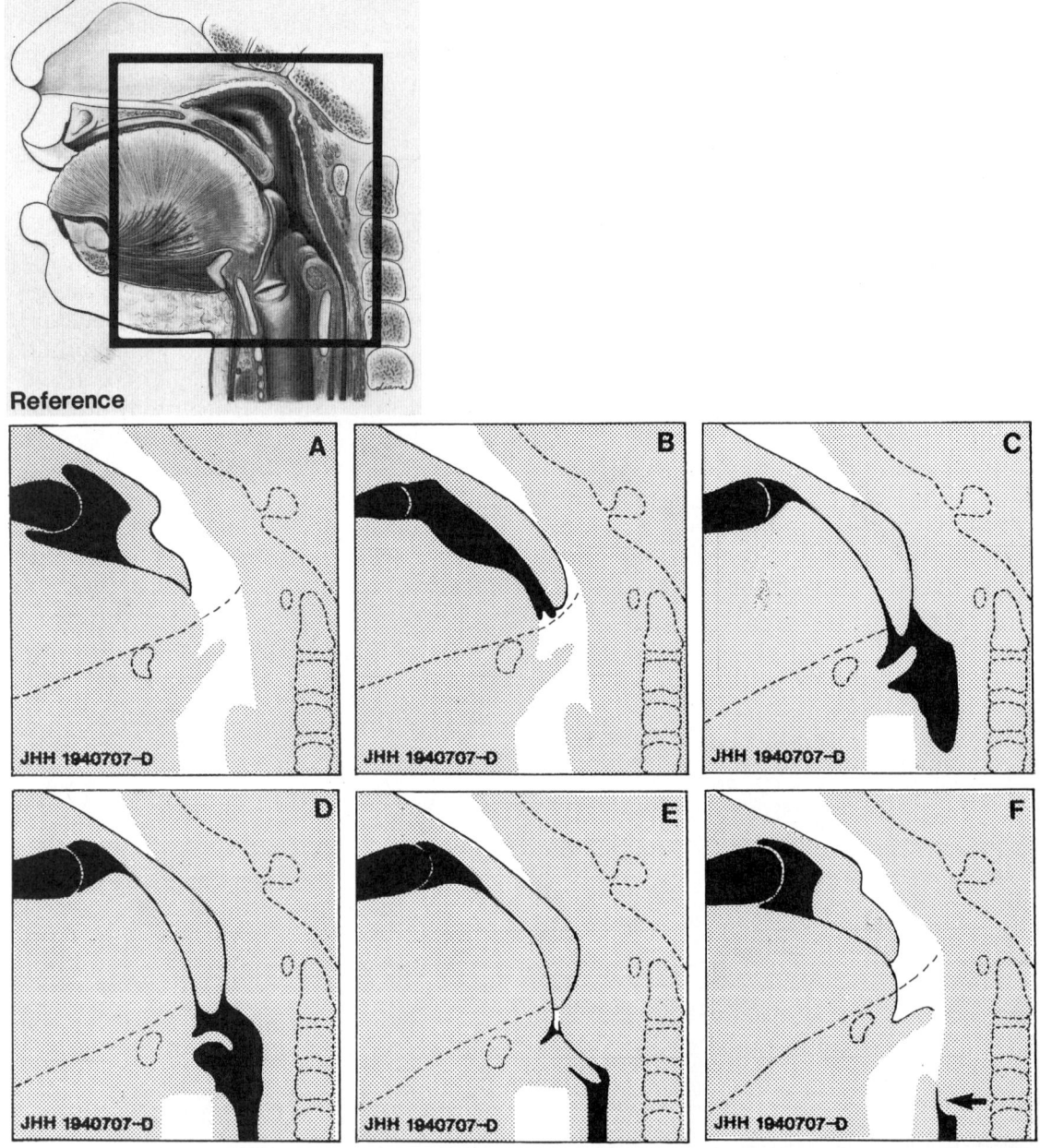

FIGURE 11.4. Drawing of normal infantile suckle feeding (lateral projections). During oral suckling, barium (black) expressed from the nipple collects posteriorly in the mouth, but is confined by the apposition of the soft palate and the tongue (A). With vigorous suckling, the soft palate configuration changes and, at times, may bow forward as the soft palate–tongue relationship is maintained. As the tongue moves the collected liquid into the pharynx (B, C), the pharyngeal swallowing sequence is initiated. The soft palate elevates, apposes the posterior pharyngeal wall, and closes off the nasopharynx. Pharyngeal contraction begins as a posterior pharyngeal wave in the superior pharyngeal constrictor. The larynx is elevating, the epiglottis is beginning to tilt, and the laryngeal vestibule is closed (C). Pharyngeal contraction, seen as a prominent posterior pharyngeal wave, transports the barium through the pharynx and the open cricopharyngeal sphincter into the esophagus (D). No barium enters the closed, elevated larynx. At the end of pharyngeal constriction, the pharynx is completely empty (E). After barium has passed into the esophagus and the cricopharyngeal sphincter has closed, the airway (white) immediately reopens (F). Note barium outlining lower margin of cricopharyngeal sphincter (arrow). (Reprinted with permission from Kramer SS. Special swallowing problems in children. *Gastrointest Radiol* 1985;10:241–250.)

11. Swallowing in Children

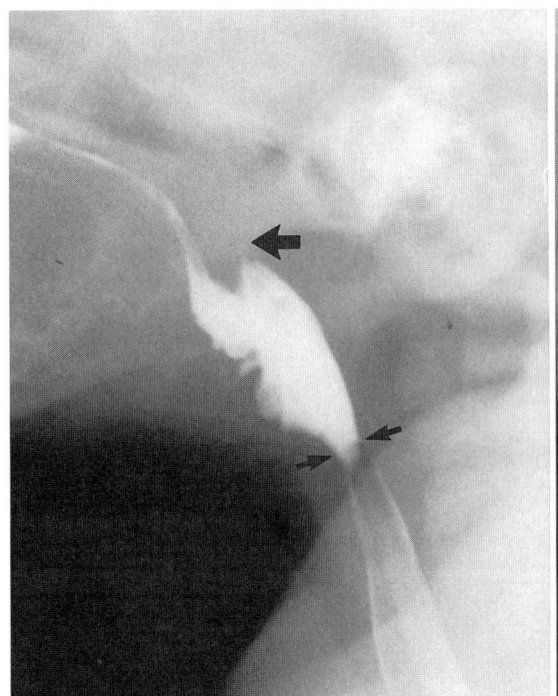
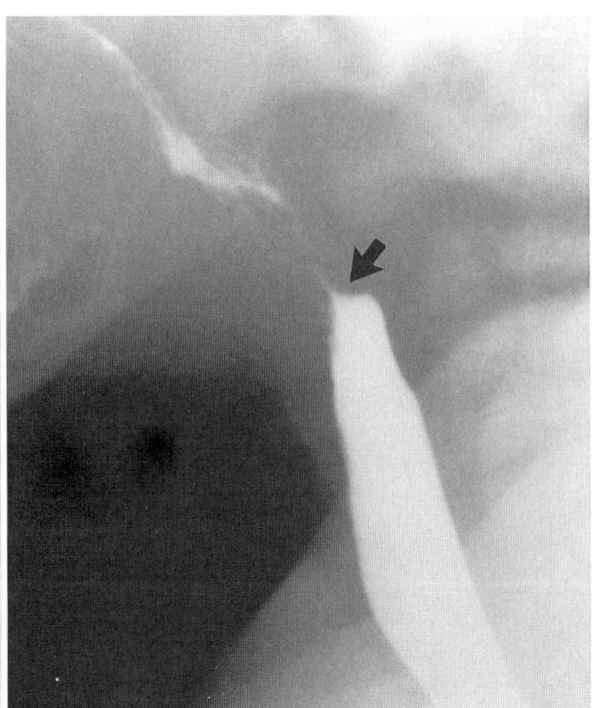
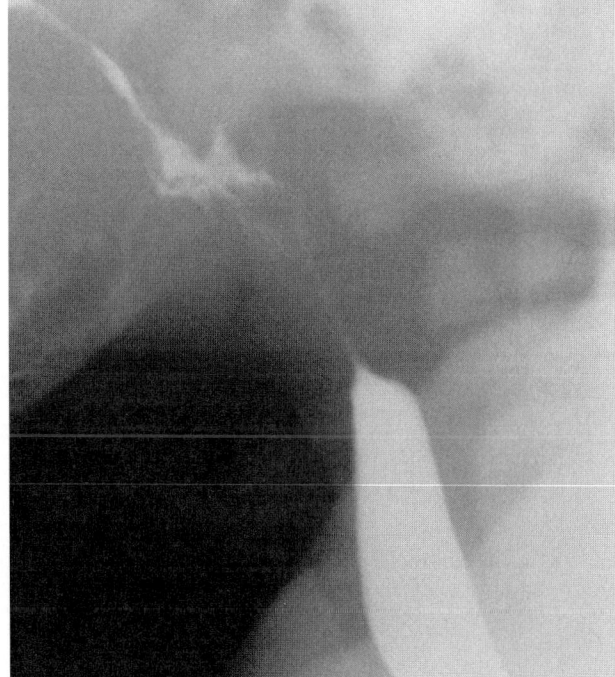

FIGURE 11.5. Spot films from fluoroscopy showing normal events in the infant's swallow. (A) The pharynx is filled and pharyngeal swallowing has begun. The soft palate is elevated, and the nasopharynx is closed. Posterior pharyngeal contraction wave has been initiated in the superior pharyngeal constrictor (large black arrow). The larynx is elevated, and the laryngeal vestibule is closed. Note the opening of the cricopharyngeal sphincter (small black arrows). (B) Pharyngeal contraction is seen as the posterior pharyngeal wave (black arrow) descends, moving the barium ahead of it through the open cricopharyngeal sphincter into the esophagus. No barium is present in the nasopharynx or larynx. (C) At the end of pharyngeal contraction, the constrictor wave has reached the cricopharyngeal sphincter, and it will continue down the esophagus as the primary wave of peristalsis. The airway has not yet reopened.

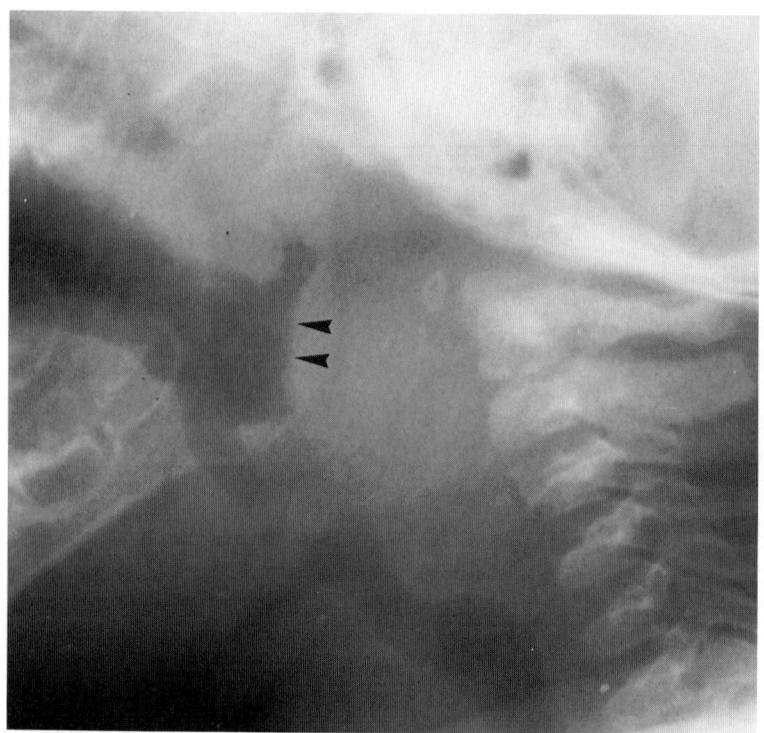

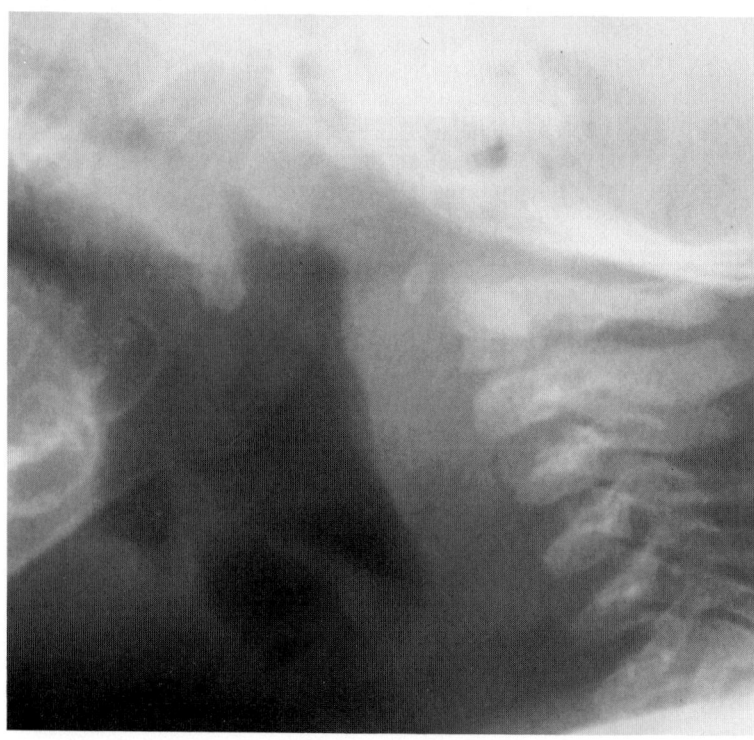

FIGURE 11.6. Spot films from fluoroscopy of a normal infant's airway. (A) The posterior pharyngeal wall (black arrowheads) has dramatically bowed forward at the end of crying. (B) An instant later, on inspiration, the pharynx is distended and the posterior wall has returned to its more familiar contour. (Reprinted with permission from Kramer SS. Radiologic examination of the swallowing impaired child. *Dysphagia* 1989;3:117–125.)

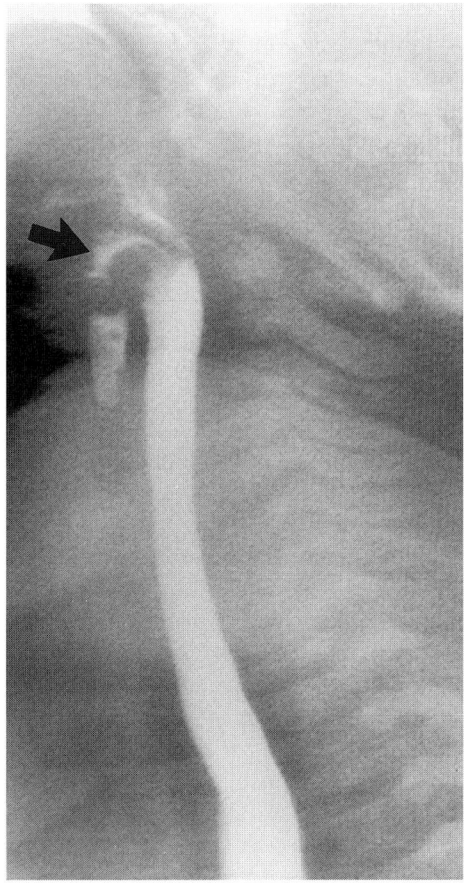

FIGURE 11.7. The column of barium in the esophagus results from rapid swallowing and summation of peristaltic waves in this infant. Laryngeal penetration (black arrow) extending below the cords is seen at the end of pharyngeal swallowing.

help the child compensate for deficits and modify negative patterns of behavior (9,29,30).

To analyze a dynamically recorded barium swallow, one must study the individual events and their coordination and timing. Multiple swallows should be reviewed, since not all swallows in a series are necessarily alike. For example, an infant may have three swallows in a row that appear perfectly normal, only to be followed by a fourth in which significant aspiration occurs. It may also be helpful to categorize abnormalities in terms of where they occur within the swallowing sequence: oral, pharyngeal, and/or esophageal phases or global (Table 11.3).

Oral Phase Abnormalities

Since so many structural and functional changes occur in the oral area, it is not surprising that the list of oral phase abnormalities in children is longer than the one for adults.

In an infant who is not sleepy, cranky, or satiated from a previous feeding, suckling deficits may appear as failure to latch onto and maintain attachment to the nipple, inability to keep the nipple properly positioned within the mouth (e.g., displacement of nipple beneath the tongue), tongue thrusting, weak or deficient tongue motion to compress the nipple, and early tiring.

Refusal of oral feedings may develop as a specific response to a type of food, a particular assessed in terms of the clinical setting, and even then the relative importance of various factors may be hard to ascertain.

Swallowing impairments seen in children are not necessarily fixed but may change and even improve with time and development. An adverse effect on swallowing performance may result from such factors as malnutrition, major stress or illness, and medications, such as seizure drugs, sedatives, and muscle relaxants. Children who are fed by gastrostomy tube because of diversions of the alimentary tract may show signs of regression in oral feeding function (28). On the other hand, oral and/or feeding therapy can play a positive role and can

TABLE 11.2. Protection of the laryngeal airway during deglutition.

Momentary suspension of respiration
Adduction of the true and false vocal cords
Valleculae and piriform sinuses = lateral food channels around the laryngeal vestibule
Elevation of the larynx
Closure of the laryngeal aditus by contraction of the oblique arytenoid and aryepiglottic muscles—the so-called laryngeal sphincter
Posterior tilt of the epiglottis
Pharyngeal contraction compressing the tilted epiglottis over the laryngeal entrance
Cough

Source: Kramer SS. Radiologic examination of the swallowing impaired child. *Dysphagia* 1989;3:117–125.

TABLE 11.3. Radiological swallowing abnormalities.

> Oral phase
>   Deficient suckling
>   Refusal of oral feeding
>   Failure to develop more mature feeding modes
>   Oral-motor dysfunction
>   Tongue abnormality
>   Premature leak into pharynx
> Pharyngeal phase
>   Delayed onset of pharyngeal swallow
>   Abnormal soft palate function
>   Nasopharyngeal reflux
>   Pharyngeal contraction/emptying deficit
>   Laryngeal penetration
>   Cricopharyngeal sphincter abnormality
> Esophageal phase
>   2° aspiration
>   Esophageal abnormality: anatomical or
>   functional gastroesophageal reflux
> Incoordination

Source: Reprinted with permission from Kramer SS. Radiologic examination of the swallowing impaired child. *Dysphagia* 1989;3:117–125.

consistency (e.g., liquids or solids), a mode of feeding, or some other specific cause, or it may be generalized. There may be an underlying functional or organic cause for such refusal that can be demonstrated by the barium study. Problems such as gastroesophageal reflux with reflux esophagitis and/or stricture, aspiration of thin liquids but not thick ones, and pharyngeal paresis exacerbated by thickened or solid boluses may be elucidated by using techniques described earlier in the section entitled "Radiological Examination Technique." Overlying feeding refusal, there may be a behavioral component associated with lack of normal oral stimulation and adverse oral hypersensitivity.

The unsuccessful development at the appropriate time of more mature oral feeding modes, such as transitional feeding or adult oral function, can occur as an isolated problem or more commonly in conjunction with other oral phase abnormalities. Occasionally a child is seen who has normal suckle feeding behavior, but at an age beyond which this should persist as the major feeding mechanism; the child has not acquired the voluntary oral functions of biting, chewing, and manipulation of a more complex diet.

Oral motor dysfunction of a generalized type is commonly seen in patients of all ages with moderate to severe cerebral palsy and mental retardation. Because of deficits in higher CNS cortical voluntary function, the child may have deficient buccal closure, resulting in drooling and abnormal tongue and jaw movements, in turn leading to difficulty in chewing, processing, and propelling liquids and solids from the anterior part of the mouth back into the pharynx. However, with intact reflex brain stem function, the pharyngeal swallowing activity may be normal, so that food placed directly into the pharynx is handled safely and effectively. An element of suckle feeding behavior may also be retained.

Tongue abnormalities include atrophy, macroglossia, ptosis associated with small mandible in Pierre-Robin syndrome (14) (Figure 11.8), and weak or abnormal motion. Rarely, masses such as cystic hygromas, hemangiomas, and teratomas can involve the tongue: after surgery, deficits may be seen.

Incomplete posterior closure of the oral cavity by apposition of the soft palate to the posterior tongue during the oral phase may result in premature leakage of material out of the mouth into the pharynx while the pharynx is serving its respiratory function. There is a great risk of aspiration in this situation. Sometimes this premature leak with its attendant incoordination between oral and pharyngeal function is difficult to differentiate from a simple delay in the onset of the pharyngeal swallowing. In each instance there is a time delay between barium reaching the pharynx and the onset of pharyngeal contraction. In the former, the tongue does not actively move the bolus posteriorly and soft palate function is abnormal as barium dribbles over the back of the tongue. In the latter, the oral phase is normal, but there is a time lag between the end of the oral phase and the beginning of the pharyngeal phase during which barium remains in the pharynx and the airway may be open.

Pharyngeal Phase Abnormalities

Nasopharyngeal reflux (Figure 11.9) results from incomplete closure of the nasopharynx at the beginning of pharyngeal swallowing. It may be due to an anatomical defect in the soft palate, such as a cleft, or it may be a functional problem caused by inadequate angulation and elevation of the soft palate to appose the posterior pharyngeal wall, limited anterior excursion of the superior pharyngeal constrictor (Passavant's cushion) to meet the soft palate, or incoordination of these functions. Small amounts of nasopharyngeal reflux may occur in premature and even normal full-term infants, usually because of transient swallowing incoordination. It may be of no clinical significance or, at times, it may be associated with infant sleep apnea (31). In older children, it is sometimes seen following adenoidectomy and in cases of nasopharyngeal masses. Patients with cleft palate or soft palate palsy/paralysis frequently have larger amounts of nasopharyngeal reflux.

Defective pharyngeal contraction and emptying (32) is seen radiographically as deficient posterior tongue thrust, a weak or disordered posterior pharyngeal stripping wave, and retention of bolus material. It should be differenti-

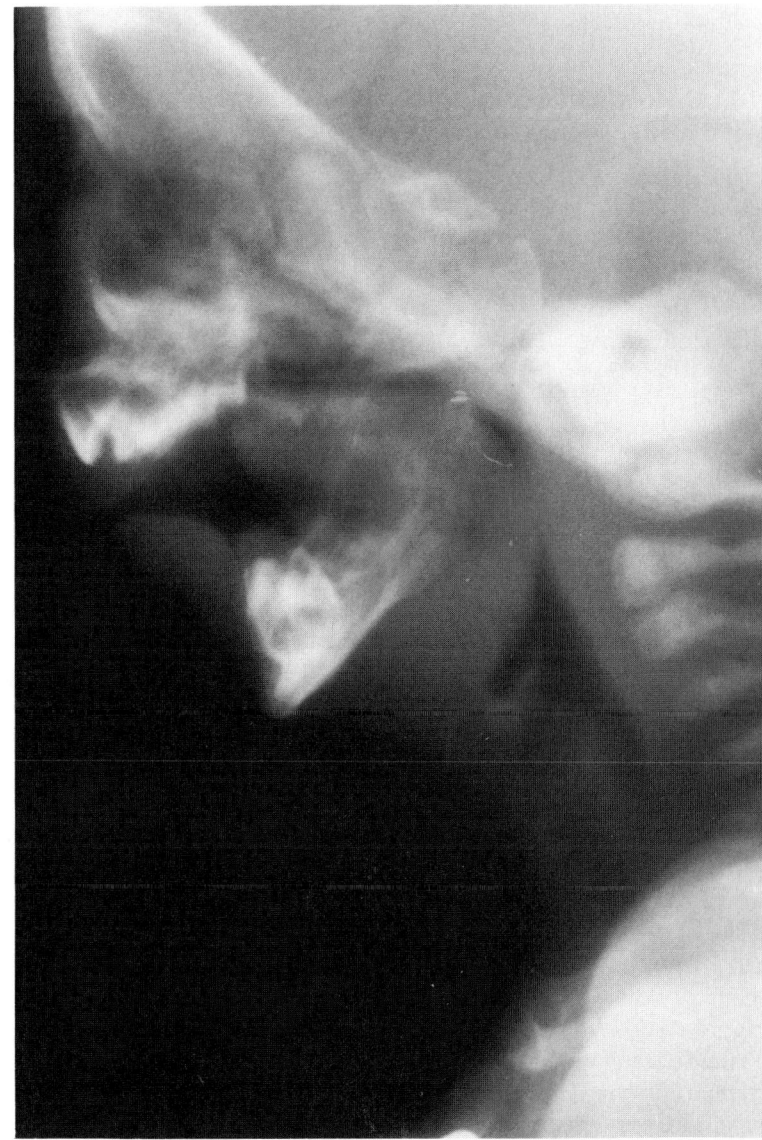

FIGURE 11.8. Pierre-Robin syndrome. Lateral radiograph of an infant demonstrates a small mandible and ptotic position of tongue, pharynx, and larynx (cf. Figure 11.2). (Reprinted with permission from Kramer SS. Special swallowing problems in children. *Gastrointest Radiol* 1985;10:241–250.)

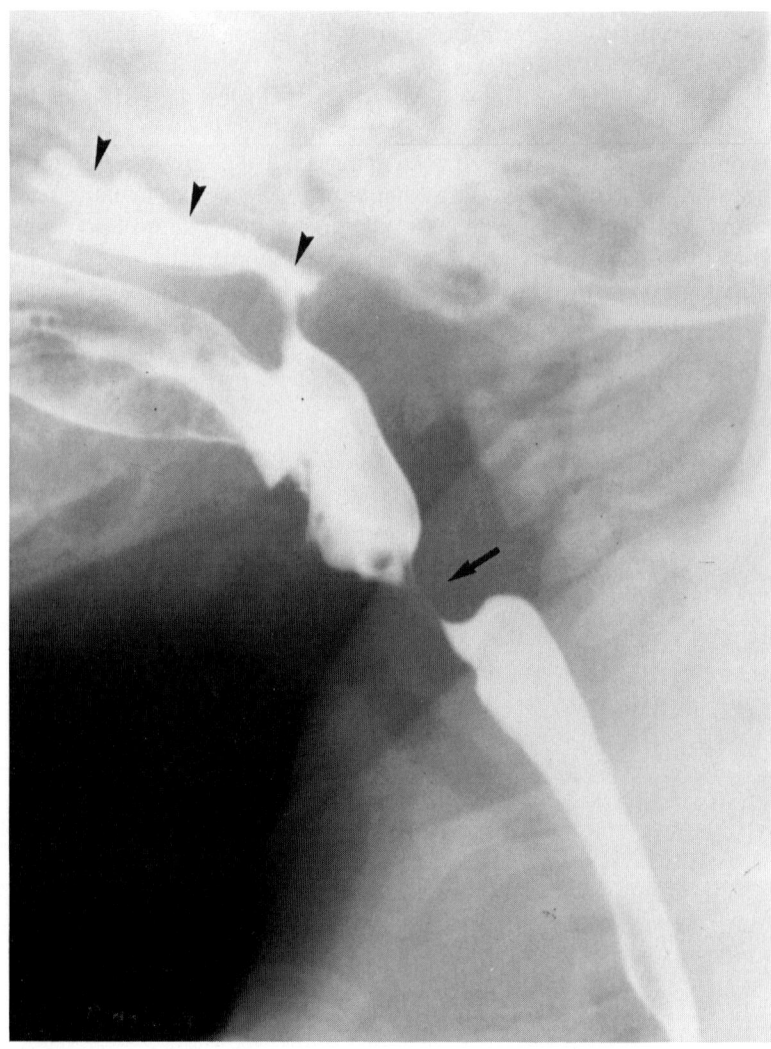

FIGURE 11.9. Nasopharyngeal reflux (black arrowheads) in a 5-month-old infant with paroxysmal cough and choking spells with feeding, accompanied by apnea and cyanosis. The prominent cricopharyngeal impression (black arrow) is associated with gastroesophageal reflux in this case. (Reprinted with permission from Kramer SS. Radiologic examination of the swallowing impaired child. *Dysphagia* 1989;3:117–125.)

ated from incomplete emptying caused by obstruction at the cricopharyngeal sphincter. Both, however, are precursors of secondary aspiration.

In normal infants, a small amount of barium may transiently enter the laryngeal aditus above the vocal cords and be promptly "squeezed" back out during pharyngeal contraction. Laryngeal penetration (Figures 11.7 and 11.10) occurs when barium directly enters an incompletely protected laryngeal airway and extends below the vocal cords, even into the trachea, during the pharyngeal swallow. Radiographically, one may see inadequate laryngeal elevation, paralysis of the vocal cords, incomplete closure of the laryngeal vestibule (the so-called laryngeal sphincter), and failure of tilt of the epiglottis.

Laryngeal penetration, which happens during pharyngeal contraction, is different from aspiration, which occurs during breathing. Material may be "aspirated" in the oral phase in instances of premature leak into the pharynx, in the pharyngeal phase when there is delayed triggering of the pharyngeal swallow after pharyngeal filling, or in the esophageal phase if there is residue in the pharynx left by inadequate pharyngeal stripping (Figure 11.11), upper esophageal sphincter obstruction, or gastroesophageal reflux resulting in esophagopharyngeal regurgitation. In all cases of airway soiling, it is important to note the presence or absence of a cough response, to estimate the extent and volume of the aspirate, and to exclude the possibility of a laryngeal cleft or tracheoesophageal fistula.

Cricopharyngeal sphincter abnormalities (33–37) include absent, incomplete, or delayed opening or early closure of the sphincter during swallowing. A prominent posterior cricopharyngeal impression may be seen, frequently in association with gastroesophageal reflux (Figure 11.9). Although physiological tonic contraction of the pharyngoesophageal segment between swallows protects the pharynx from regurgitated esophageal contents, this mechanism sometimes fails. Webs or lateral pharyngeal pouches are seen in the same vicinity in rare instances.

Esophageal Phase Abnormalities

Anatomical and functional abnormalities of the esophagus, which interfere with normal swal-

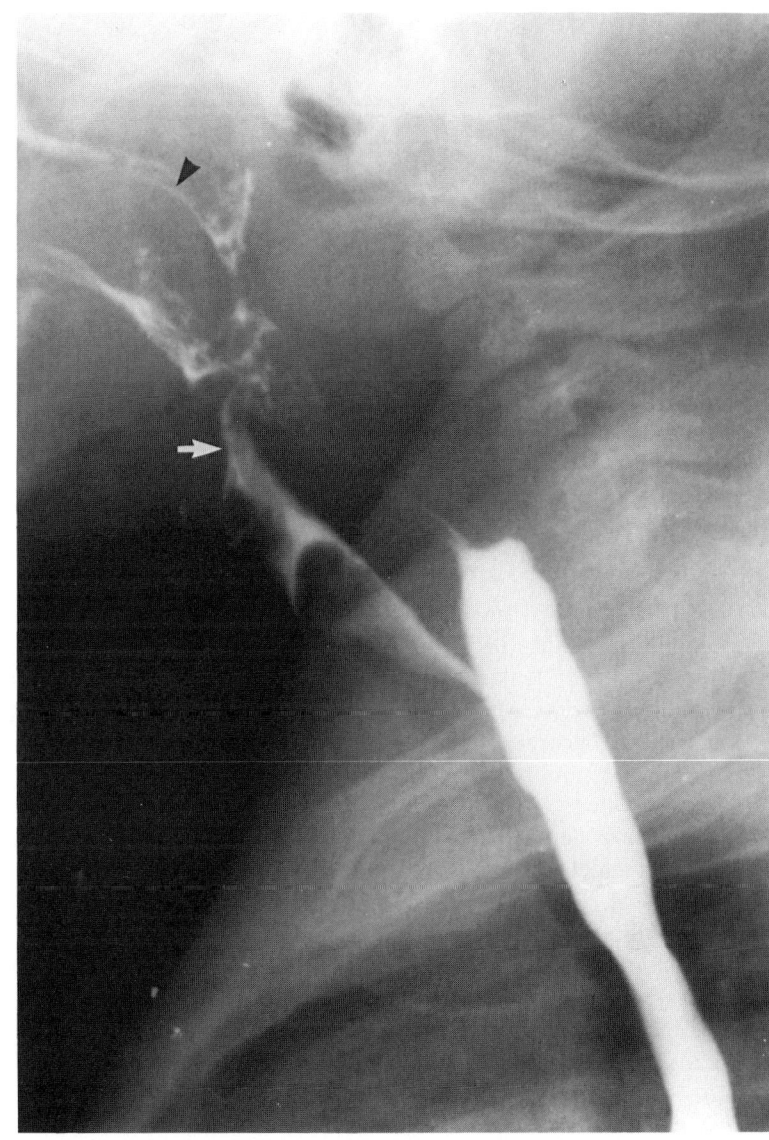

FIGURE 11.10. Direct laryngeal penetration (white arrow) during swallow and nasopharyngeal reflux (black arrowhead) have occurred during a barium examination in a neurologically impaired 10-month-old infant. (Reprinted with permission from Kramer SS. Special swallowing problems in children. *Gastrointest Radiol* 1985;10:241–250.)

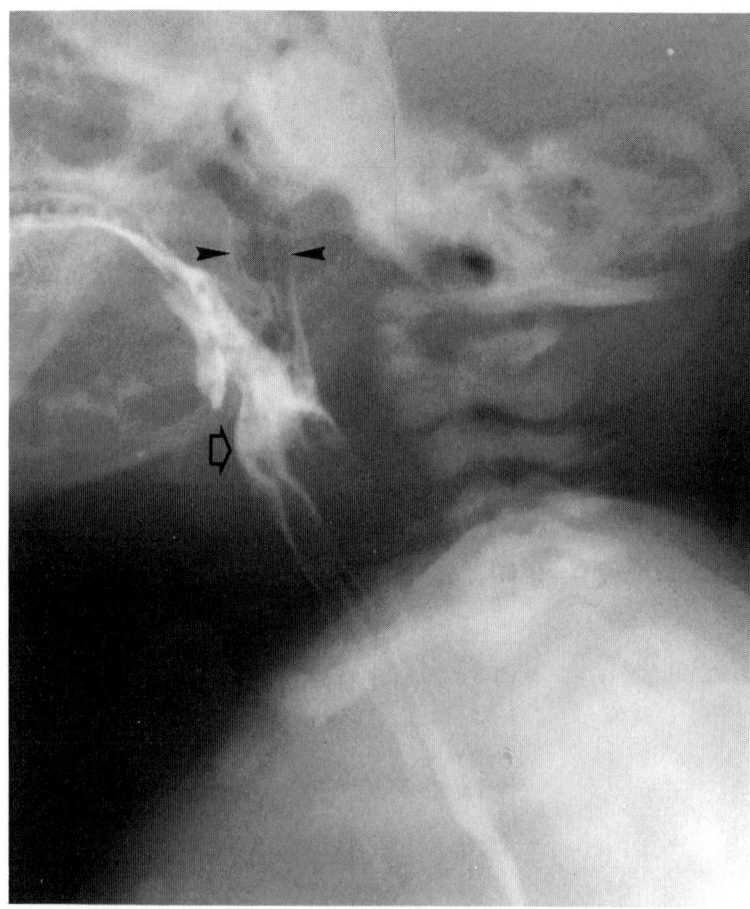

FIGURE 11.11. Abnormal swallowing function has resulted in secondary aspiration in a brain-damaged 8-day-old infant. The nasopharynx (between black arrowheads) and larynx (open arrow) are open as the infant "breathes in" barium remaining in the pharynx after the swallow. (Reprinted with permission from Kramer SS. Radiologic examination of the swallowing impaired child. *Dysphagia* 1989;3:117–125.)

lowing performance and can lead to overflow aspiration, are well depicted by barium examination. They include lye stricture, abnormalities following repair of esophageal atresia/tracheoesophageal fistula (disordered peristalsis, recurrent fistula or leak, and anastomotic or reflux-induced stricture) (38) (Figure 11.12), and achalasia. Gastroesophageal reflux is by far the most common and controversial late esophageal stage event to complicate swallowing (2,6,30).

Aspirated material, either swallowed food or refluxed gastric contents, can affect the respiratory tract either by stimulating receptors in the mucosa, which by vagal pathways leads to reflex apnea, laryngospasm, or bronchospasm (2,6), or by directly interfering with function through the chemical/physical nature or volume of the aspirate. As an example of the latter effect, large particles may lodge in the larynx and cause a choking episode or asphyxia. Smaller particles, which may reach the bronchi, can result in atelectasis, air trapping, or focal inflammation. Aspirated liquids, depending on composition, volume, and host defenses, can damage the airways more peripherally or even cause aspiration pneumonia; recurrent injury may lead to bronchiectasis and recurrent pneumonia. Many of these complications of aspiration are best portrayed by radiographic techniques.

Other Imaging Studies (7)

Upper Gastrointestinal (UGI) Series

The remainder of the upper gastrointestinal tract, including the esophagus, stomach, duodenum, and proximal jejunum, may be examined, usually as a separate fluoroscopic study. Esophageal anatomy and mucosal pattern, peristalsis, gastroesophageal reflux (GER), hiatal hernia, gastric and duodenal anatomy, gastric emptying, inflammatory lesions, malrotation, and other obstructing lesions can be assessed by this technique.

Nuclear Medicine Studies

The technetium (^{99m}Tc) labeled milk scan can demonstrate and quantitate pharyngeal and esophageal transit, GER episodes occurring and clearing during the study, and gastric emptying (39). Occasionally, aspiration of ingested or refluxed material may be documented.

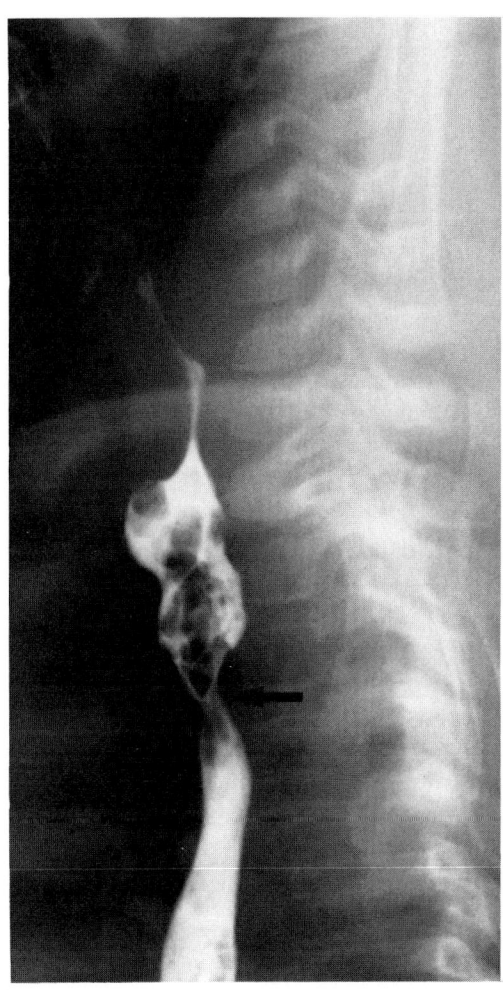
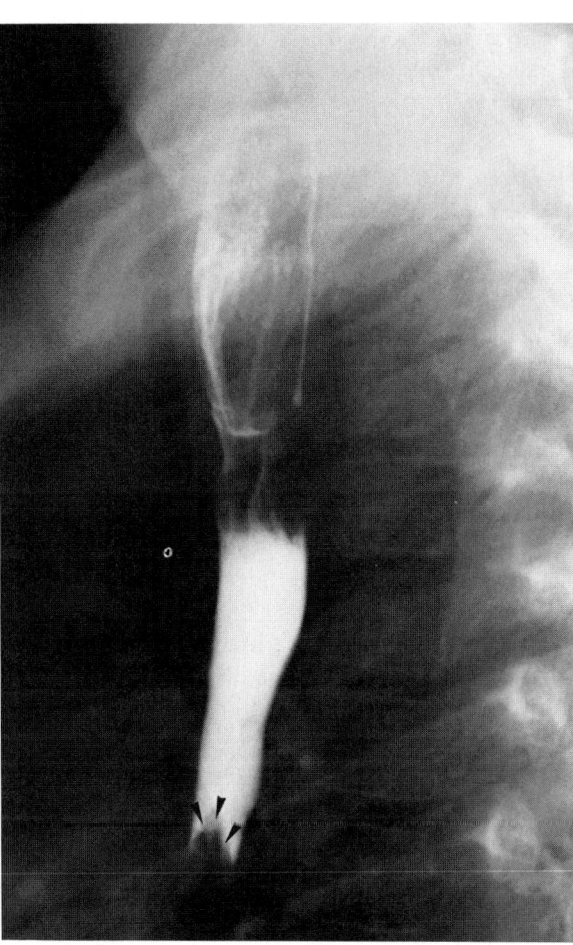

FIGURE 11.12. Lateral views from barium esophagograms performed on two different children who have had esophageal atresia and tracheoesophageal fistula repairs. Each child has nonopaque foreign matter impacted at an esophageal stricture. (A) Sunflower seeds are causing a partial obstruction at the strictured site of the original esophageal anastomosis (arrow). (B) The anastomosis in the midesophagus is widely patent, but inspissated food has resulted in complete obstruction at a stricture in the lower esophagus caused by reflux esophagitis (arrowheads). (Reprinted with permission from Kramer SS. Pediatric radiology corner: complications following esophageal atresia repair. *Dysphagia* 1989;3:155–156.)

Ultrasound Examination

Noninvasive ultrasonography can be used to image the oral cavity. From the submental approach, the transducer can demonstrate the motion of the tongue and floor of the mouth in several planes during feeding (40,41). Observations made with this technique have added to our understanding of oral motor function, peristaltic tongue motion during suckle feeding, and the coordination of suckling, swallowing, and breathing (42). However, acoustic shadowing from bones and intraluminal air limits visualization of the pharynx, and ultrasonography remains primarily a research tool.

Other Diagnostic Studies (7)

pH Probe Study

Many children with neuromuscular dysfunction and swallowing impairment also have gastroesophageal reflux. It may manifest itself by further complicating swallowing function, vomiting or regurgitation, refusal of feeds, gastrointestinal bleeding, or respiratory problems including recurrent pneumonia or tracheobronchitis (43). Bronchospasm, laryngospasm, and apnea (44) have been linked to GER as a result of either aspiration or the stimulation of vagally mediated irritant receptors.

The pH probe study is readily available and is a more sensitive test for the occurrence and severity of GER than a UGI series. Endoscopy and biopsy are the gold standard for the diagnosis of reflux esophagitis.

Manometry

Manometry has been used to document esophageal motor function, and more recently to study pharyngeal peristalsis and upper esophageal sphincter responsiveness with the aid of a specially designed catheter or probe. Intraluminal pressure recordings are correlated to provide a picture of motor activity and coordination during swallowing. This procedure is moderately invasive, technically demanding, and requires sophisticated equipment and trained personnel (45). It has had limited clinical applications in children.

Fiberoptic Endoscopic Swallowing Evaluations

Fiberoptic endoscopic evaluations have been used to assess pharyngeal anatomy and pharyngeal swallowing function (46,47) and to perform sensory testing in the larynx and pharynx (48). The presence of retained secretions or inflammation, the movement of the pharyngeal walls and larynx, the timing of pharyngeal swallowing events, and laryngeal penetration or aspiration can be documented. Postswallow residue, aspiration, and cough reflex can be noted, along with the effects of therapeutic maneuvers, such as a change in feeding consistencies and patient positioning. This examination is invasive, requires special equipment and experienced personnel, and does not evaluate the oral phase. Its applications in children have so far been limited.

Managing Feeding Problems (49)

Because feeding difficulties in children usually result from the interaction of multiple factors, managing them can be difficult, time-consuming, and frustrating. Effective treatment (8,50) usually requires intervention from more than one therapeutic discipline. The treatment team, including the child's caregiver, needs to prioritize the goals of treatment and outline an integrated plan to approach these goals. The primary care provider, with input from the team, oversees the plan and monitors progress toward the goals. This is done in the context of the child's medical, nutritional, and developmental well-being.

Treatment should focus on (1) minimizing factors identified during the assessment as contributing to the feeding dysfunction and (2) facilitating positive practice. Components of a successful treatment strategy include minimizing negative medical influences, optimizing positioning for feeding, facilitating oral-motor function, improving the mealtime environment, being consistent, and constantly monitoring the child's progress.

Common Medical Conditions Contributing to Poor Feeding

Gastroesophageal reflux can interfere with feeding success in multiple ways: decreased intake associated with discomfort from reflux of larger intragastric volumes and reflux esophagitis, increased losses from emesis, adverse influence on respiratory function, restriction of oral-motor pattern, and limitations on body positioning. A number of therapeutic modalities, including proper positioning, meal modification, medications, and surgery, may be needed to control these difficulties (51). The goal of each of these interventions is to protect the esophagus from reflux of stomach acid, either by decreasing the amount of food in the stomach at any one time or by decreasing the amount of acidic stomach juices that are excreted.

Constipation may also interfere with feeding because of slowed motility, increased intra-abdominal pressure, and the possibility of increasing GER.

Respiratory compromise may interfere with feeding (52). Therapies include adequate oxygenation for "work" of feeding and the use of the easiest textures for the child to facilitate intake.

Proper Positioning for Feeding

Feeding is a flexor activity that requires good breathing support. Appropriate positioning maximizes the child's ability to both flex and breathe (53). The child should be firmly supported through the hips and trunk to provide a stable base. The head and neck should be aligned in a neutral position, which decreases extension through the oral musculature while maintaining an open airway. Such positioning allows improved coordination and more control of the steps in oral-motor preparation and transport. This in turn results in more positive feedback to the child and caregiver from good feeding experiences (54).

Optimization of Oral-Motor Function

Facilitating jaw and lip closure when necessary may help make the child's oral feeding pattern more effective, as well as accustom the child to the proper position for accepting food (55). Spoon placement with gentle pressure on the midtongue region can help remind the child to keep the tongue inside the mouth. Chewing may be enhanced by placing food between the upper and lower back teeth. This encourages the child to move the jaw and use the tongue in an effort to dislodge the food.

Food textures can be manipulated to facilitate safe, controlled swallowing (56). Thickening of liquids slows their rate of flow, allowing more time for the child to organize and initiate a swallow. Thickening agents or instant pudding powders can transform any thin liquid into a nectar-, honey-, or milk shakelike consistency. This provides children who have difficulty drinking more options to ensure adequate hydration. Almost any food can be chopped fine or puréed to a texture that the child may more competently manage.

It is important to remember that the primary goal of eating is to achieve adequate nutrition. Thus, when a child is first learning to accept higher texture foods, these foods should be presented during snacktime, when volumes are smaller. At mealtimes, easier textures should be used to ensure consumption of adequate calories during the transition period.

Making the "Work" of Mealtimes More Inviting

Eating requires more coordination among muscle groups than any other motor activity. Therefore, it is important to make eating as easy as possible (57). This can be accomplished by increasing the child's focus on the meal and including foods in each meal that are more desirable and easier for the child to control (58). Let the child know that mealtime is coming so he or she can prepare for the "work" to be done. This may entail a premeal preparatory routine or relaxation therapy followed by oral stimulation to get the needed muscles ready for eating. Children with feeding difficulties usually eat better in one-on-one situations or in small groups, because there is less distraction, and they are better able to focus on the eating process. Undivided attention also makes mealtimes more reinforcing.

A number of adaptive devices can promote independence in feeding. These include bowls with high sides, spoons with built-up or curved handles, and cups with rocker bottoms. The satisfaction children get from eating can be increased by social attention during the meal or by providing a favorite food after the meal is completed.

Summary

Pediatric feeding problems often occur in the presence of neuromuscular impairment, anatomical anomalies, or syndromes. They are frequently complicated by the demands of growth and development, high nutritional needs, growing anatomical structures, and a maturing central nervous system. In infants and young children with dysphagia, feeding skills must be learned without a foundation of existing skills. This task is often made more difficult by the child's inability to communicate clinical information or fully comprehend instructions. The fluoroscopic examination provides the best demonstration of the swallowing mechanism and, therefore, plays a central role in the diagnostic evaluation of any child with a swallowing impairment. Most pediatric feeding difficulties are complex and necessitate a multidisciplinary approach by specialists from different disciplines to correctly diagnose the contributing factors, appreciate the problem's effect on the patient's daily life, and construct a successful treatment plan.

References

1. Kramer SS. On the care and feeding of children [editorial]. *Dysphagia* 1989;3:109–110.
2. Tuchman DN. Cough, choke, sputter: the evaluation of the child with dysfunctional swallowing. *Dysphagia* 1989;3:111–116.
3. Kramer SS. Special swallowing problems in children. *Gastrointest Radiol* 1985;10:241–250.
4. Kosko JR, et al. Differential diagnosis of dysphagia in children. *Otolaryngol Clin North Am* 1998;31:435–450.
5. Kramer SS. Radiologic examination of the swallowing impaired child. *Dysphagia* 1989;3:117–125.
6. Loughlin GM. Respiratory consequences of dysfunctional swallowing and aspiration. *Dysphagia* 1989;3:126–130.
7. Kramer SS, Eicher PS. The evaluation of pediatric feeding abnormalities. *Dysphagia* 1993;8:215–224.
8. Stevenson RD, Allaire JH. The development of normal feeding and swallowing. *Pediatr Clin North Am* 1991;38:1439–1453.
9. Christenson JR. Developmental approach to pediatric neurogenic dysphagia. *Dysphagia* 1989;3:131–134.
10. Bosma JF. Physiology of the mouth, pharynx, and esophagus: physiology of the mouth. In: Paparella MA, Shumrick DA, eds. *Otolaryngology*. Philadelphia: WB Saunders; 1980:319–331.
11. Bosma JF, Donner MW. Physiology of the mouth, pharynx, and esophagus: physiology of the pharynx. In: Paparella MA, Shumrick DA, eds. *Otolaryngology*. Philadelphia: WB Saunders; 1980:332–345.
12. Jones B, Kramer SS, Donner MW. Dynamic imaging of the pharynx. *Gastrointest Radiol* 1985;10:213–224.
13. Ardran GM, Kemp FH. The mechanism of changes in form of the cervical airway in infancy. *Med Radiogr Photogr* 1968;44:26–38.
14. Bosma J. Oral and pharyngeal development and function. *J Den Res* 1963;42:375–380.
15. Bosma JF. Anatomic and physiologic development of the speech apparatus. In: Tower DB, ed. *The Nervous System*. Vol 3. New York: Raven Press; 1975:469–481.
16. Bosma JF. Introduction to the symposium. In: Bosma JF, Showacre J, eds. *Symposium on Development of Upper Respiratory Anatomy and Function: Implications for Sudden Infant Death Syndrome*. Washington, DC: US Government Printing Office; 1976:5–49.
17. Ardran GM, Kemp FH, Lind J. A cineradiographic study of bottle feeding. *Br J Radiol* 1958;31:11–22.
18. Bosma JF. Postnatal ontogeny of performances of the pharynx, larynx, and mouth. *Am Rev Respir Dis* 1985;131(suppl):S10–S15.
19. Bosma JF. Development of feeding. *Clin Nutr* 1986;5:210–218.

20. Bosma JF. Oral-pharyngeal interactions in feeding. Paper presented at: Symposium on Dysphagia; February 27, 1986; the Johns Hopkins Medical Institutions.
21. Logan WJ, Bosma JF. Oral and pharyngeal dysphagia in infancy. *Pediatr Clin North Am* 1967; 14:47–61.
22. Illingworth RS. Sucking and swallowing difficulties in infancy: diagnostic problem of dysphagia. *Arch Dis Child* 1969;44:655–665.
23. Ardran GM, Kemp FH. Some important factors in the assessment of oropharyngeal function. *Dev Med Child Neurol* 1970;12:158–166.
24. Fisher SE, Painter M, Milmoe G. Swallowing disorders in infancy. *Pediatr Clin North Am* 1981;28: 845–853.
25. Franken EA. Swallowing disorders. In: *Gastrointestinal Imaging in Pediatrics.* Harper & Row: New York; 1982:26–32.
26. Gryboski J, Walker WA. Suck and swallow. In: *Gastrointestinal Problems in the Infant.* Philadelphia: WB Saunders; 1983:12–29.
27. Cohen SR. Difficulty with swallowing. In: Bluestone CD, Stool SE, eds. *Pediatric Otolaryngology.* Philadelphia: WB Saunders; 1983: 903–911.
28. Monahan PS, Shapiro B, Fox C. Effect of tube feeding on oral function. *Dev Med Child Neurol* 1988;57(suppl):7.
29. Morris SE. Developmental implications for the management of feeding problems in neurologically impaired infants. *Semin Speech Lang* 1985;6:293–315.
30. Morris SE. Development of oral-motor skills in the neurologically impaired child receiving non-oral feedings. *Dysphagia* 1989;3:135–154.
31. Plaxido DT, Loughlin GM. Nasopharyngeal reflux and neonatal apnea. *Am J Dis Child* 1981;135:793.
32. Ardran GM, et al. Congenital dysphagia resulting from dysfunction of the pharyngeal musculature. *Dev Med Child Neurol* 1965;7:157–166.
33. Margulies SI, et al. Familial dysautonomia: a cineradiographic study of the swallowing mechanism. *Radiology* 1968;90:107–112.
34. Gyepes MT, Linde LM. Familial dysautonomia: the mechanism of aspiration. *Radiology* 1968;91: 471–475.
35. Bishop HC. Cricopharyngeal achalasia in childhood. *J Pediatr Surg* 1974;9:775–778.
36. Giedion A, Nolte K. The nonobstructive pharyngo-esophageal cross roll. *Ann Radiol* 1973;161:129–135.
37. Utian HL, Thomas RG. Cricopharyngeal incoordination in infancy. *Pediatrics* 1969;43:402–406.
38. Kramer SS. Pediatric radiology corner: complications following esophageal atresia repair. *Dysphagia* 1989;3:155–156.
39. Heyman S, Eicher PS, Alavi A. Radionuclide studies of the upper gastrointestinal tract in children with feeding disorders. *J Nucl Med* 1995;36: 351–354.
40. Smith WL, et al. Physiology of sucking in the normal term infant using real-time ultrasound. *Radiology* 1985;156:379–381.
41. Bosma JF, et al. Ultrasound demonstration of tongue motions during suckle feeding. *Dev Med Child Neurol* 1990;32:223–229.
42. Yang WT, et al. Ultrasound assessment of swallowing in malnourished disabled children. *Br J Radiol* 1997;70:992–994.
43. Bagwell CE. Gastroesophageal reflux in children. In: *Surgery Annual;* 1995:133–163.
44. Thach BT. Reflux associated apnea in infants: evidence for a laryngeal chemoreflex. *Am J Med* 1997;103(5A):120S–124S.
45. Staiano A, et al. Disorders of upper esophageal sphincter motility in children. *J Pediatr Gastroenterol Nutr* 1987;6:892–898.
46. Leder SB. Serial fiberoptic endoscopic swallowing evaluations in the management of patients with dysphagia. *Arch Phys Med Rehab* 1998;79: 1264–1269.
47. Leder SB, Karas DE. Fiberoptic endoscopic evaluation of swallowing in the pediatric population. *Laryngoscope* 2000;110:1132–1136.
48. Link DT, et al. Pediatric laryngopharyngeal sensory testing during flexible endoscopic evaluation of swallowing: feasible and correlative. *Ann Otol Rhinol Laryngol* 2000;109:899–905.
49. Arvedson JC. Management of pediatric dysphagia. *Otolaryngol Clin North Am* 1998;31:453–477.
50. Sonies BC. Swallowing disorders and rehabilitation techniques. *J Pediatr Gastroenterol Nutr* 1997;25:S32–S33.
51. Lewis ME, et al. Impact of nutritional rehabilitation on gastroesophageal reflux in neurologically impaired children. *J Pediatr Surg* 1994;29:167–170.
52. Timms BJM, et al. Increased respiratory drive as an inhibitor of oral feeding of preterm infants. *J Pediatr* 1993;123:127–131.
53. Larnert G, Ekberg O. Positioning improves the oral and pharyngeal swallowing function in children with cerebral palsy. *Acta Paediatr* 1995;84: 689–692.

54. Kerwin ME, Osborne M, Eicher PS. Effect of position and support on oral-motor skills of a child with bronchopulmonary dysplasia. *Clin Pediatr* 1994;33:8–13.
55. Gisel EG, et al. Oral motor skills following sensorimotor therapy in two groups of moderately dysphagic children with cerebral palsy. *Dysphagia* 1996;11:59–71.
56. Gisel EG. Oral motor skills following sensorimotor intervention in the moderately eating-impaired child with cerebral palsy. *Dysphagia* 1994;9:180–192.
57. Kerwin ME, et al. The costs of eating: a behavioral economic analysis of food refusal. *J Appl Behav Anal* 1995;28:245–260.
58. Luiselli JK. Oral feeding treatment of children with chronic food refusal and multiple developmental disabilities. *Am J Mental Retard* 1994;98:646–655.

12
Aging and Neurological Disease

BRONWYN JONES

Does aging affect the pharynx? Can the same standards be applied to a 70-year-old swallow as to a 20-year-old swallow? Can laryngeal penetration and retention in the pharynx be normal findings in an 80-year-old? What exactly is aging, and how does it affect the swallow?

Aging

Aging, according to *Stedman's Medical Dictionary* (26th edition, p. 38) is "the process of growing old, especially by failure of replacement of cells in sufficient number to maintain full functional capacity" and also "the gradual deterioration of a mature organism from time-dependent irreversible changes in structure that are intrinsic to the particular species, and that eventually lead to decreased ability to cope with the stresses of the environment, thereby increasing the probability of death."

So, how can these definitions apply to the swallowing process, namely, oral, pharyngeal, laryngeal, and esophageal function and structure?

What Is Presbyphagia?

It is important to think about swallowing in the elderly (presbyphagia) (1) under two separate categories:

1. The effects of the normal aging process on the organs of swallowing (primary presbyphagia)
2. The effects of other diseases that afflict the aged (such as cerebrovascular accident and Parkinson's disease) on swallowing (secondary presbyphagia)

Sheth and Diner (2) have discussed this concept in depth in a recommended review in the journal, *Dysphagia*.

The question is, When does "aging" begin?

There are genetic syndromes in humans with many features of accelerated aging, such as Down's syndrome and progeria (3). In this context, it is thought that motoneuron aging is programmed genetically, but that secondary factors may influence the time course (e.g., exhaustion of motoneurons following increased metabolic demands).

Experimentally, electrical stimuli of low, gradually increasing intensity were applied to single motor units and the results compared at different ages (4). It was found that there is little loss of functioning motoneurons before the age of 60 years but there is a striking and progressive depletion subsequently. Assuming that the concept of stress-induced exhaustion is correct, motoneurons will age faster also in conditions in which there is partial denervation such as following poliomyelitis (i.e., the "post-polio syndrome"). Motoneuron disease (amyotrophic lateral sclerosis, or Lou Gehrig's disease) may actually represent an accelerated form of aging affecting the neuromuscular system.

Prevalence

Prevalence studies for dysphagia conducted in general hospitals and nursing homes have yielded surprisingly high numbers, namely, 12 to 20% in a general hospital and 50 to 90% in a nursing home (5). Although swallowing impairment occurs in all age groups, the elderly clearly are the largest group affected. As individuals survive longer owing to improved life support systems and refined surgical techniques in head and neck cancer, more and more people will develop degenerative disorders or postoperative swallowing difficulties.

Experimental Studies

There are some experimental data and clinical observations of aging in the muscles and nerves of the head and neck in swallowing in the elderly (6,7).

It has been observed that the number of nerve terminal branches per end plate at the neuromuscular junction of muscles involved in continuous repetitive activity, such as the diaphragm, appear to be less affected by aging than the less frequently recruited motor innervation of limb muscles (8).

It was suggested (8) that "muscle activity may therefore play a major role in determining how end-plate morphology changes in response to aging. Indirect evidence obtained from regenerating tissue supports this hypothesis" (e.g., electrical stimulators and forced exercise have been shown to be associated with increased sprouting of nerve terminals). It is conceivable that the repetitive activity of the tongue and pharynx during swallowing, breathing, and speech can be compared with these observations made on the diaphragm.

Changes in the Mouth with Aging (Table 12.1)

Tongue position and movements are often altered in older people (9). The anterior position of the tongue associated with altered speech, dysphagia, and traumatic bite injuries in the elderly has been attributed to changes in the function of the suspensory muscles of the tongue (9,10). The tongue and hyoid bone are low in position owing to ptosis and weakness of suprahyoid musculature.

Changes in lip posture may be one of the reasons for drooling of saliva, not uncommon in older persons (9). Saliva output itself is altered by aging, xerostomia being a common problem. The senses of taste and smell are also blunted, resulting in decreased appeal of food (11). Changes and limitation of mastication may result from temporomandibular joint disease (12) or from poor dentition.

In a longitudinal study of oral health in 863 healthy veterans, masticatory muscle function did not change significantly with aging in those who had natural teeth or fixed replacement for missing teeth. The number of chewing strokes necessary to prepare food for swallowing, however, did increase significantly with age (13).

Lingual-palatal closure pressure at the tongue tip, and 3 and 6 cm, respectively, from the tip, during dry swallows and swallowing of water, mashed potatoes, and honey were measured in a young control group and in an elderly group (14). It was found that oral peristaltic wave amplitude for all bolus variables was significantly lower and the duration of peristaltic waves at all sites was generally longer with aging. On the other hand, consistency-dependent modulatory feedback between the oral cavity and the brain stem swallowing centers appeared to be preserved in the elderly, since in both the younger control group and in the elderly the amplitude of the wave was significantly increased with mashed potatoes and honey over the height with water, and the increases were not significantly different between young and old.

Changes in the Pharynx with Age (Table 12.1)

Upward movemen of the larynx and hyoid bone are an important component of safe swallowing. Decreased excursion due to sus-

TABLE 12.1. Changes in swallowing with aging.

	Radiological observations	Changes
Oral phase	Ptosis of tongue and hyoid bone	Lack of connective tissue support of hyoid and dysfunction of tongue suspensory muscles
	Time needed for bolus preparation prolonged	Poor or absent dentition Temporomandibular joint abnormalities Altered, ineffective tongue movements Increased number of chewing strokes
	Swallow initiation delayed	Diminished salivation Abnormal tongue motility Reduced sensory perception
	Leakage	Neurological sensory/motor impairment of tongue and palate
Pharyngeal phase	Larynx/hyoid bone elevation diminished	Lack of connective tissue support of larynx and epiglottis, often associated with voice changes
	Laryngeal closure impaired	Increase in fatty deposits and atrophy of intrinsic laryngeal muscles
	Pharyngeal cavity enlarged	Laxity and atrophy of pharyngeal boundaries (muscles and connective tissue)
	Retention of bolus in squared valleculae	Diminished pharyngeal constrictor function
	Signs of oropharyngeal compensation observed in some patients	Loss of connective tissues and subepiglottic fatty tissue
Esophageal phase	Impaired peristalsis; wave absent or markedly reduced in amplitude	Localization of lesion causing motility disturbance of presbyesophagus unknown
	Segmental aperistalsis	Decrease in intramural ganglion cells in Auerbach's plexus
	High incidence of nonperistaltic contractions and tertiary waves	*Note*: Presbyesophagus is (1) only rarely seen in persons under age 70 and is (2) usually asymptomatic.
	Esophagus sometimes dilated and air filled, lacking intrinsic tone	
	Delayed esophageal emptying	
	Compression by tortuous descending aorta or aberrant arteriosclerotic artery (subclavian)	

pensory muscle aging may set the stage for bolus penetration into the larynx. Laxity of connective tissue surrounding the larynx and trachea may lead to ptosis, with bolus retention in the valleculae and piriform sinuses. Similarly, muscle atrophy may prevent the soft palate from making contact with Passavant's cushion. The epiglottis becomes less pliable with advancing age, consistent with the description of breakdown of elastic fibers (15) and regressive changes of extrinsic and intrinsic muscles of the larynx (16). The epiglottis may fail to fold backward to cover the laryngeal aditus completely.

The laryngeal surface epithelium appears to become less sensitive to aspirated material with increasing age (17,18). Experimentally, when a chemical irritant (anhydrous ammonia) was used in randomized concentrations, it was found that the median threshold for coughing (due to aspiration) increased sixfold from the second to the eighth and ninth decades of life (17). This decrease in sensitivity associated with loss of the protective cough reflex explains why silent aspiration seems to occur more often in older people. Moreover, the protective airway reflex can be further aggravated by neurodepressant medications (7).

Borgstrom and Ekberg found defective closure of the laryngeal vestibule (i.e., laryngeal penetration) during swallowing in 70 of 101 patients over the age of 80 (19). No respiratory consequence is mentioned in this report. Thus the significance of laryngeal penetration in older people is unknown.

On the other hand, Borgstrom and Ekberg also studied the speed of peristalsis in populations of various ages (under 40, between 50 and 60, and over 75 years of age) and found no significant changes with increasing age (20).

Tracy et al. in 1989 studied the effects of increasing age and increasing bolus volumes on various parameters of the swallow in a combined videofluoroscopic and manometric study of 24 normal volunteers (21). Increasing age was associated with an increase in the duration of pharyngeal swallow delay and a decrease in duration of pharyngeal swallow response, duration of cricopharyngeal (CP) opening, peristaltic amplitude, and peristaltic velocity. Increasing bolus size (maximum of 20mL) resulted in shortening of the oral transit time (increasing bolus volume resulted in the bolus head being held sequentially more posteriorly in the mouth) and increased duration of CP opening.

Radiographic Observations

So how do all these scientific facts translate into radiographic observations. What is the spectrum of findings that can be normal for someone of 70 years of age versus those in a person only 30 years old?

Ekberg and Feinberg studied 56 patients with a mean age of 83 years who had no symptoms of dysphagia or eating difficulty (22). Normal swallow, as defined in the young, was found in only 16% of cases! Oral "abnormalities" (difficulty ingesting, controlling, and delivering the bolus relative to initiation of pharyngeal swallow) were seen in 63%. Pharyngeal "dysfunction" (retention of bolus, paresis) or lingual or pharyngeal constrictor paresis was seen in 25%. Pharyngoesophageal segment "abnormalities" were seen in almost 40% of cases (mostly CP muscle dysfunction). Esophageal "abnormalities" were seen in 36% (mostly motor abnormalities).

Similarly Robbins et al. in a combined videofluoroscopic and manometric study evaluated 80 normal volunteers stratified by gender and age into four age groups (23). Total duration of oropharyngeal swallow was significantly longer in the oldest group, primarily due to delay in initiation of maximal hyolaryngeal excursion. Females had a longer time of upper esophageal sphincter (UES) opening. Not affected by age or gender were UES pressure, amplitude of pharyngeal pressures, duration of peak pharyngeal pressures, and rate of propagation of contraction. Subsequently, Frederick et al. evaluated 110 patients with videoradiography (aged 19–84 years) (24). They categorized patients into three groups: less than 40 years, 40 to 60 years, and greater than 60 years. There was a significant increase in the prevalence (23, 36, and 57%) and severity of functional abnormalities of the pharynx in older patients. Laryngeal penetration, aspiration, pharyngeal retention, and cricopharyngeal bar were the most common findings in the two older groups.

Thus, it appears that "normal" in the older patient may include findings that would be considered abnormal in those under 40 years of age.

Changes in the Esophagus with Age (Table 12.1)

The term "presbyesophagus" has been coined for motility changes in the elderly observed radiographically or with manometry. These changes may be dramatic with a "corkscrew" appearance on barium swallow, but they may be asymptomatic, as well (25). The incidence of nonperistaltic contractions, tertiary waves, delayed esophageal emptying, and esophageal dilatation increases with age. In one radiological study, 90% of nonagenarians had impaired esophageal motility, with one third having complete loss of the primary wave (26). Another study, by Mandelstam and Lieber, reported similar observations: primary peristaltic waves were absent or markedly reduced in amplitude in 50% of octogenarians and in 80% of nonagenarians (27).

A manometric study by Ren et al. examined the effect of aging on secondary esophageal peristalsis induced by either balloon distension or air distension (28). Frequency of secondary peristalsis and lower esophageal sphincter (LES) relaxation in response to air distension was significantly lower in the elderly than in the young.

Innervation to the esophagus is supplied by the vagus nerve with smooth muscle supplied via the myenteric plexus (29). The reduction in number of esophageal ganglion cells in Auerbach's plexus may be responsible for the motility changes of the esophagus in the elderly (30).

Absent or diminished amplitude of esophageal contraction (31) and nonperistaltic esophageal contractions encourage stasis of liquids and food or displacement of bolus in a cephalad direction against the cricopharyngeal sphincter, occasionally associated with regurgitation into the pharynx. This regurgitation may be silent or symptomatic, and it may lead to functional or, in time, to morphological changes such as lateral pharyngeal pouches.

Lower esophageal sphincter response to swallowing in the elderly has been reported variably as normal (31) and reduced (32). The lower esophageal sphincter high-pressure zone may also be displaced higher into the thorax. The latter observation probably explains the increased incidence of gastroesophageal reflux in the elderly (33).

Neurological Disease and the Pharynx (34,35) (Table 12.2)

It is important to distinguish between patients whose difficulty in drinking or eating is due to a variety of causes such as limb weakness or incoordination, or cognitive disorders such as decreased attention span, and patients with true dysphagia due to intrinsic oral or pharyngeal problems. Very important therapeutic decisions rest on this differentiation.

Normal swallowing requires finely tuned coordination between many cranial nerves and the muscles supplied by those nerves. Afferent sensory input to the brain tells us not only about bolus size and where the bolus is in the mouth, but also the characteristics of that bolus, including consistency, shape, texture, and taste. Neuromuscular disorders can cause swallowing problems by affecting either afferent or efferent impulses and by an abnormality at many levels (i.e., from the cerebral cortex, the basal ganglia, the cranial nerve nuclei, the cranial nerves, the neuromuscular junction, and the muscles themselves) (34–36).

Dysphagia may be a major or a minor symptom of a neuromuscular process. Sometimes, it can be the presenting, predominant, or only complaint. For example, the acute onset of dysphagia may signal a focal brain stem stroke either de novo or as a perioperative complication, presumably as the result of a low-flow state during anesthesia, or an arrhythmia. At the Johns Hopkins Swallowing Center, approximately 30% of our patients have an underlying neurological disease and in 10% of these, dysphagia was the predominant symptom, overshadowing other symptoms and signs such as limb weakness.

Classically symptoms or decompensation with *liquids* point toward a neuromuscular problem, whereas problems with solids indicate a structural narrowing such as a web, ring, stricture, or cancer.

Neuromuscular disorders result in weakness and/or incoordination of the muscles involved in a swallow. As a result, radiographic findings indicating *decompensation* are seen such as tremor or myoclonus, loss of the bolus in and from the mouth, nasopharyngeal regurgitation, laryngeal penetration or aspiration (silent or with reflexive cough), pharyngeal paresis with retention in valleculae and piriform sinuses, and prominence of the cricopharyngeus.

When reviewing the videofluoroscopic swallowing study (VFSS), it should be determined

TABLE 12.2. Neurodegenerative and vascular disorders associated with dysphagia prevalent in the elderly.

Disorders	Radiological observations
Diseases of the brain and brain stem	
Vascular disorders	
Bilateral cortical stroke	Aphagia
Unilateral cortical stroke (preliminary data)	Swallow may be preserved (brain stem receives input from opposite hemisphere)
	Unilateral tongue weakness and poor oral bolus control may be observed
	Impairment may not be characteristic
Left side	Impaired oral stage function; difficulty initiating coordinated swallows (apraxia)
Right side	Pharyngeal pooling; airway penetration and aspiration
Brain stem stroke	
Pseudobulbar palsy (upper motor neurons) (corticobulbar tract, upper motoneuron disease in upper brain stem)	Swallow abnormal in bilateral involvement; oral phase most affected
Bulbar palsy (lower motor neurons) (lower brain stem nuclei, cranial nerves, n-m junction, muscles, lower motoneuron disease)	Weakness and atrophy; pharyngeal phase most impaired; complete swallowing incoordination; pharyngoesophageal segment does not relax on time; often no swallow at all
Wallenberg syndrome (unilateral vertebral artery occlusion)	Bilateral pharyngeal paresis
Intracranial hemorrhage (subdural, subarachnoid, intraparenchymal)	Findings in oropharynx depend on location and extent of bleeding, and complications (e.g., mass effect, raised intracranial pressure)
Multiple sclerosis	
Multifocal white matter lesions, course relapsing and remitting, may be steadily progressive	Findings as in bilateral corticobulbar lower brain stem lesions; severity of dysphagia varies with disease remission or exacerbation
Amyotrophic lateral sclerosis (ALS)	
Commonest form of motoneuron disease	Considerable oropharyngeal muscle atrophy;
Upper and lower motor neurons in brain stem affected	CP segment relaxation maintained
Common cause of insidious dysphagia in the elderly	Signs of compensation may be present
Movement disorders and neurodegenerative diseases	
Parkinson's disease (Degeneration of dopamine-producing neurons in substantia nigra)	Primarily difficulty with oral initiation
May represent example of premature aging	
Less common	
Spinocerebellar degeneration	Oral phase impairment
Progressive supranuclear palsy	Feeding and swallowing impairment depending on facial, oral, lingual, or palatopharyngeal muscle involvement
Huntington's disease	
Alzheimer's disease	
Dystonia and dyskinesia	
Infections	
Poliomyelitis	Residual dysphagia following acute infection of motor neurons; pharyngeal dysfunction may slowly worsen owing to progressive postpolio muscle atrophy
Neurosyphilis	Dysphagia and swallowing impairment depending on site of CNS involvement
Encephalitis, meningitis	
Medication effects	
Antibiotics, immuno- and CNS-suppressive drugs	May mimic or worsen underlying neurological impairment; pharyngeal constriction frequently affected

12. Aging and Neurological Disease

TABLE 12.2. *Continued*

Disorders	Radiological observations
Diseases of cranial nerves Involving muscles of cranial nerves V (jaw), VII (face), IX/X (palate, pharynx, and larynx), and XII (tongue) Nerves may be interrupted along their course by trauma, neoplasms, infections, and inflammatory and immune-mediated disorders	Oropharyngeal impairment (nerve palsies) depending on selection and degree of nerve involvement by trauma or disease process
Diseases of the neuromuscular junction Myasthenia gravis	Various degrees of generalized pharyngeal muscle weakness with features of increasing fatigue during swallowing
Eaton-Lambert syndrome (in setting of malignancy)	Generalized pharyngeal impairment; sluggish contractions during swallowing
Familial dysautonomia (Riley-Day syndrome)	Delay in cricopharyngeal sphincter relaxation with airway penetration
Diseases of the muscle Polymyositis, dermatomyositis Sarcoid myopathy Metabolic myopathy Cortisone myopathy Mitochondrial myopathy (ragged red fiber disease) Dysthyroid myopathy Muscular dystrophy	Sluggish pharyngeal contraction Tongue/palate usually involved Pharyngoesophageal segment relaxes on time, closes early
Myotonic dystrophy	Oropharyngeal muscles usually uniformly involved; sluggish pharyngeal contractions; chilled barium aggravates changes
Duchenne's muscular dystrophy Oculopharyngeal dystrophy	Pharyngeal retention; aspiration likely

Source: Developed and modified after Buchholz (34).

what organs are weak, whether there is any sign of atrophy, and whether the process is focal or global. Occasionally the findings will suggest a specific neurological process (especially when combined with the physical finding: e.g., oral decompensation or tremor with a normal pharynx and an impassive facies is suggestive of Parkinson's disease).

Neurological Diseases

Cerebrovascular Accident (CVA, Stroke)

Depending on the site of the ischemic or hemorrhagic damage and the size of the deficit, CVAs can result in dysphagia. It has been reported that dysphagia occurs to some extent in 25 to 50% of CVAs (37–39). Recovery can parallel the recovery of limb weakness, or the patient may recover physical limb strength and not recover normal swallow. Classically, there was thought to be bilateral representation of swallowing in the cerebral cortex, and it was formerly thought that since each corticobulbar tract supplies both sides of the brain stem with cortical input, a unilateral CVA should not result in dysphagia.

More recent work by Robbins et al. challenged the theory of bilateral representation of swallowing (40,41). These authors studied a group of patients with unilateral cortical strokes (defined by computed tomography) and compared the findings of infarcts in the right cerebral cortex with those of the left. Initiation of pharyngeal swallow was delayed in all patients. However, left cortical stroke dysphagia was characterized by impaired oral function, difficulty initiating coordinated motor activity, and apraxia, whereas pharyngeal pooling, penetration, and aspiration were prominent in right cortical stroke patients. Further studies with more sensitive imaging modalities, such as magnetic resonance imaging (MRI), are in progress to determine if these preliminary findings are indeed valid.

Even MRI, however, may be negative in stroke. At least two papers from the early 1990s address the problem of either focal brain stem stroke, dysphagia, and negative MRI scans (42) or stroke with negative MRI imaging (43).

Wallenberg's syndrome is a stroke involving the lateral aspect of the medulla in the distribution of the posterior inferior cerebellar artery (lateral medullary infarction). Traditional teaching has been that the pharyngeal paresis that resulted was unilateral. Two studies, however, demonstrated that in fact the deficit is bilateral (44,45). More recently, aphagia was reported following acute lateral medullary infarction (46).

Occasionally it is possible to differentiate between a *pseudobulbar dysphagia* (cranial nerve nuclei or above), resulting in increased tone, and a *bulbar dysphagia* (cranial nerve nuclei, nerves, neuromyonal junction or muscle), which may be associated with atrophy of prevertebral soft tissues and hyporeflexia or decreased tone. Usually, however, the differentiation is not possible on the basis of a radiographic study alone.

Amyotrophic Lateral Sclerosis (ALS) (36)

Amyotrophic lateral sclerosis is also known as motor neuron disease and Lou Gehrig's disease. Among the neurological causes of oropharyngeal swallowing impairment, motor neuron disease frequently causes dysphagia, which can rapidly progress like the disease itself. Bulbar palsy alone, pseudobulbar palsy alone, or a combination of the two can be seen in this disorder. In addition to dysphagia, airway protection and speech are usually impaired, with early onset of dysarthria and episodes of choking. Muscle atrophy of tongue, palate, and pharyngeal constrictors is usually pronounced, together with various degrees of pharyngeal paralysis and suspensory muscle weakness resulting in a low hyoid position (Figure 12.1). Failure of the larynx to close and the epiglottis to invert leads to airway penetration or aspiration relatively early in the disease (Figure 12.2). To maintain airway and swallowing, the patient often compensates by holding the head and neck in sustained extension ("swan neck position"). Because of the rapid progression of the disease and the need for swallowing therapy intervention or feeding recommendations, several examinations may be necessary.

Multiple Sclerosis (MS)

In multiple sclerosis dysphagia is frequent. Oropharyngeal swallowing may be vastly impaired. Corresponding to the course of the disease itself, swallowing impairment in MS is relapsing and remitting.

The radiographic appearance depends on the location and extent of the foci of demyelinization; lesions are usually localized in the white matter of the brain in a periventricular distribution and are randomly scattered through the brain stem, spinal cord, and cerebellar peduncles. Abnormalities may vary from difficulty initiating swallow to episodes of choking on liquids to holdup of solid particles in the pharynx. Sensory loss may lead to underestimation of the severity of disease, and even in the presence of severe decompensation, symptoms, including silent aspiration, may be minimal or absent (47).

Neurodegenerative Disorders

Parkinson's disease (PD) is associated with dysphagia in as many as 50% of patients. Symptoms may be mild, with decompensation seen on radiographic studies. Although oral phase abnormalities are characteristic, the pharynx may be involved. Delay or inability to form a bolus, squeezing of the bolus between tongue and palate, piecemeal deglutition, and hesitancy to propel the bolus into the pharynx are characteristic observations in Parkinson's disease (48). Airway penetration, aspiration, and pooling of contrast medium in valleculae and piriform sinuses following a delayed swallowing reflex may be seen.

Leopold and Kagel studied 72 patients with Parkinson's disease and found "pre-pharyngeal dysphagia" in 48 patients (49). Dysphagia symptoms were present in 82%. Impaired mastication and oral preparatory lingual movements were the most common abnormalities reported, but other findings included jaw rigidity, impaired head and neck posture, impulsive feeding, and impaired amount regulation.

These authors also studied the intrinsic and extrinsic laryngeal muscles in PD and found both defective closure of the larynx and defective elevation of the larynx in 59 of 72 patients (81.9%) (50).

Cricopharyngeal dysfunction has been noted in Parkinson's disease in a report of 5 patients by Born et al. (51). A CP myotomy was performed in 4 of the 5 patients with excellent results.

Esophageal abnormalities have been reported on manometry in over 60% of patients in one study of 18 patients (52). Findings included repetitive contractions, simultaneous contractions, reduced LES pressure, and high-amplitude contractions.

One of the treatments for advanced PD is pallidotomy, a unilateral surgical procedure creating a lesion in the globus pallidus. Worsening or new onset of dysphagia has been reported following this procedure (53).

Other Neurodegenerative Conditions

Progressive supranuclear palsy (PSP) is another neurodegenerative syndrome with features similar to Parkinson's disease but with a more rapid decline than is associated with Parkinson's disease. Dysphagia is a common feature in this syndrome. Neumann et al. reported 14 patients with PSP and dysphagia; VFSS was performed in 10 of 14 (54). Both oral and pharyngeal findings were present in all patients, including poor oral control and premature leakage, with delayed initiation of pharyngeal swallow and decreased pharyngeal contraction, laryngeal penetration, or even aspiration. Interestingly, lingual tremor was absent in all 10 patients, unlike the findings in Parkinson's disease.

Other authors have studied patients with PSP and found oral and pharyngeal abnormalities in both groups (55,56).

Other neurodegenerative disorders associated with dysphagia and/or feeding difficulty include Huntington's disease (HD) and Alzheimer's disease (AD), both of which are compounded by dementia.

Kagel and Leopold reported a 16-year experience with 35 patents with HD and found a high incidence of multiple abnormalities including tachyphagia, deficient mastication, and whole-bolus swallowing (57,58). Horner et al. reported on observations in 25 patients with moderate or severe Alzheimer's disease and observed a trend toward an increased incidence of aspiration in patients with more severe dementia (59).

Infections

Viral infections of the nervous system may produce dysphagia. Bulbar poliomyelitis, a viral infection of motor neurons, presents with pharyngeal muscle paralysis and disturbance of aspiration and vasomotor control due to lesions in the medullary reticular formation, including the region of the nucleus ambiguus. Acute infections are very low in countries where vaccination is widespread, but there has been a resurgence in areas that do not practice vaccination. However, residua of previous epidemics can be seen in patients with postpolio syndrome and/or progressive muscle atrophy (60,61).

It is important to differentiate the "postpolio syndrome" (PPS) from "progressive postpolio muscular atrophy" (PPMA). The former term refers to symptoms experienced by survivors of the poliomyelitis virus infection. A minority of patients have progressive symptoms with ongoing denervation of muscle, which results in progressive pain, weakness, and wasting—this is true PPMA.

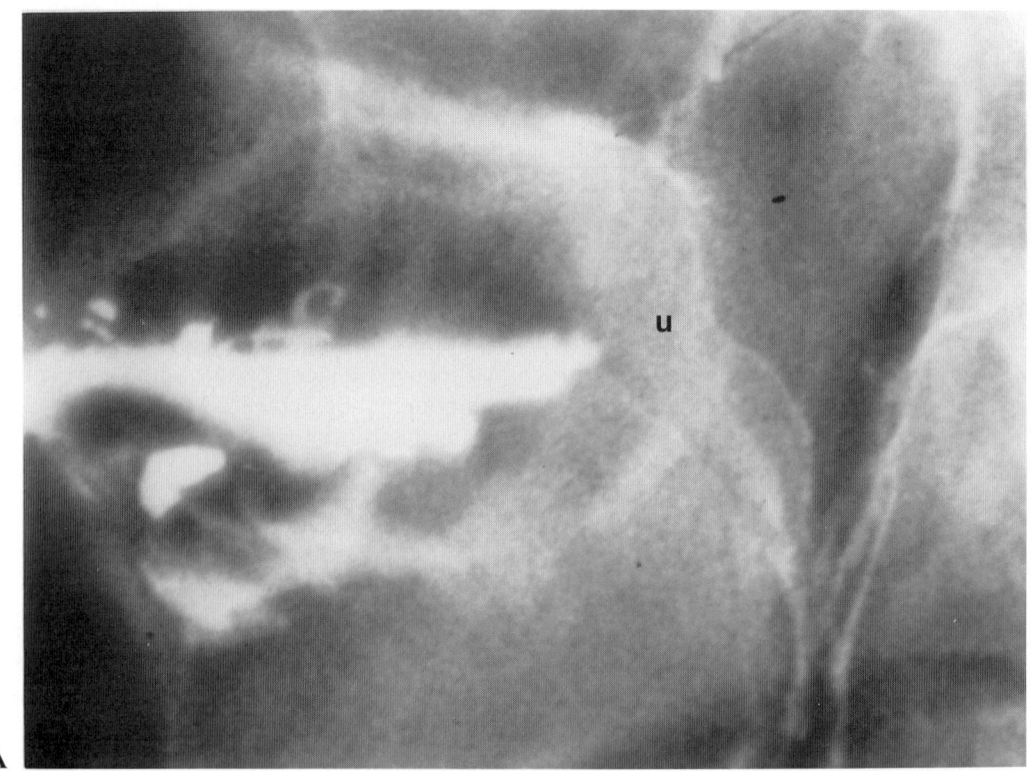

A
B

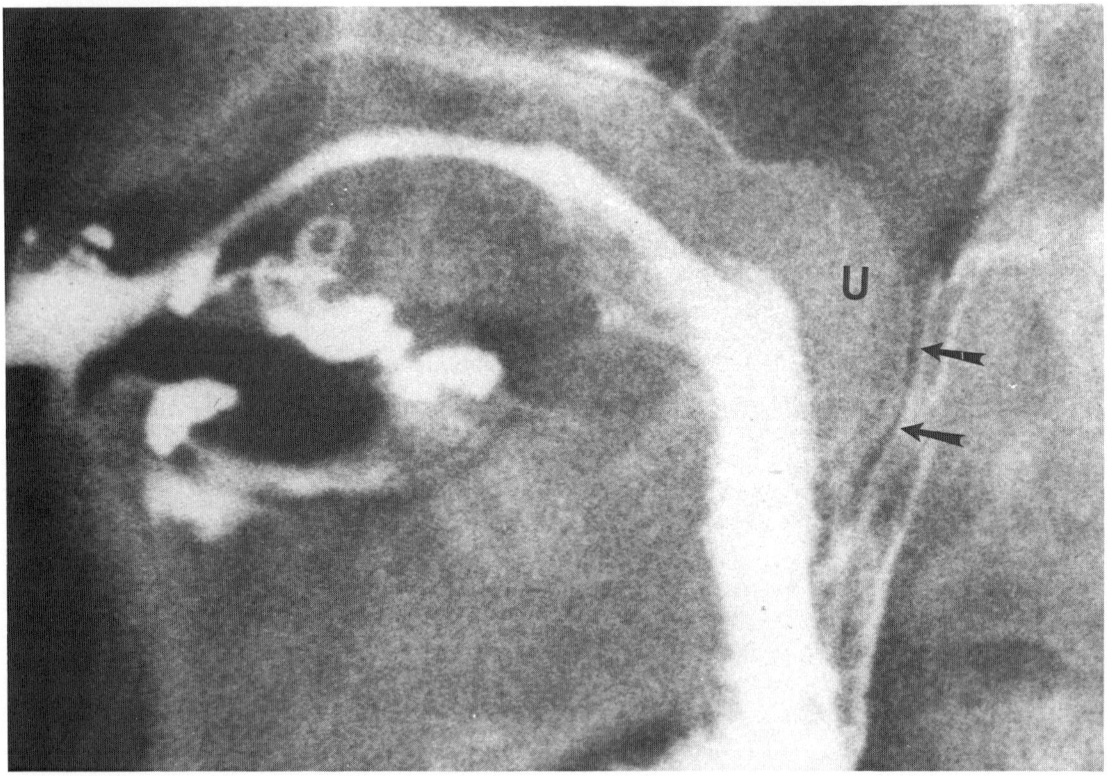

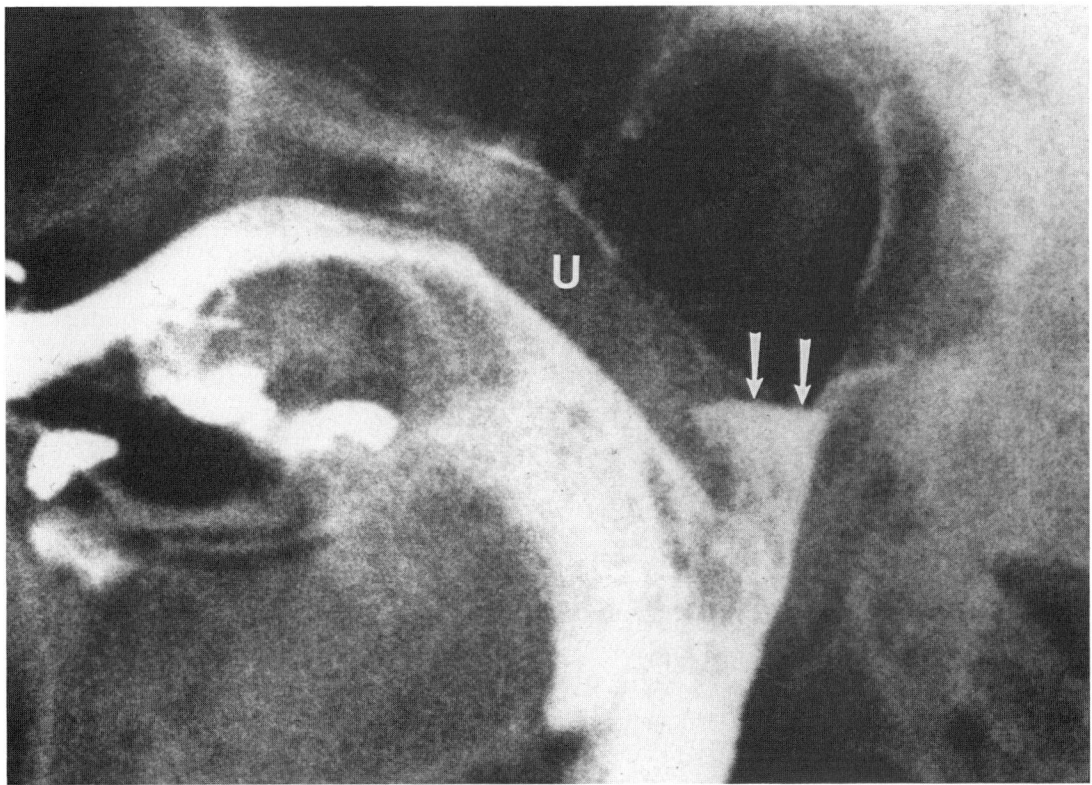

C

FIGURE 12.1. Soft palate abnormalities in a patient with advanced amyotrophic lateral sclerosis. (A) There is atrophy of the tongue and soft palate, and there is compensatory kinking of the uvula (U) to maintain bolus within the mouth. (B) As bolus leaves the mouth, there is curling of the soft palate (U), a sign of weakness. Note, also, the lack of formation of Passavant's cushion; air seen between the incompletely elevated soft palate and the posterior pharyngeal wall (arrows). (C) The weakened soft palate (U) fails to remain elevated, flopping back against the back of the tongue, with resultant nasopharyngeal regurgitation. Note the air/barium level in the nasopharynx in this upright patient (arrows).

Sonies and Dalakas evaluated 32 patients with a remote history of poliomyelitis and new onset of weakness in limbs (62). Fourteen of these patients had new onset of dysphagia; 18 were asymptomatic for swallowing. These authors found some abnormalities on sonography and VFSS in almost all patients, even in those who were asymptomatic for dysphagia.

Another study reviewed the VFSS in 20 patients with a remote history of poliomyelitis and recent or progressive dysphagia (63). Radiographic abnormalities were found in varying degrees in all but one patient. Findings included atrophy of prevertebral tissues, unilateral or bilateral weakness of the tongue or soft palate, paresis or paralysis of the pharyngeal constrictors, absence of epiglottic tilt, poor laryngeal elevation and closure, and laryngeal penetration or aspiration, often silent. In addition, structural diseases such as Zenker's diverticulum or stricture or hiatal hernia, contributed to the dysphagia in a significant number of patients.

Myasthenia and Myasthenia-Related Disorders

Myasthenia gravis (64) and the Eaton-Lambert myasthenic-myopathic syndrome (65) are myoneuronal junction disorders with diminished release or inadequate binding of acetylcholine,

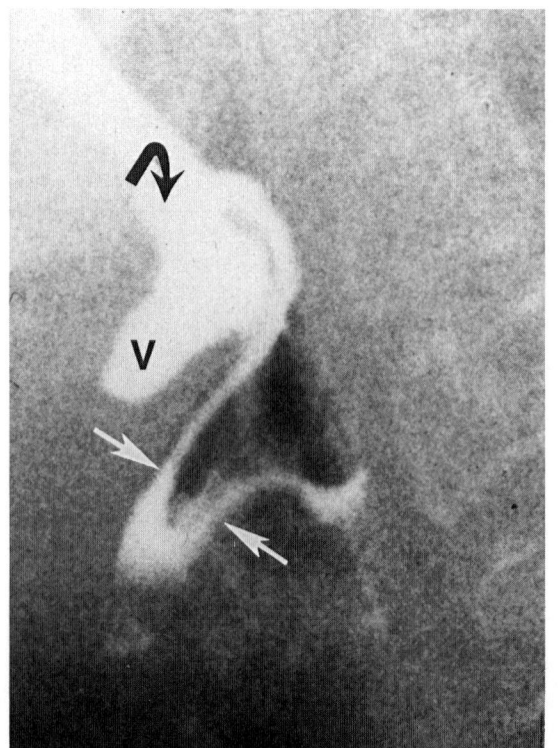
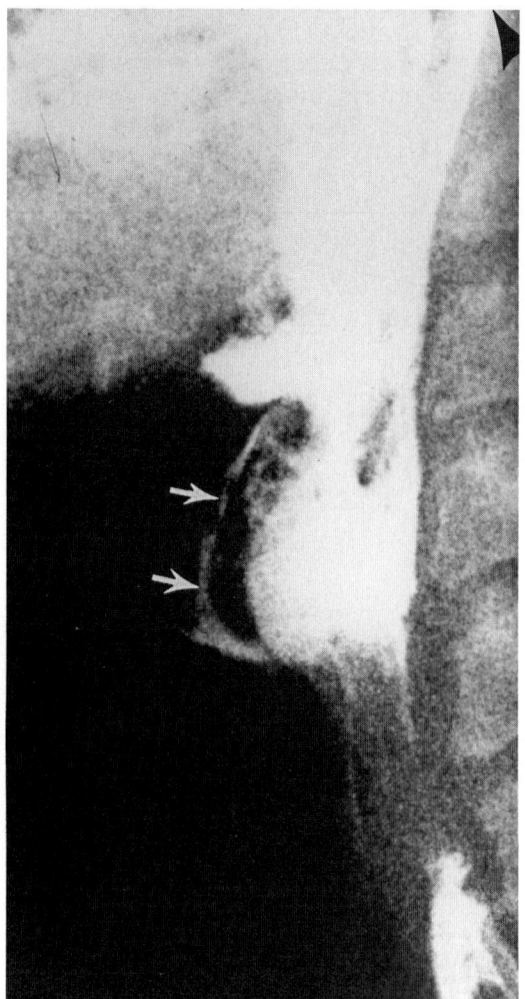
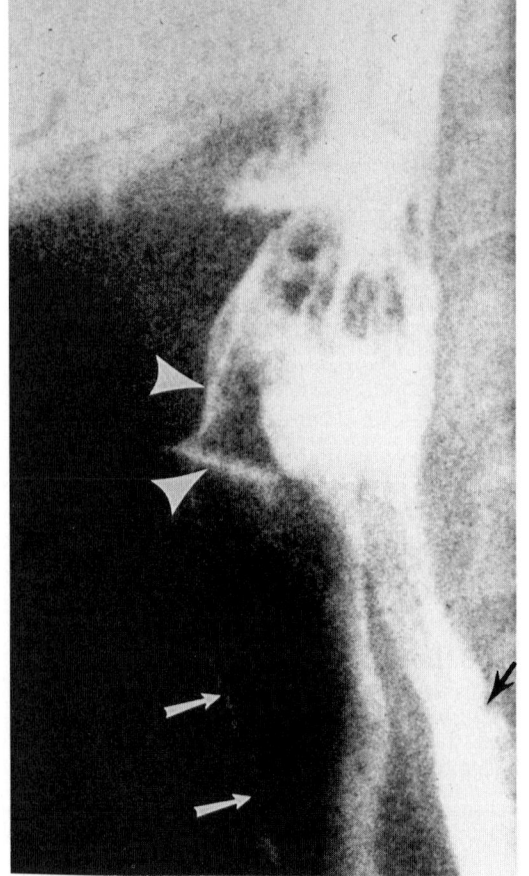

FIGURE 12.2. Multiple signs of decompensation in a patient with advanced amyotrophic lateral sclerosis. (A) There is leakage of contrast over the back of the tongue (curved arrow) into the valleculae (V) with extension over the back of the epiglottis into the open vestibule of the larynx (arrows). (B) A large bolus is seen in the valleculae and piriform sinuses. Nasal regurgitation is evident superiorly (arrowhead), and there is penetration into the open larynx (arrows). Bolus from a previous swallow can be seen passing through into the cervical esophagus. (C) There is no evidence of a pharyngeal stripping wave. The cricopharyngeus is open (black arrow), and there is laryngeal penetration (arrowheads) and aspiration down into the trachea (white arrows).

which may lead to muscle weakness. In addition to ocular and proximal limb muscles, the pharynx is frequently involved. Symmetrical weakness of pharyngeal constrictors increases with activity. Fatigue or decompensation during continuous swallowing of several ounces of a liquid can suggest the diagnosis during radiographic observation.

Dysphagia may be the presenting symptom in the Eaton-Lambert syndrome, together with diplopia and dysarthria. However, muscles of the trunk, pelvis, and shoulder girdle primarily become weak and fatiguable. Although the syndrome is observed most often with oat cell carcinoma of the lung, it may also be associated with carcinoma of the breast, prostate, stomach, and rectum (65).

Myopathy

Myopathies prominently affecting bulbar muscles may be due to inflammatory disease (polymyositis, dermatomyositis, sarcoidosis) (66,67), metabolic and endocrine in origin (68–70) (mitochondrial or ragged red fiber disease, dysthyroid myopathy due to hypo- or hyperthyroidism), induced by a prolonged course of steroid medication, or due to muscular dystrophy. The latter category includes myotonia dystrophica (71) resulting in pharyngeal and esophageal motor abnormalities and oculopharyngeal dystrophy in which difficulty in swallowing and bilateral ptosis and change in voice are associated (72).

Some manometric studies have been performed in patients of French-Canadian ancestry with oculopharyngeal muscular dystrophy (OPMD) (73). Castell et al. studied 11 patients with OPMD and found pharyngeal abnormalities in 9. Abnormalities included low pharyngeal pressures, poor pharyngeal contraction, and abnormal UES relaxation. Surprisingly, however, these authors also found esophageal abnormalities in 10 of the 11 patients, the most common of which were simultaneous contractions and incomplete lower esophageal sphincter relaxation.

Subsequently, Perie et al. studied 22 patients with OPMD and dysphagia by several means, including endoscopy, VFSS, and manometry (74).

Cricopharyngeal myotomy resulted in improvement in 10 of 12 patients, but this procedure was felt to be contraindicated with pharyngeal aperistalsis.

Medications

Medications may induced or aggravate an existing myasthenia gravis, or induce myopathy or neuropathy involving the pharynx. Many drugs in current clinical use may interfere with neuromuscular transmission, among them antibiotics such as neomycin, streptomycin, and certain tetracyclines (75,76), procainamide (77), and immunosuppressant agents such as ACTH, prednisone, and azathioprine (78,79). Antipsychotic and antidepressant medications may produce extrapyramidal symptoms of the Parkinsonian type (80) or muscle spasm and dystonia. Near-fatal and fatal choking episodes have been correlated with the development of tardive dyskinesia on antipsychotic medications (81).

Other drugs may unmask a latent neuromuscular disease (78). For example, we have seen at least two patients with dysphagia on benzothiaprine whose disease and VFSS improved after cessation of the medication (82) and severe dysphagia has been associated with tranquilizer use (83,84).

Ideally, administration of any medications known to affect the swallow should be temporarily suspended several days prior to evaluation of swallowing function.

References

1. Kashima HK. Presbyphagia, introduction. In: Goldstein JC, Kashima HK, Koopmann CF, eds. *Geriatric Otorhinolaryngology*. Toronto: Brian C Decker; 1989.
2. Sheth N, Diner WC. Swallowing problems in the elderly. *Dysphagia* 1988;2(4):209–215.
3. Giaquinto S. *Aging and the Nervous System*. New York: John Wiley & Sons; 1988.
4. McComas AF, Lipton ARM, Sica REP. Motoneuron disease and aging. *Lancet* 1973;2: 1477–1480.
5. Groher ME, Bukatman R. The prevalence of swallowing disorders in two teaching hospitals. *Dysphagia* 1986;1:3–6.

6. Malmgren LT. Aging related changes in peripheral nerves in the head and neck. In: Goldstein JC, Kashima HK, Koopmann CF, eds. *Geriatric Otorhinolaryngology*. Toronto: Brian C Decker; 1989.
7. Pontoppidan H, Beecher HK. Progressive loss of protective reflexes in the airway with the advance of age. *JAMA* 1960;174:2209–2213.
8. Rosenheimer JL, Smith DO. Differential changes in the endplate architecture of functionally diverse muscles during aging. *J Neurophysiol* 1985;53:1567–1581.
9. Baum BJ, Bodner L. Aging and oral motor function: evidence for altered performance among older persons. *J Den Res* 1983;62:2–6.
10. Kaplan H. The oral cavity in geriatrics. *Geriatrics* 1971;26:96–102.
11. Rolls BJ. Regulation of food and fluid intake in the elderly. *Ann N Y Acad Sci* 1989;561:217–225.
12. Osterberg T, Carlsson G. Symptoms and signs of mandibular dysfunction in 70-year-old men and women in Gothenburg, Sweden. *Commun Den Oral Epidemiol* 1979;7:315–321.
13. Feldman RS, Kapur KK, Alman JE, et al. Aging and mastication changes in performance and in the swallowing threshold with natural dentition. *J Am Geriatr Soc* 1980;28(3):96–102.
14. Shaker R, Dodds WJ, Hogan WJ, et al. Effect of aging on swallow-induced lingual palatal closure pressure. *Gastroenterology* 1989;96:A464.
15. Ferreri G. Senescence of the larynx. *Ital Gen Rev Otorhinolaryngol* 1959;1:640–709.
16. Kahane JC. Postnatal development and aging of the human larynx. *Semin Speech Lang* 1983;4:189–203.
17. Erskine RJ, Murphy PJ, Langton JA, Smith G. Effect of age on the sensitivity of upper airway reflexes. *Br J Anaesth* 1993;70(5):574–575.
18. Aviv JE. Effects of aging on sensitivity of the pharyngeal and supraglottic areas. *Am J Med* 1997;103(5A):74S–76S.
19. Borgstrom PS, Ekberg O. Pharyngeal dysfunction in the elderly. *J Med Imaging* 1988;2:74–81.
20. Borgstrom PS, Ekberg O. Speed of peristalsis in pharyngeal constrictor musculature: correlations to age. *Dysphagia* 1988;2:140–144.
21. Tracy JF, Logemann JA, Kahrilas PJ, Kobara M, Krugler C. Preliminary observations on the effects of age on oropharyngeal deglutition. *Dysphagia* 1989;4:90–94.
22. Ekberg O, Feinberg MJ. Altered swallowing function in elderly patients without dysphagia: radiologic findings in 56 cases. *AJR Am J Roentgenol* 1991;156(6):1181–1184.
23. Robbins J, Hamilton JW, Lof GL, Kempster GB. Oropharyngeal swallowing in normal adults of different ages. *Gastroenterology* 1992;103(3):823–829.
24. Frederick MG, Ott DJ, Grishaw EK, Gelfand DW, Chen MY. Functional abynormalities of the pharynx: a prospective analysis of radiographic abnormalities relative to age and symptoms. *Am J Roentgenol* 1996;166(2):353–357.
25. Hellemans J, Vantrappen G. Presbyesophagus. In: *Diseases of the Esophagus*. Berlin, Heidelberg, New York: Springer-Verlag; 1974:372–378.
26. Zboralske FF, Amberg KR, Soergel KH. Presbyesophagus: cine-radiographic manifestations. *Radiology* 1964;82:463–467.
27. Mandelstam P, Lieber A. Cineradiographic evaluation of the esophagus in normal adults. *Gastroenterology* 1970;58:32–39.
28. Ren J, Shaker R, Kusano M, Podvrsan B, Metwally N, Dua KS, Sui Z. Effect of aging on the secondary esophageal peristalsis: presbyesophagus revisited. *Am J Physiol* 1995;268(5 pt 1):G772–G779.
29. Geokas MC, Conteas CN, Majundar APN. The aging gastrointestinal tract, liver, and pancreas. *Clin Geriatr Med* 1985;1:177–205.
30. Eckardt VF, LeCompte PM. Histology of esophageal smooth muscle and Auerbach's plexus in elderly persons. *Gastroenterology* 1977;72:1055.
31. Hollis JB, Castell DO. Esophageal function in elderly men: a new look at presbyesophagus. *Ann Intern Med* 1974;80:371.
32. Khan TA, Shragge RW, Crispin JS, Lind JF. Esophageal motility in the elderly. *Am J Dig Dis* 1977;22:1049–1054.
33. Soergel KH, Zboralske FF, Amberg JR. Presbyesophagus: esophageal motility in nonagenarians. *J Clin Invest* 1964;43:1472–1479.
34. Buchholz D. Neurologic causes of dysphagia. *Dysphagia* 1987;1:152–156.
35. Kirshner S. Causes of neurogenic dysphagia. *Dysphagia* 1989;3:184–188.
36. Silbiger ML, Pikheney R, Donner MW. Neuromuscular disorders affecting the pharynx: cineradiographic analysis. *Invest Radiol* 1967;2:442–448.
37. Veis SL, Logemann JA. Swallowing disorders in persons with cerebrovascular accident. *Arch Phys Med Rehab* 1985;66:372–375.
38. Gordon C, Hewer RL, Wade DT. Dysphagia in acute stroke. *Br Med J* 987;295:411–414.

39. Nilsson H, Ekberg O, Olsson R, Hindfelt B. Dysphagia in stroke: a prospective study of quantitative aspects of swallowing in dysphagic patients. *Dysphagia* 1998;13(1):32–38.
40. Robbins JA, Levine RL. Swallowing after unilateral stroke of the cerebral cortex: preliminary experience. *Dysphagia* 1988;3:11–17.
41. Robbins JA, Levine RL, Maser A, Rosenbek JC, Kempster GB. Swallowing after unilateral stroke of the cerebral cortex. *Arch Phys Med Rehabil* 1993;74(12):1295–1300.
42. Buchholz DW. Clinically probable brainstem stroke presenting primarily as dysphagia and nonvisualized by MRI. *Dysphagia* 1993;8(3):235–238.
43. Alberts MJ, Faulstich ME, Gray L. Stroke with negative brain magnetic resonance imaging. *Stroke* 1992;23(5):663–667.
44. Neumann S, Buchholz D, Wuttge-Hannig A, Hannig C, Prosiegel M, Schröter-Morasch H. Bilateral pharyngeal dysfunction after lateral medullary infarction (LMI). *Dysphagia* 1994;9:263.
45. Neumann S, Buchholz D, Jones B, Palmer J. Pharyngeal dysfunction after lateral medullary infarction is bilateral: review of 15 additional cases. *Dysphagia* 1995;10:136.
46. Buchholz D, Neumann S. Aphagia due to pharyngeal constrictor paresis from acute lateral medullary infarction. *Dysphagia* 1999;14(3):187.
47. Daly DD, Code CF, Anderson HA. Disturbances of swallowing and esophageal motility in patients with multiple sclerosis. *Neurology* 1962;59:250–256.
48. Lieberman AN, Horowitz L, Redmond P, Pachter L, Lieberman I, Leibowitz M. Dysphagia in Parkinson's disease. *Am J Gastroenterol* 1980;74:157–160.
49. Leopold NA, Kagel MC. Pharyngo-esophageal dysphagia in Parkinson's disease. *Dysphagia* 1997;12(1):11–18.
50. Leopold NA, Kagel MC. Laryngeal deglutition movement in Parkinson's disease. *Neurology* 1997;48(2):373–376.
51. Born LJ, Harned RH, Rikkers LF, Pfeiffer RF, Quigley EM. Cricopharyngeal dysfunction in Parkinson's disease: role in dysphagia and response to myotomy. *Mov Disord* 1996;11(1):53–58.
52. Bassotti G, Germani U, Pagliaricci S, Plesa A, Giulietti O, Mannarino E, Morelli A. Esophageal manometric abnormalities in Parkinson's disease. *Dysphagia* 1998;13(1):28–31.
53. Neumann S, Buchholz D, Reich S, Goldberg P, Purcell L, Lenz F, Jones B. Dysphagia following pallidotomy for Parkinson's disease. *Dysphagia* 1997;12:110.
54. Neumann S, Reich S, Buchholz D, Purcell L, Jones B. Progressive supranuclear palsy (PSP): characteristics of dysphagia in 14 patients. *Dysphagia* 1996;11:164.
55. Johnston BT, Castell JA, Stumacher S, Colcher A, Gideon RM, Li Q, Castell DO. Comparison of swallowing function in Parkinson's disease and progressive supranuclear palsy. *Mov Disord* 1997;12(3):322–327.
56. Leopold NA, Kagel MC. Dysphagia in progressive supranuclear palsy: radiologic features. *Dysphagia* 1997;12(3):140–143.
57. Leopold NA, Kagel MC. Dysphagia in Huntington's disease. *Neurology* 1985;42:57–60.
58. Kagel MC, Leopold NA. Dysphagia in Huntington's disease: a 16-year retrospective. *Dysphagia* 1992;7:106–114.
59. Horner J, Alberts MJ, Dawson DV, Cook GM. Swallowing in Alzheimer's disease. *Alzheimer Dis Assoc Disord* 1994;8(3):177–189.
60. Dalakas MC, Elder G, Hallett M, Ravits J, Baker M, Papadopoulos N, Albrecht P, Sever J. A long-term follow-up study of patients with post-poliomyelitis neuromuscular symptoms. *N Engl J Med* 1986;314:959–963.
61. Cashman NR, Maselli R, Wollmann RL, Roos R, Simon R, Antel JP. Late denervation in patients with antecedent paralytic poliomyelitis. *N Engl J Med* 1987;317:7–12.
62. Sonies BC, Dalakas MC. Dysphagia in patients with the post-polio syndrome. *N Engl J Med* 1991;324:1162–1167.
63. Jones B, Buchholz DW, Ravich WJ, Donner MW. Swallowing dysfunction in the postpolio syndrome: a cinefluorographic study. *AJR Am J Roentgenol* 1992;158:283–286.
64. Murray JP. Deglutition in myasthenia gravis. *Br J Radiol* 1962;35:43–52.
65. Eaton LM, Lambert EH. Electromyography and electric stimulation of nerves and diseases of motor unit: observations on myasthenia syndrome associated with malignant tumors. *JAMA* 1957;163:1117.
66. Jacob H, Berkowitz D, McDonald E, Bernstein L, Beneventano T. The esophageal motility disorder of polymyositis: a prospective study. *Arch Intern Med* 1983;143:2262–2264.
67. Merieux P, Verity M, Clements P, Paulus H. Esophageal abnormalities and dysphagia in polymyositis and dermatomyositis: clinical,

radiographic, and pathologic features. *Arthritis Rheum* 1983;26:961–968.
68. Riminton DS, Chambers ST, Parkin PJ, Pollock M, Donaldson IM. Inclusion body myositis presenting solely as dysphagia. *Neurology* 1993; 43(6):1241–1243.
69. Buchholz DW, Neumann S, Ravich W, O'Brien R, Jones B. Inclusion body myositis presenting as dysphagia: report of 3 cases. *Dysphagia* 1997; 12:110.
70. Houser SM, Calabrese LH, Strome M. Dysphagia in patients with inclusion body myositis. *Laryngoscope* 1998;108(7):1001–1005.
71. Siegel CL, Hendrix TR, Harvey JC. The swallowing disorder in myotonia dystrophica. *Gastroenterology* 1966;50:541–550.
72. Duranceau A, Jamieson G, Clermont RJ. Oropharyngeal dysphagia in patients with oculopharyngeal muscular dystrophy. *Can J Surg* 1978;21:326–329.
73. Castell JA, Castell DO, Duranceau CA, Topart P. Manometric characteristics of the pharynx, upper esophageal sphincter, esophagus, and lower esophageal sphincter in patients with oculopharyngeal muscular dystrophy. *Dysphagia* 1995;10(1):22–26.
74. Perie S, Eymard B, Laccourreye L, Chaussade S, Fardeau M, Lacau St Guily J. Dysphagia in oculopharyngeal muscular dystrophy: a series of 22 French cases. *Neuromuscul Disord* 1997;7(1): S96–S99.
75. McQuillen MP, Cantor HE, O'Rourke JR Jr. Myasthenic syndrome associated with antibiotics. *Arch Neurol* 1968;18:402–415.
76. Pittinger CB, Eryase Y, Adamson R. Antibiotic induced paralysis. *Anesth Analg* 1970;49:487.
77. Miller CD, Oleshansky MA, Gibson KF, Cantilena LR. Procainamide-induced myasthenia-like weakness and dysphagia. *Ther Drug Monit* 1993;15(3):251–254.
78. Swift TR. Disorders of neuromuscular transmission other than myasthenia gravis. *Muscle Nerve* 1981;4:334.
79. Adams RD, Victor M. *Principles of Neurology*. 4th ed. New York: McGraw Hill; 1989.
80. Leopold NA. Dysphagia in drug-induced parkinsonism: a case report. *Dysphagia* 1996;11(2): 151–153.
81. Bazemore PH, Tonkonogy J, Ananth R. Dysphagia in psychiatric patients: clinical and videofluoroscopic study. *Dysphagia* 1991;6(1):2–5.
82. Buchholz D, Jones B, Neumann S, Ravich W. Benzodiazepine-induced pharyngeal dysphagia: report of two probable cases. *Dysphagia* 1995; 10:142.
83. Hughes TA, Shone G, Lindsay G, Wiles CM. Severe dysphagia associated with major tranquilizer treatment. *Postgrad Med J* 1994;70 (826):581–583.
84. Dantas RO, Nobre Souza MA. Dysphagia induced by chronic ingestion of benzodiazepine. *Am J Gastroenterol* 1997;92(7):1194–1196.

13
Dysphagia in AIDS

MAYA D. MEUX AND SUSAN D. WALL

Since the onset of the acquired immunodeficiency syndrome (AIDS) epidemic, complaints of dysphagia have been noted among these patients. Dysphagia is noted both early and late among patients with human immunodeficiency virus (HIV) disease, and it has been described in prospective studies in up to 47% of AIDS patients (1). These patients frequently are infected with opportunistic organisms and/or have opportunistic neoplasms, any of which can involve the oral cavity, hypopharynx, or esophagus, and result in dysphagia. Because of the location, infection and early tumor may cause symptomatology that would otherwise not be notable in more distal sites of the gastrointestinal tract. Furthermore, some AIDS-related infections and/or neoplasms of the gastrointestinal tract may be treated with subsequent palliation of the patient's discomfort. Dysphagia and odynophagia are symptoms that can decrease food intake significantly, thereby worsening the nutritional status of the patient. Correct diagnosis of the cause of these symptoms may have important prognostic consequences (2). Therefore, to detect pathology that might be treatable, it is important for the radiologist to respond to complaints of dysphagia with an evaluation of swallowing function as well as morphology of the oral cavity, hypopharynx, and esophagus. This is important because in contrast to other causes of debilitation in AIDS, dysphagia and odynophagia frequently are symptoms of treatable disorders of the esophagus (2).

The gastrointestinal tract is one of the major target organs for both opportunistic pathogens and opportunistic neoplasms in patients with AIDS. Kaposi's sarcoma and non-Hodgkin's lymphoma are the most frequently noted neoplasms. Opportunistic pathogens include *Candida albicans*, cytomegalovirus (CMV), herpes simplex virus, *Cryptospiridium*, *Mycobacterium tuberculosis*, *Mycobacterium avium-intracellulare*, *Isospora belli*, and *Torulopsis glabrata* (1). All these except *I. belli* have been noted in the oral cavity, hypopharynx, or esophagus in patients with HIV disease. Common presenting symptomatology includes dysphagia, odynophagia, dysphonia, and/or hoarseness. Dysphagia can result from inflammation, ulceration, stricture, mass, and/or a motility disturbance involving the esophagus. In patients with AIDS, esophageal symptoms are the second most common manifestation of gastrointestinal disease, and it has been estimated that 40 to 50% of HIV-infected patients will have symptoms of esophageal disease during the course of their illness (3–5). It is important to consider the coexistence of different etiological agents when one is evaluating patients with esophageal symptoms, since approximately 25% of patients will have more than one isolate on examination (6,7). Esophageal symptoms have also been attributed to the following etiological agents: the HIV virus, Epstein-Barr virus, lymphomatoid granulomatosis, *Pneumocystis carinii*, and *Cryptococcus neoformans* (8).

The epidemic of AIDS is no longer restricted to large cities with a high proportion of intravenous drug users or homosexual men. Currently, it affects all geographic areas of the United States, with an increasing number of women and children being diagnosed (9), and is noted throughout the United States. New drug regimens are responsible for improved patient survival. As long-term survival improves, it is increasingly important that physicians have an understanding of the gastrointestinal (GI) and abdominal diseases that afflict the AIDS patient (10,11). The majority of these individuals exhibit GI symptoms at some point during their illness, and the initial AIDS-defining illness, usually an opportunistic infection or malignancy, may involve the GI tract or abdomen (9). Symptoms associated with swallowing are common.

Often the radiographic manifestations of HIV/AIDS are the first indicator of the diagnosis. Hence, it is appropriate for radiologists everywhere to be cognizant of its manifestations. Opportunistic infection or neoplasms of the esophagus, oral cavity, or hypopharynx are well-known early complications of the syndrome, and they have notable radiographic manifestations. In general, the clinical and radiological investigation of patients with HIV/AIDS should be tailored to evaluate specific clinical signs or symptoms. Barium studies are useful in the evaluation of patients with symptoms referable to the GI tract (e.g., dysphagia and odynophagia, diarrhea, or GI hemorrhage) and are advantageous in that they are noninvasive. Double-contrast barium studies provide an excellent depiction of mucosal detail and allow better evaluation of both mucosal and submucosal abnormalities than is obtained with single-contrast radiography. Advantages of barium esophagography versus endoscopy include lower cost, less risk to the patients with virtually no morbidity or mortality, no need for sedation, and less risk to health care workers. However, there are advantages of endoscopy, including greater sensitivity and the ability to obtain tissue samples for cytology and culture (1,2). Endoscopy may be necessary subsequent to a barium examination that demonstrates pathology to confirm a diagnosis prior to the institution of therapy or to exclude the presence of more than one etiology. However, some entities, such as *Candida* esophagitis, are so characteristic that they do not require confirmatory endoscopy.

Opportunistic Neoplasms

Kaposi's Sarcoma

Kaposi's sarcoma (KS) is the most common malignancy in AIDS followed by non-Hodgkin's lymphoma (5) and is noted frequently as an opportunistic tumor in patients with HIV disease. Commonly, particularly in homosexual men, KS involves the gastrointestinal tract (12). Some investigators have noted that at some stage of their illness, 38% of patients with AIDS will develop KS and two thirds of these will have involvement of the head and neck with or without other sites (5). The condition tends to develop in patients with CD4 counts below 200 cells/μL (1). Dysphagia is a common presenting complaint, but odynophagia, dysphonia, and hoarseness can be present. This tumor was noted to be present in the luminal gastrointestinal tract at the time of diagnosis or early thereafter in about 50% of patients with cutaneous disease in the early years of the AIDS epidemic. However, a decreasing incidence has been noted in recent years, now more often approaching about one third of such patients. Occasionally gastrointestinal lesions can precede cutaneous disease. Although early Kaposi's sarcoma elsewhere in the gastrointestinal tract often is asymptomatic (13,14), small nodular lesions in the oropharynx or hypopharynx can produce symptoms because of their location (15). Very early lesions of Kaposi's sarcoma in the gastrointestinal tract are not detectable on double-contrast barium radiography because lesions at this stage are macular. Biopsy at this time often gives false negative results because the forceps of the flexible fiberoptic endoscope do not reach the submucosa where the tumor originates. In one study, only 23% of endoscopic biopsy specimens were positive (9). However, diagnosis is readily made by experienced endoscopists using visual inspection because the appearance is characteristic. Typically, there are multiple flat, red-purple or violaceous lesions varying in size from a few millimeters to 1 to 2 cm (14). As the disease progresses, the lesions become nodular and then are well demonstrated on barium radiography (Figure 13.1) (16–20). With good double-contrast technique, central umbilication may be seen, but "target" or "bull's-eye" lesions are only occasionally present, especially in the oropharynx or hypopharynx. Furthermore, this finding should not be required for the radiographic diagnosis of gastrointestinal Kaposi's sarcoma here, in the esophagus, or in the more distal luminal gastrointestinal tract. Advanced disease is demonstrated on double- or single-contrast barium radiography by the presence of bulky and often coalescent nodular lesions (Figure 13.2) (15) or irregular fold thickening (9). The differential diagnosis includes coaptation artifact, lymphoma, carcinoma, and candidiasis.

The nodular lesions of Kaposi's sarcoma in the oral cavity and hypopharynx (Figure 13.3) can be demonstrated by asking the patient to swallow a high-density barium suspension and performing a modified Valsalva maneuver. Computed tomographic (CT) scanning of the hypopharynx will demonstrate multiple soft tissue masses distorting the structure of the hypopharynx (Figure 13.4) (15). Obliteration of parapharyngeal spaces will be noted when large coalescent lesions are present (Figure 13.5).

If the typical nodular lesions for Kaposi's sarcoma are noted in the hypopharynx and/or esophagus, it may be appropriate to look elsewhere in the gastrointestinal tract for additional lesions. Multifocal disease of the upper and/or lower gastrointestinal tract frequently is seen in patients with AIDS, and this has been noted in as many as 65 to 70% of cases referred for barium evaluation of the gastrointestinal tract (19). Multifocal disease (three or more sites) can be due to multiple sites of opportunistic tumor, multiple opportunistic infections, and/or coexistent opportunistic tumor and opportunistic infection.

Since even small lesions of early Kaposi's sarcoma in the oropharynx and/or hypopharynx cause symptoms because of their location,

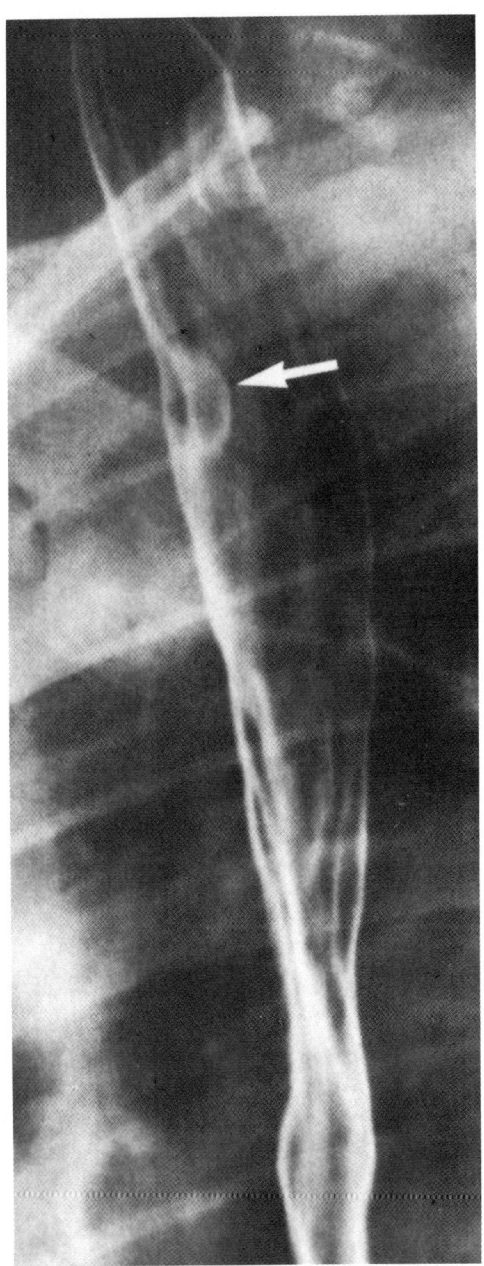

FIGURE 13.1. Early Kaposi's sarcoma is manifested by this single, smooth tumor nodule (arrow) in the proximal esophagus in a patient with AIDS and dysphagia. (Reprinted with permission from Megibow AJ, Wall SD, Balthazar EJ, Rybak BJ. Gastrointestinal radiology in AIDS patients. In: Federle M, Megibow AJ, Naidich DP, eds. *Radiology of AIDS*, New York: Raven Press; 1988:77–105.)

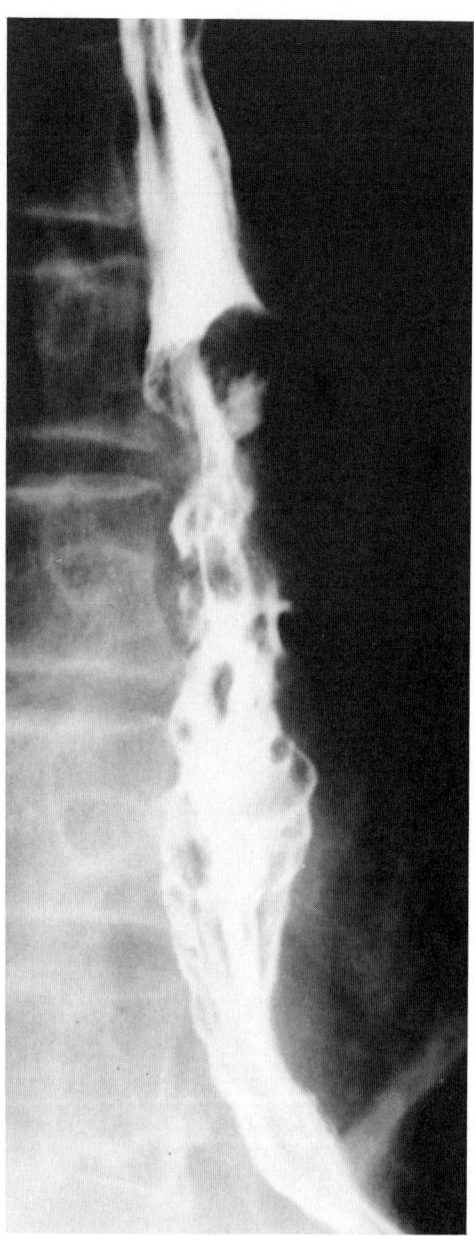

FIGURE 13.2. Advanced Kaposi's sarcoma is manifested by multiple bulky confluent tumor nodules in the mid- and distal esophagus in this patient with AIDS and severe dysphagia.

these patients may present with dysphagia, odynophagia, dysphonia, and/or hoarseness. Pharyngography will demonstrate well-defined nodular lesions (Figure 13.6). They may be present at the base of the tongue, posterior oral cavity, hypopharynx, valleculae, and/or piriform sinuses. Pharyngography, which has proven to be a useful screening examination in patients with HIV disease and symptoms associated with AIDS (15), often is preferable to laryngoscopy for several reasons. For instance, barium pharyngography can demonstrate the full extent of disease better than can direct visualization at laryngoscopy, since large lesions preclude a complete assessment of the caudal extent of tumor. Radiographic examination in such a case can more accurately define the required radiation port for therapy if indicated. Also, pharyngography is more easily tolerated by the patient, and it is less time-consuming. Furthermore, laryngoscopy is a more invasive procedure, and there is more risk to the examiner of exposure to the patient's body fluids. Barium pharyngography requires neither the operating room nor general anesthesia or sedation, and so is less expensive and safer than indirect laryngoscopy. Finally, concurrent examination of the upper gastrointestinal tract can be performed readily in association with barium pharyngography.

Oral, pharyngeal, or hypopharyngeal lesions of Kaposi's sarcoma may be treated for local palliation with radiation or chemotherapy, with consequent regression of tumor bulk (Figure 13.6C). However, the former treatment has limited use because of the severe inflammatory response of the mucosa in patients with HIV disease. It may be indicated in selective cases, and in some situations it can temporarily improve quality of life. Both endoscopic laser therapy or injection sclerotherapy hold promise for treatment of bulky tumors (20).

Lymphoma

Lymphoma is the second most common malignant neoplasm in AIDS patients, with non-Hodgkin's lymphoma (NHL) being more common than either Hodgkin's lymphoma (21) or Burkitt's lymphoma. Unlike KS, which has a higher frequency in homosexual men, AIDS-related NHL occurs in all AIDS risk groups. The AIDS-related lymphomas (ARL) can involve any segment of the GI tract, and multifocal disease is not uncommon (9). Lymphoma has been noted in the oral cavity and hypopharynx less frequently than has Kaposi's sarcoma. Also, it has only infrequently been seen in the esophagus. Prior case reports have described ulcerated lesions as being characteristic of lymphomatous involvement (6). The most common radiographic patterns for esophageal lymphoma include a large intramural mass, polypoid masses with or without ulcerations, and ulcerated stenosis. Sabate et al. described two cases of primary esophageal lymphoma in AIDS patients, both with complaints of dysphagia, manifested by circumferential infiltration of the esophageal wall with associated ulcerations (22). Esophageal stricture has also been described (23). Symptoms of lymphoma can be similar to those of involvement by KS.

There have been occasional reports of other unusual tumors and tumorlike lesions in the esophagus of patients with HIV disease, such as the two patients with squamous cell carcinoma of the esophagus reported by Frager et al. (24) and the inflammatory fibroid polyp described by Simmons et al. (25). One patient developed a focal flat lesion that simulated segmental

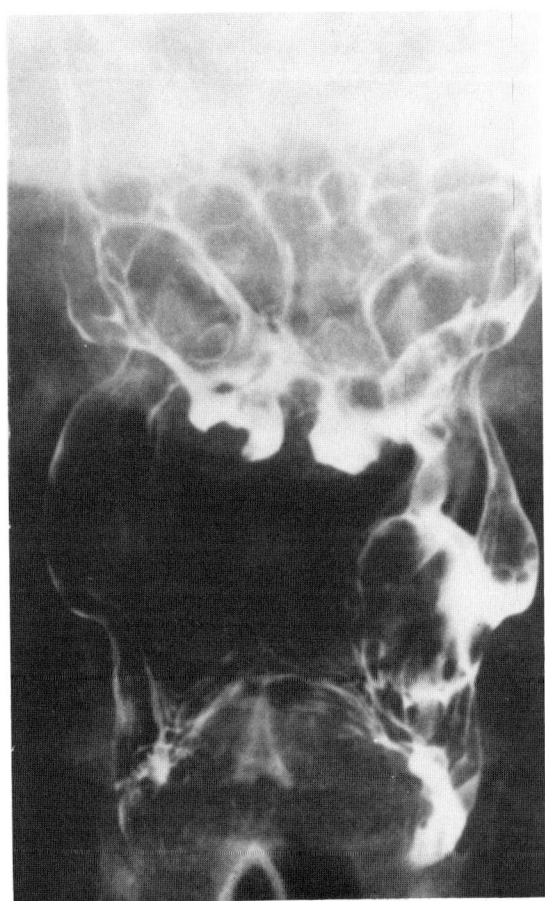
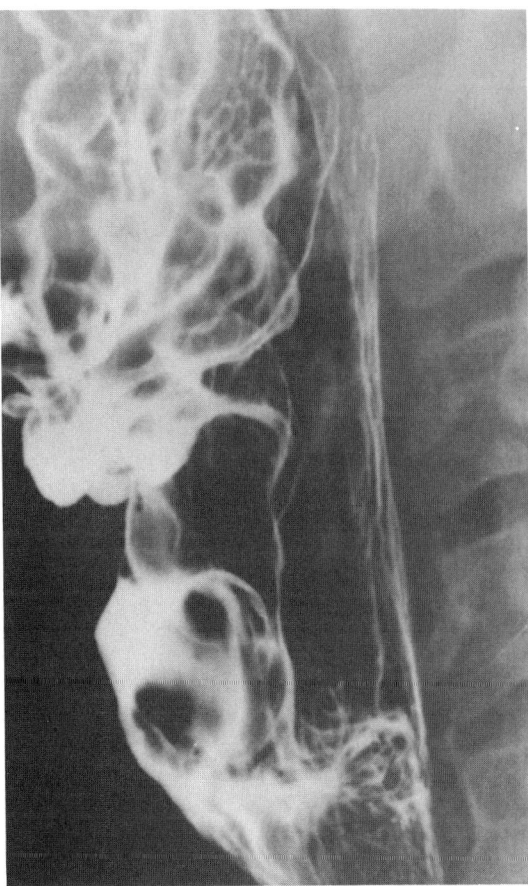

FIGURE 13.3. A 38-year-old homosexual man with dysphagia and Kaposi's sarcoma. (A) Anteroposterior and (B) oblique views of pharynx demonstrate multiple large nodular submucosal lesions involving the anterior oropharynx and base of the tongue. The valleculae are deformed, and there is a 2.5cm lesion in the left piriform sinus. (Reprinted with permission from Emery CD, Wall SD, Federle MP, Sooy CD. Pharyngeal Kaposi's sarcoma in patients with AIDS. *AJR Am J Roentgenol* 1986;147:919–922.)

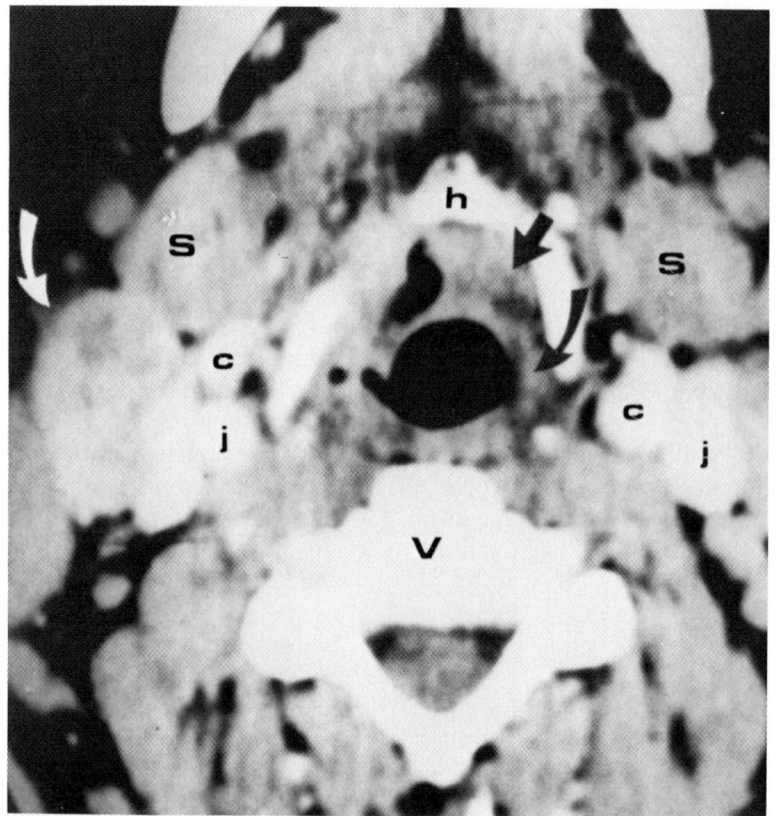
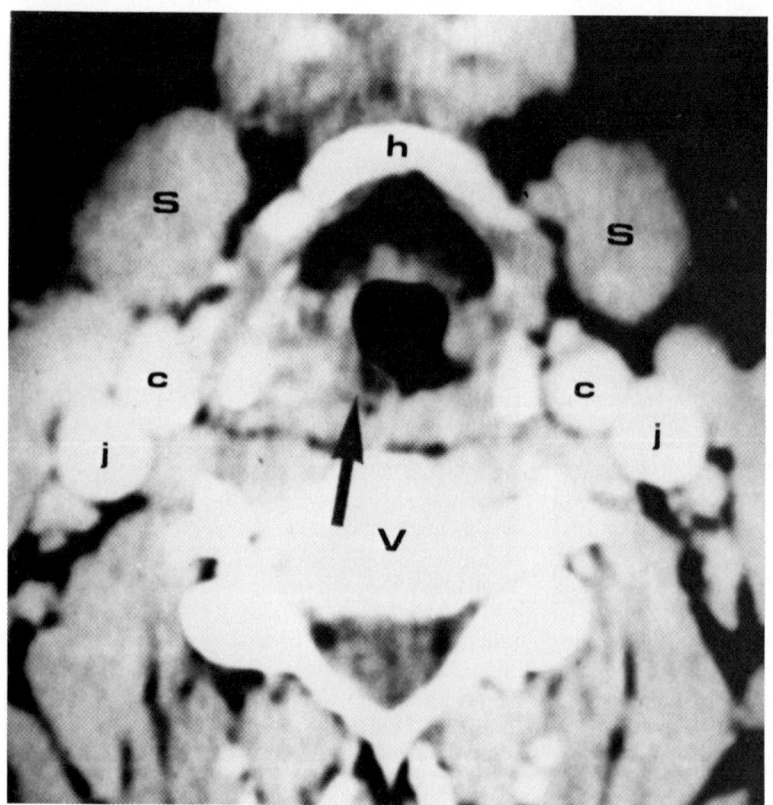

FIGURE 13.4. A 31-year-old homosexual man with Kaposi's sarcoma and dysphagia. (A) Computed tomography of the neck demonstrates obliteration of the left vallecula (straight arrow) and orifice of the left piriform sinus (curved black arrow). Curved white arrow indicates large lymph node with heterogeneous enhancement from intravenous contrast material. (B) At the level of the hyoid bone (h), there is thickening of the aryepiglottic fold with narrowing of the laryngeal vestibule (arrow) and infiltration of the parapharyngeal spaces bilaterally. V, vertebral body; S, submandibular gland; c, carotid artery; j, internal jugular vein. (Reprinted with permission from Emery CD, Wall SD, Federle MP, Sooy CD. Pharyngeal Kaposi's sarcoma in patients with AIDS. *AJR Am J Roentgenol* 1986;147:919–922.)

esophagitis, and the other had a superficial spreading carcinoma that mimicked diffuse esophagitis (Figure 13.7).

Opportunistic Infections

Candida

Dysphagia is a very common presenting complaint in patients with HIV disease and opportunistic infection (26). The esophagus is the most common site of infection in candidiasis, and *Candida* infection is the most common cause of esophagitis in AIDS patients (6,8,9, 20,27–29). Esophageal candidiasis is the AIDS-defining event in 13% of patients, and 22% develop it during the course of disease (30). Esophageal candidiasis occurs with increasing frequency as the CD4 count drops below 200 cells/μL (9).

The radiographic findings of *Candida* esophagitis vary according to the duration and severity of the infection. The earliest abnormality observed is disordered primary and secondary peristalsis. This can range from a mildly dilated aperistaltic esophagus to spasm with multiple nonpropulsive tertiary contractions. The esophagus may appear normal in structure if there is only superficial involvement of the mucosa. The most common detectable lesions found early in the course of the disease are

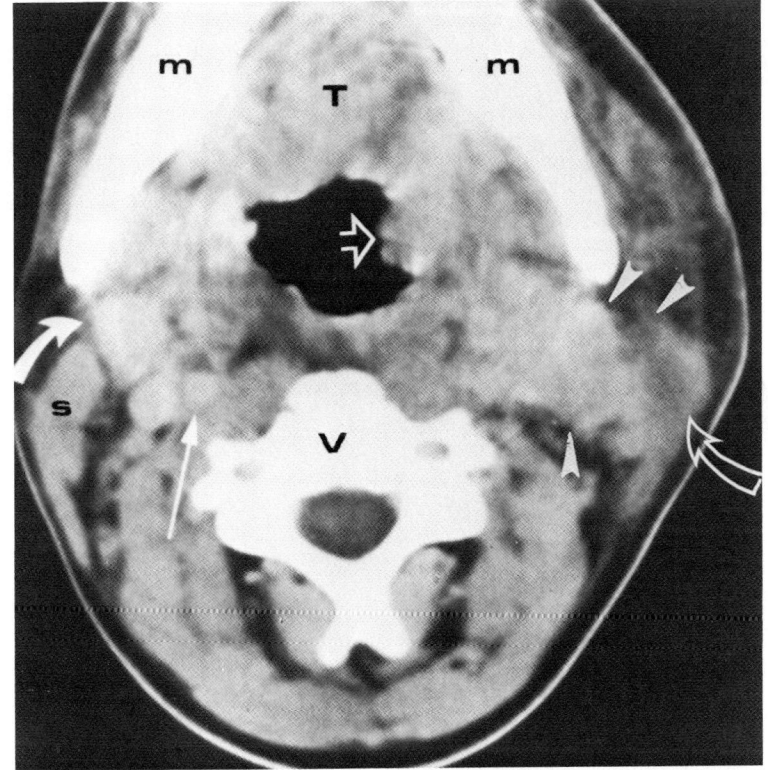

FIGURE 13.5. A 22-year-old homoxexual man with Kaposi's sarcoma and dysphagia. Computed tomography of the neck demonstrates bilateral parapharyngeal space infiltration by Kaposi's sarcoma (open straight arrow). Note tumor extension on the left about the carotid sheath into the sternocleidomastoid muscle (open curved arrow). Ill-defined but enlarged submandibular gland (arrowheads) on the left was biopsy sample of positive for Kaposi's sarcoma. Curved arrow indicates right submandibular gland; straight arrow indicates right carotid artery. V, vertebral body; T, tongue; m, mandible; s, submandibular gland. (Reprinted with permission from Emery CD, Wall SD, Federle MP, Sooy CD. Pharyngeal Kaposi's sarcoma in patients with AIDS. *AJR Am J Roentgenol* 1986;147:919–922.)

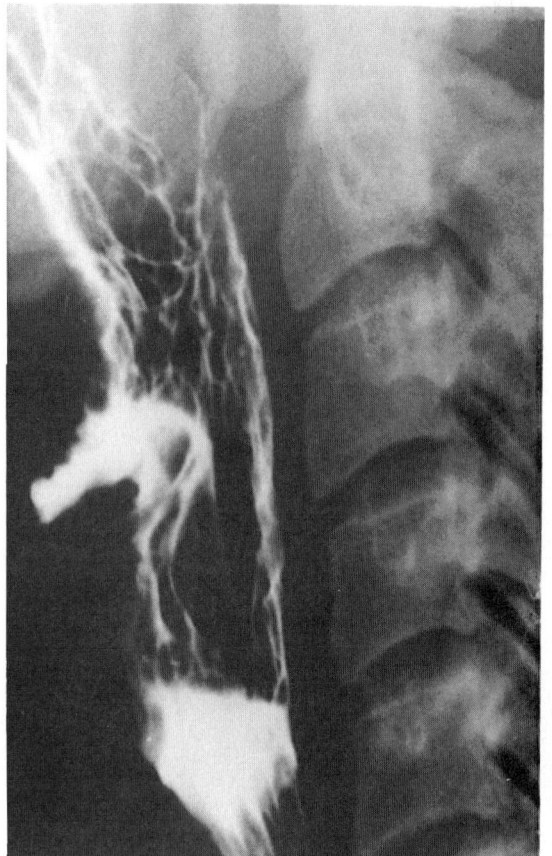
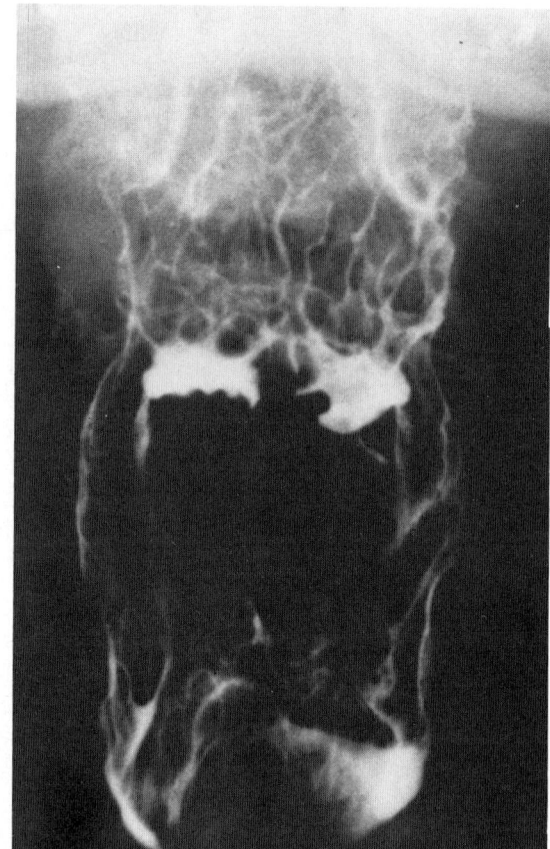
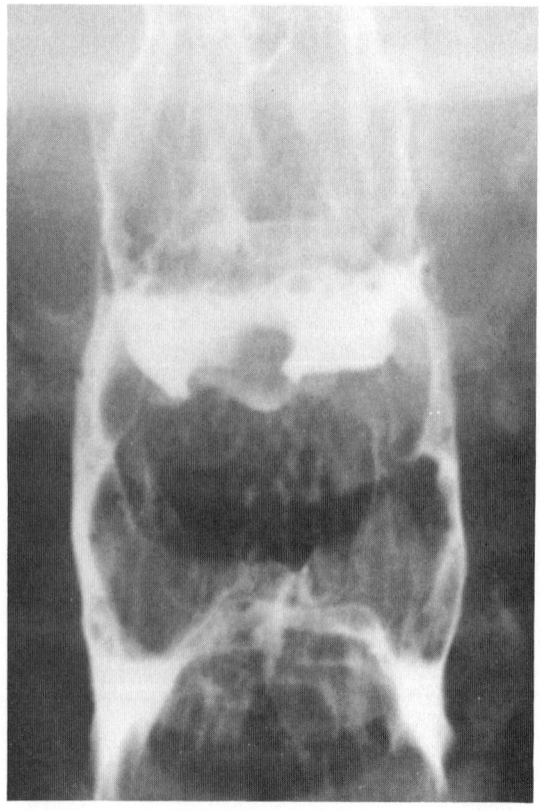

FIGURE 13.6. A 30-year-old homosexual man with oral Kaposi's sarcoma and dysphagia. (A) Lateral and (B) anteroposterior views of the pharynx demonstrate multiple small coalescent nodules of Kaposi's sarcoma in the oroparynx and hypopharynx with deformity of the valleculae and piriform sinuses. (C) Reevaluation 10 months later after local radiation treatment shows fewer lesions and less distortion of the valleculae and piriform sinuses. (Reprinted with permission from Emery CD, Wall SD, Federle MP, Sooy CD. Pharyngeal Kaposi's sarcoma in patients with AIDS. *AJR Am J Roentgenol* 1986;147:919–922.)

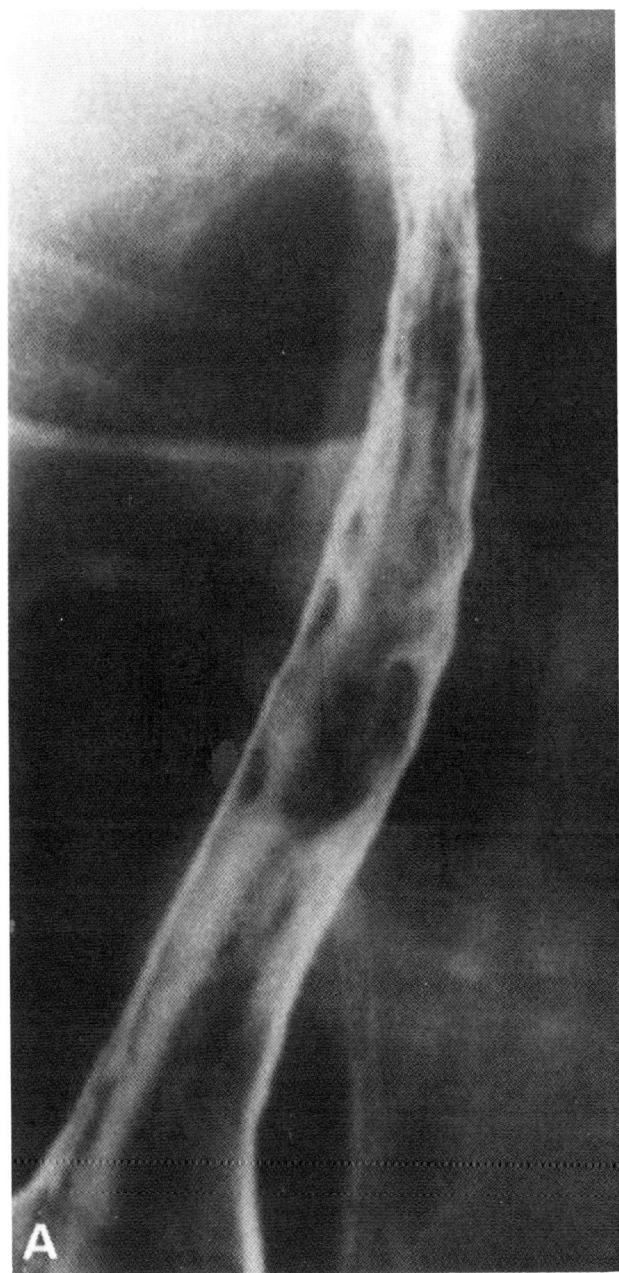 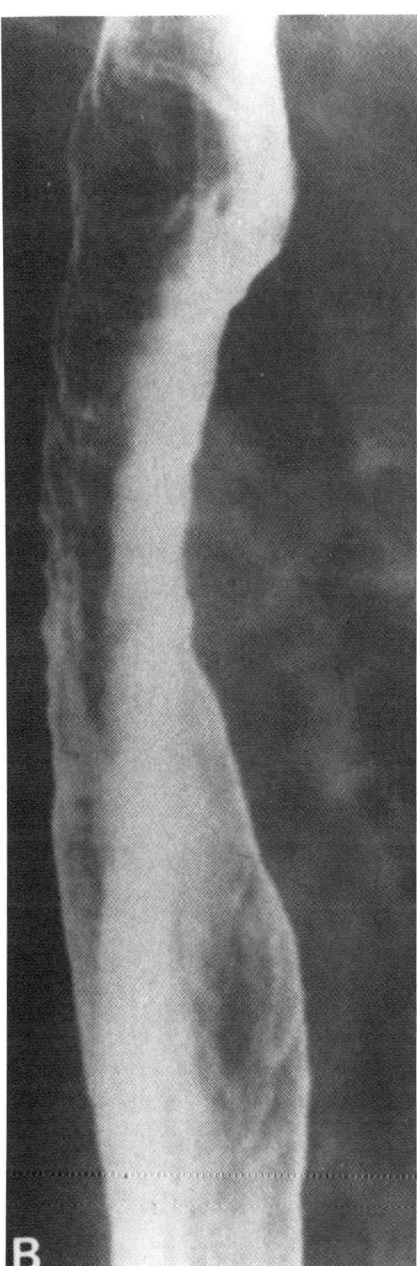

FIGURE 13.7. Double-contrast views of the proximal and midesophagus in a patient with AIDS and dysphagia demonstrate diffuse nodularity of the mucosa without ulceration. Findings were caused by a superficially spreading carcinoma mimicking esophagitis. (Reprinted with permission from Frager DH, Wolf EF, Competiello LS, Frager JD, Klein RS, Beneventano TC. Squamous cell carcinoma of the esophagus in patients with acquired immunodeficiency syndrome. *Gastrointest Radiol* 1988;13: 358–360.)

small mucosal plaques causing filling defects that usually are oriented along the long axis of the esophagus. They are best demonstrated on double-contrast images. These plaques may result in subtle irregularity of the esophageal contour (9,29). Thickened folds (>2–3 mm), a hazy-appearing granular mucosa, and/or abnormal motility may be seen, but these are nonspecific findings. Narrowing of the esophageal lumen may occur as a result of edema and pseudomembrane formation. A cobblestone pattern seen as nodular filling defects is produced by inflammation and edema of the submucosa and lamina propria. With disease progression, barium esophagography reveals extensive plaque formation that produce the classic "shaggy" mucosal appearance (Figure 13.8) (9,20), caused by barium coating within the interstices of confluent plaques and pseudomembranes. In most cases, *Candida* esophagitis produces diffuse mucosal abnormalities, involving most of the thoracic esophagus. When segmental disease occurs, the midesophagus and distal esophagus are more often involved (29). Occasionally, an isolated lesion of *Candida* organisms and denuded necrotic mucosa is noted that can simulate the appearance of a mass. In rare cases of chronic esophageal candidiasis, gastric bezoars due to *Candida* fungus balls may develop (9). Small or discrete ulcers are atypical manifestations of candidiasis, and in general, they suggest a viral, idiopathic, peptic, or neoplastic etiology (8,29). Barium can dissect beneath plaques, producing intramural tracts. Strictures, though uncommon, may develop as a complication of severe esophageal candidal infection, and occasionally these appear abrupt, annular, or asymmetric, simulating a malignancy (29).

Radiographic confirmation (without endoscopy) of clinically suspected *Candida* esophagitis has become increasingly common, and it frequently serves as the basis for extensive therapy. Contrast studies are particularly useful when platelet counts preclude biopsy, perforation is suspected, and/or an esophageal stricture is present (31). Furthermore, radiographic reexamination is a good monitor of response to therapy. Typically patients improve following the proper antifungal therapy and

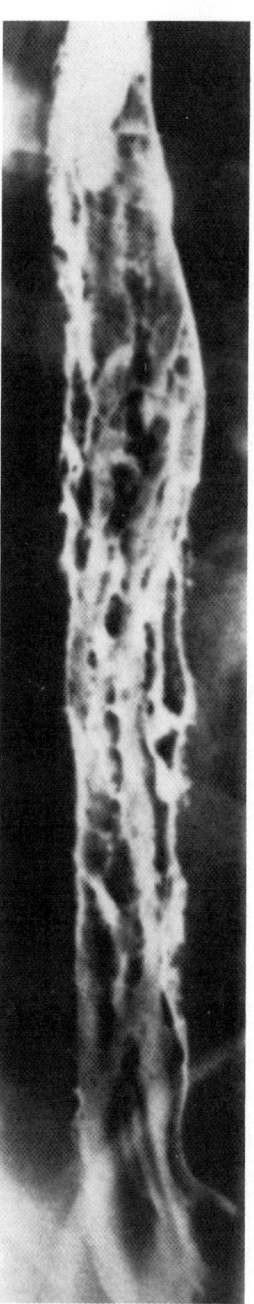

Figure 13.8. Diffuse nodular irregularity and shagginess of the esophagus is demonstrated on this barium esophagram of a patient with AIDS. Findings are representative of severe monilial esophagitis. (From Megibow AJ, Wall SD, Balthazar EJ, Rybak BJ. Gastrointestinal radiology in AIDS patients. In: Federle M, Megibow AJ, Naidich DP, eds. *Radiology of AIDS*. New York: Raven Press; 1998:77–105.)

should be followed to complete radiographic and clinical resolution. If the patient fails therapy, endoscopy is warranted to exclude a coexistent infection or neoplasm (9).

Wilcox et al., who performed endoscopy on patients who failed to respond to empiric oral antifungal therapy, found a specifically treatable cause other than *Candida* in 80% of patients, with esophageal ulceration being the most common finding (4). Based on their study, endoscopy is recommended for patients with persistent esophageal symptoms despite a 1-week course of standard dose of empiric oral antifungal therapy, particularly for those with worsening odynophagia and those with a CD4 count below 100 cells/mm^3. In patients with a CD4 count exceeding 100 cells/mm^3, long duration of symptoms, or dysphagia without odynophagia, and normal endoscopic examination, a barium study to evaluate for a motility disorder or gastroesophageal reflux may be warranted (32).

Levine et al. evaluated the radiographic findings of AIDS patients with opportunistic esophagitis. After correlation of the radiographic findings with those on endoscopy, autopsy, and/or clinical course, they concluded that fungal and viral esophagitis can be differentiated with double-contrast esophagography (33). Radiographic differentiation is possible when a grossly irregular or "shaggy" mucosa is apparent, indicating *Candida* infection. Conversely, discrete ulcerations upon a background of normal mucosa are more typical of cytomegalovirus or herpes simplex infection. Other infectious etiologies with a similar morphological appearance include HIV and, less commonly, *Mycobacterium avium-intracellulare* (34,35).

Cytomegalovirus

Nearly ubiquitous in patients with AIDS (36), CMV is the most common life-threatening opportunistic infection in these patients; CMV infections develop when the CD4 count is less than 100 cells/μL (9,37). Abnormalities that are related to the severity of infection and level of immune compromise, are produced by CMV esophagitis, which is associated with a poor prognosis (9,38). With early disease, superficial erosions and shallow ulcerations may occur. With more severe disease, patients may develop solitary or multiple deep ulcers. Primarily, CMV infects endothelial cells and mesenchymal cells, with epithelial cells less frequently involved. The result of CMV infection is a vasculitis of the submucosal capillaries and venules, producing thrombosis, ischemia, and necrosis (9).

Balthazar et al. have described the radiographic findings of CMV esophagitis in patients with HIV disease (39,40). Typical radiographic findings were those of focal, discretely marginated diamond-shaped ulcers surrounded by a well-defined peripheral lucency representing a zone of edema (Figure 13.9). This was most representative of CMV esophagitis when seen against a background of normal esophageal mucosa. A characteristic finding is the presence of a giant (>2 cm) flat ovoid ulcer located in the distal esophagus (29). Occasionally, Balthazar et al. noted clustered superficial aphthous lesions producing a localized granular appearance (39,40). Of particular interest is the high incidence of ulceration noted at the gastroesophageal junction, with occasional extension of this process into the proximal stomach. Such large ulceration generally produced thickening of the folds of the esophagus as well as the gastric fundus (9,29). On CT scanning, thickening of the abdominal portion of the esophagus was noted as well as increased density of the lesser omental fat. In an endoscopic study of 33 patients, Wilcox et al. found esophageal disease due to CMV infection to be highly variable in appearance (41). Multiple ulcers were found in 58% of patients, and they were the most common endoscopic finding. Giant ulcers were found in 28%, with 43% of the lesions less than 1 cm in greatest dimension. Diffuse erosive disease was found in 6% of the patients. The majority of lesions were located in the mid- to distal esophagus.

When the superficial esophageal ulcers of CMV infection are small, they may be identical in appearance to herpetic ulcerations, although they tend not to be as numerous. There are other diagnostic considerations when these lesions enlarge into giant ulcers (29). For

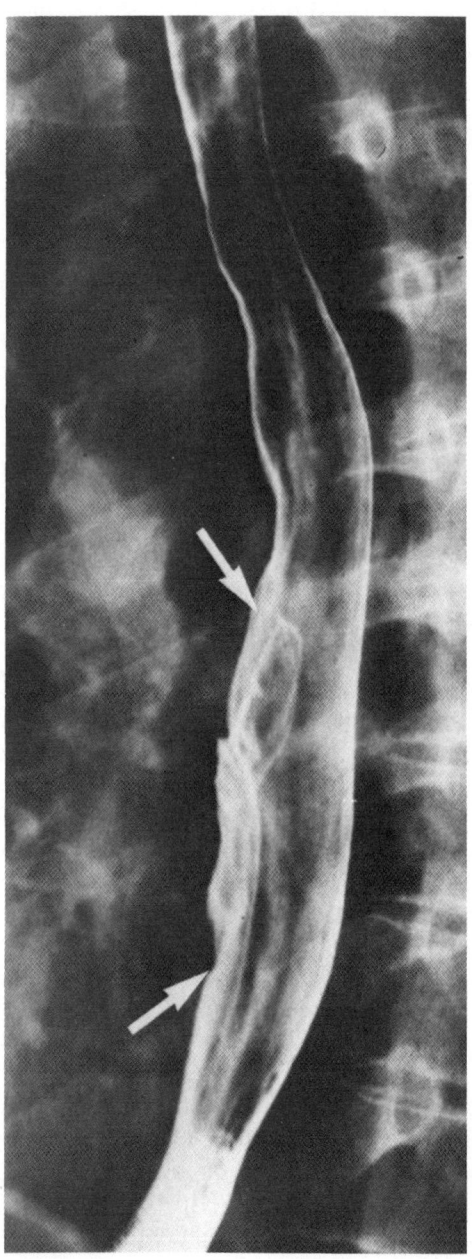

FIGURE 13.9. Double-contrast barium esophagogram demonstrates giant ulceration (arrows) of CMV esophagitis. Note the background of normal mucosa. (Reprinted with permission from Megibow AJ, Wall SD, Balthazar EJ, Rybak BJ. Gastrointestinal radiology in AIDS patients. In: Federle M, Megibow AJ, Naidich DP, eds. *Radiology of AIDS*. New York: Raven Press; 1998:77–105.)

instance, the radiographic appearance can be similar to the large flat ulcerations associated directly with HIV itself, and definitive diagnosis requires endoscopic biopsy and histopathological evaluation (9,29). Other etiologies of giant esophageal ulcers include *Candida*, *Mycobacterium avium-intracellulare*, and *Mycobacterium tuberculosis*. Noninfectious causes of large ulcers include reflux esophagitis and drug-induced esophagitis. Peptic ulcerations usually are adjacent to the esophagogastric junction and may be associated with a hiatal hernia or gastroesophageal reflux. Clinical history will aid in identifying medication-induced ulcerations (29). Medications that have been associated with esophageal ulcerations in HIV-infected patients include zalcitabine (ddC) and zidovudine (AZT) (3,20). Double-contrast radiography is important in the evaluation of the aforementioned findings in the hypopharynx and esophagus.

Herpes Simplex Virus

Herpes simplex virus 1 is a frequent inhabitant of the salivary glands of adults, and therefore, saliva serves as the source of autoinoculation as well as transmission to others (29). The initial HSV infection results from direct inoculation of the virus through mucous membranes. The virus reaches the nerve root ganglion via the afferent nerve and persists in a latent state. When reactivated, the virus undergoes replication and travels back along the efferent nerve to the mucous membrane, where clinically apparent lesions develop. Viral reactivation frequently occurs when the CD4 count decreases below 50 cells/µL. This virus is a frequent cause of esophagitis in immunosuppressed individuals and is an AIDS-defining condition (9,42). The clinical presentation is indistinguishable from that of *Candida* esophagitis, with most patients complaining of odynophagia or dysphagia (9).

Manifestations of HSV esophagitis, seen to best advantage on double-contrast barium esophagograms, include multiple shallow ulcers [0.3–2.0cm in diameter (2)] that are diffusely scattered and separated by normal intervening mucosa (Figure 13.10). Herpes ulcers may, however, be clustered together, occurring most commonly in the midesophagus. These ulcers typically have a diamond or stellate configuration, and they demonstrate a thin lucent halo of edema. With advanced cases of HSV esophagitis, diagnosis becomes increasingly difficult because there is progression to plaquelike defects, nodularity with cobblestoning, and a grossly irregular esophageal contour identical to findings seen in *Candida* esophagitis. Reported complications include stricture formation, esophageal perforation with tracheoesophageal fistula formation, fatal hemorrhage, and diffuse visceral dissemination. The differential diagnosis includes CMV esophagitis, HIV esophagitis, reflux esophagitis, acute corrosive ingestion, acute radiation esophagitis, drug-induced esophagitis, and Crohn's disease. Most of these conditions may be excluded on the basis of the patient's clinical history (29).

Mycobacterium Tuberculosis

Previously, tuberculous involvement of the esophagus was considered to be a rare finding on autopsy. The resurgence of systemic tuberculosis that has been associated with the AIDS epidemic combined with aggressive endoscopic diagnosis has resulted in an increase in the number of cases over the past decade (31). Tuberculosis occurs with increased frequency as the CD4 counts fall below 400 cells/µL and extrapulmonary manifestations occur in approximately 40 to 80% of AIDS patients when CD4 counts fall below 200 cells/µL (9). In tuberculous esophagitis, the esophagus is secondarily involved via several pathways. Local extension from, or extrinsic compression by (43), adjacent infected necrotic mediastinal nodes is the most common route. Less commonly, there may be extension from tuberculosis of the larynx, pharynx, or spine. Also, esophageal infection can occur by swallowing coughed-up infected sputum. This often is superimposed on a fixed mucosal lesion such as carcinoma or a stricture. Finally, hematogenous spread can occur from miliary tuberculosis. Primary esophageal tuberculosis is rare (29).

Patients with tuberculous esophagitis may be asymptomatic, or they may complain of dys-

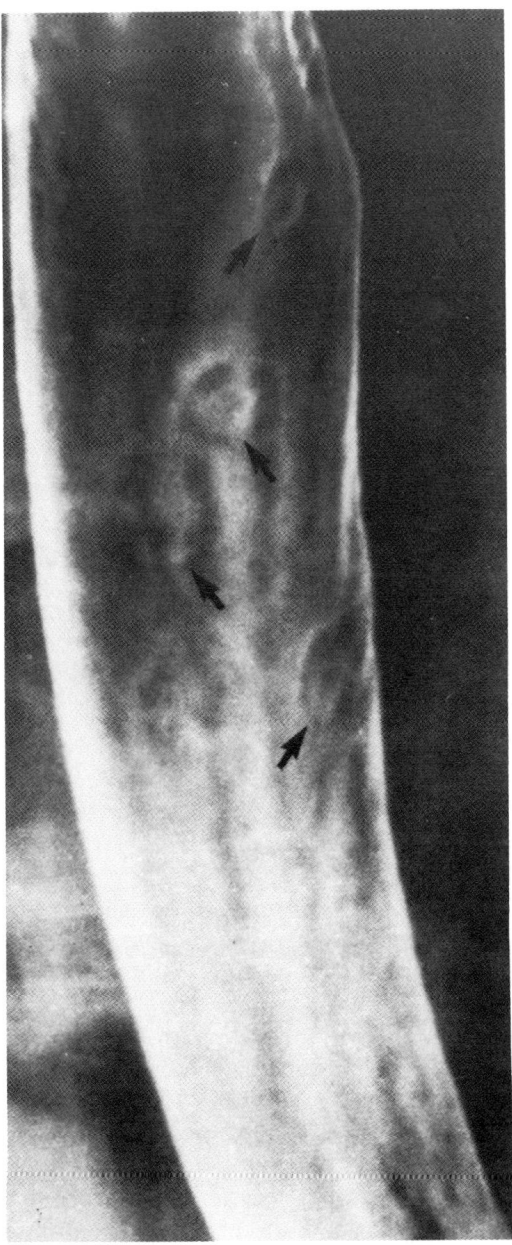

FIGURE 13.10. Double-contrast esophagogram in a patient with AIDS and dysphagia demonstrates multiple discrete, superficial ulcers (arrows) on a background of normal mucosa. Findings are representative of herpes esophagitis, which resolved both clinically and radiographically after treatment with acyclovir. (Reprinted with permission from Leving MS, Woldenberg R, Herlinger H, Laufer I. Opportunistic esophagitis in AIDS: radiographic diagnosis. *Radiology* 1987;165:815–820.)

phagia or chest pain. Barium esophagography may demonstrate focal extrinsic mass impression from adjacent mediastinal adenopathy, ulcerations that tend to be deep, and both sinus tract and fistula formation (29). Fistula formation tends to occur in the midesophagus, where the infected mediastinal lymph nodes are most commonly located (9). Traction diverticula and strictures are findings of chronic tuberculous esophagitis. Esophageal carcinoma, bronchogenic carcinoma, and metastatic mediastinal adenopathy may cause identical findings on the esophagogram. The differential diagnosis includes other rare opportunistic infections such as actinomycosis esophagitis, which may also cause deep intramural sinus tracts as well as fistula formation (29). In addition, HIV-related ulcers have been associated with fistula formation (9). Very rarely, Crohn's disease of the esophagus may demonstrate similar findings (29).

Human Immunodeficiency Virus

In addition to the numerous opportunistic infections that ultimately affect patients with AIDS, it has become clear that infection with human immunodeficiency virus (HIV) itself may produce disease (9). During the past decade, giant esophageal ulcers have been encountered with increasing frequency in HIV-positive patients soon after infection occurs. At first these ulcers were thought to be caused by CMV. More recently, electron microscopy and in situ hybridization techniques have implicated HIV itself as a cause of the ulcers (44). Soon after HIV seroconversion, some patients develop an acute febrile, mononucleosislike illness. Patients may experience a host of symptoms including sore throat, malaise, and myalgias, and may complain of symptoms related to involvement of the gastrointestinal tract including odynophagia, dysphagia, nausea, and/or diarrhea. Odynophagia in this setting often is related to primary HIV ulceration of the esophagus. HIV-related ulcers can occur either during acute HIV infection when there is transient immunosuppression or after AIDS has developed. Endoscopy and radiography have demonstrated discrete esophageal ulcers that tend to be large (>2 cm) and shallow (9,45,46).

Multiple ulcers may be present, and fistula formation can occur. The background esophageal mucosa tends to be normal (9). Because CMV ulcers in the esophagus may produce the same radiographic findings as HIV-related ulcers, endoscopy is required to differentiate these lesions. This is important because the treatment regimen is quite different, and it is not possible to differentiate these diagnoses by barium esophagography. Gancyclovir, a potentially toxic drug, is used to treat CMV esophagitis, while HIV-related ulcers usually are treated with steroids (44,46). It is also important to exclude the diagnosis of tuberculous esophagitis, which also can result in large ulcers and fistula formation. It is notable also that the HIV ulcer that occurs soon after seroconversion often resolves spontaneously.

Of note, occasional but uncommon cases of discrete esophageal ulceration in HIV patients have been found to be due to *Mycobacterium avium-intracellulare* or gram-positive cocci, presumably group B streptococcal infection (47). Megibow et al. have encountered three patients with HIV disease and severe esophagitis manifested by deep ulceration that coalesced into intramural sinus tracts paralleling the long axis of the esophagus, and in one patient actinomycosis was identified as the etiological agent (47).

Risks and Risk Prevention

The human immunodeficiency virus, which is the causative organism of AIDS, is transmitted via three routes: exchange of blood, body fluids, or tissues by means other than sexual contact; sexual contact; and perinatal infection. Because of the first route, some health workers are at risk to exposure of HIV infection in the workplace (48). This includes those who are exposed to blood or body fluids or various sharp instruments such as needles and scalpels (48). Regarding such individuals, the medical literature has focused primarily on surgical, pathology, emergency, and dental staff. However, many diagnostic and therapeutic procedures performed by radiologists have the potential to expose them and their associates to the body fluids of patients with HIV disease (48). Consequently, infection control practices must be reviewed continually by all departments of radiology. And education programs regarding the prevention of transmission of infectious diseases should be part of a scheduled, ongoing in-service training for all members of a radiology department.

Heller et al. summarized this issue and concluded that "the cornerstone of infection control practice is 'body substance precautions'" (49). The potential for a false negative report is the most important reason for not recommending that patients be screened for HIV positivity on a general basis. This is especially important in the patient who has been exposed to HIV, currently is asymptomatic, and has not converted to HIV positivity. Therefore, Heller et al. have provided a list of seven recommendations pertinent to radiology departments that are based on the publications of the Centers for Disease Control (50) and authorities on AIDS (51). Because of their importance, they are summarized here.

1. Education of all personnel regarding transmission of HIV infection should be regularly updated.

2. Appropriate barrier precautions (e.g., gloves, glasses, etc.) should be used by all personnel involved in procedures that have potential for contact with body fluids.

3. Needles should never be recapped, and containers should be readily available for disposal of sharp instruments.

4. Personnel with dermatitis or open skin lesions should not participate in procedures that have potential for contact with body fluids.

5. Airway ventilation devices should be available in every room to prevent the need for emergency mouth-to-mouth resuscitation.

6. Routine cleaning measures should be employed: a freshly prepared solution of sodium hypochlorite (1:10 dilution of household bleach) will kill the virus rapidly.

7. If a health care worker is exposed to the virus, the supervisor in Occupational Health Service for the hospital should be notified promptly. The worker should be offered counseling and periodic HIV testing, and the patient should be asked to consent to testing.

Summary

Swallowing difficulties in patients with HIV disease can be due to opportunisic tumor (usually Kaposi's sarcoma) or opportunistic infections, of which there are several, *Candida* being the most common. The radiographic evaluation of these patients can be particularly helpful regarding diagnosis, treatment planning, and response to therapy. The findings on barium esophagography and/or CT, which have the advantage of being noninvasive, can be revealing both in regard to possible etiology and in regard to extent of disease. Radiologists need to be aware of the patterns of the various disease processes that occur in these patients as well as the proper procedures to ensure protection against transmission of communicable disease.

References

1. Martinez EJ, Nord HJ, Cooper BG. Significance of solitary and multiple esophageal ulcers in patients with AIDS. *South Med J* 1995; 88:626–629.
2. Raufman JP. Odynophagia/dysphagia in AIDS. *Gastroenterol Clin North Am* 1988;17:599–614.
3. Shapiro BD, Ehrenpreis ED, Tomaka FL, Bonner GF, Secrest KM, Cheney LM. Idiopathic midesophageal stricture: a new cause of dysphagia in a patient with AIDS. *South Med J* 1997; 90:80–82.
4. Wilcox CM, Straub RF, Alexander LN, Clark WS. Etiology of esophageal disease in human immunodeficiency virus-infected patients who fail antifungal therapy. *Am J Med* 1996;101: 599–604.
5. Goldberg AN. Kaposi's sarcoma of the head and neck in acquired immunodeficiency syndrome. *Am J Otolaryngol* 1993;14:5–14.
6. Marnejon T, Scoccia V. The coexistence of primary esophageal lymphoma and *Candida glabrata* esophagitis presenting as dysphagia and odynophagia in a patient with acquired immunodeficiency syndrome. *Am J Gastroenterol* 1997; 92:354–356.
7. Bonacini M, Young T, Laine L. The causes of esophageal symptoms in human immunodeficiency virus infection. A prospective study of 110 patients. *Arch Intern Med* 1991;151:1567–1572.
8. Bonacini M, Laine LA. Esophageal disease in patients with AIDS: diagnosis and treatment.

Gastrointest Endosc Clin N Am 1998;8:811–823.
9. Redvanly RD, Silverstein JE. Intra-abdominal manifestations of AIDS. *Radiol Clin North Am* 1997;35:1083–1125.
10. Noyer CM, Simon D. Oral and esophageal disorders. *Gastroenterol Clin North Am* 1997;26:241–257.
11. Wilcox CM, Monkemuller KE. Diagnosis and management of esophageal disease in the acquired immunodeficiency syndrome. *South Med J* 1998;91:1002–1008.
12. Neville CR, Peddada AV, Smith D, Kagan AR, Frost DB, Sadoff L. Massive gastrointestinal hemorrhage from AIDS-related Kaposi's sarcoma confined to the small bowel managed with radiation. *Med Pediatr Oncol* 1996;26:135–138.
13. Gottlieb MS, Groopman JE, Weinstein WM, Fahey JL, Detels R. The acquired immunodeficiency syndrome. *Ann Intern Med* 1983;99:208–220.
14. Friedman SL, Wright TL, Altman DF. Gastrointestinal Kaposi's sarcoma in patients with acquired immunodeficiency syndrome. Endoscopic and autopsy findings. *Gastroenterology* 1985;89:102–108.
15. Emery CD, Wall SD, Federle MP, Sooy CD. Pharyngeal Kaposi's sarcoma in patients with AIDS. *AJR Am J Roentgenol* 1986;147:919–922.
16. Hill CA, Harle TS, Mansell PW. The prodrome, Kaposi sarcoma, and infections associated with acquired immunodeficiency syndrome: radiologic findings in 39 patients. *Radiology* 1983;149:393–399.
17. Rose HS, Balthazar EJ, Megibow AJ, Horowitz L, Laubenstein LJ. Alimentary tract involvement in Kaposi sarcoma: radiographic and endoscopic findings in 25 homosexual men. *AJR Am J Roentgenol* 1982;139:661–666.
18. Wall SD, Friedman SL, Margulis AR. Gastrointestinal Kaposi's sarcoma in AIDS: radiographic manifestations. *J Clin Gastroenterol* 1984;6:165–171.
19. Wall SD, Ominsky S, Altman DF, et al. Multifocal abnormalities of the gastrointestinal tract in AIDS. *AJR Am J Roentgenol* 1986;146:1–5.
20. Wilcox CM. Esophageal disease in the acquired immunodeficiency syndrome: etiology, diagnosis, and management. *Am J Med* 1992;92:412–421.
21. Gelb AB, Medeiros LJ, Chen YY, Weiss LM, Weidner N. Hodgkin's disease of the esophagus. *Am J Clin Pathol* 1997;108:593–598.
22. Sabate JM, Franquet T, Palmer J, Monill JM. AIDS-related primary esophageal lymphoma. *Abdom Imaging* 1997;22:11–13.
23. Cappell MS, Botros N. Predominantly gastrointestinal symptoms and signs in 11 consecutive AIDS patients with gastrointestinal lymphoma: a multicenter, multiyear study including 763 HIV-seropositive patients. *Am J Gastroenterol* 1994;89:545–549.
24. Frager DH, Wolf EL, Competiello LS, Frager JD, Klein RS, Beneventano TC. Squamous cell carcinoma of the esophagus in patients with acquired immunodeficiency syndrome. *Gastrointest Radiol* 1988;13:358–360.
25. Simmons MZ, Cho KC, Houghton JM, Levine CD, Javors BR. Inflammatory fibroid polyp of the esophagus in an HIV-infected individual: case study. *Dysphagia* 1995;10:59–61.
26. Federle MP. A radiologist looks at AIDS: imaging evaluation based on symptom complexes. *Radiology* 1988;166:553–562.
27. Frager DH, Frager JD, Brandt LJ, et al. Gastrointestinal complications of AIDS: radiologic features. *Radiology* 1986;158:597–603.
28. Wilcox CM, Alexander LN, Clark WS, Thompson SE III. Fluconazole compared with endoscopy for human immunodeficiency virus–infected patients with esophageal symptoms. *Gastroenterology* 1996;110:1803–1809.
29. Yee J, Wall SD. Infectious esophagitis. *Radiol Clin North Am* 1994;32:1135–1145.
30. Hood SV, Hollis S, Percy M, Atkinson G, Williams K, Denning DW. Assessment of therapeutic response of oropharyngeal and esophageal candidiasis in AIDS with use of a new clinical scoring system: studies with D0870. *Clin Infect Dis* 1999;28:587–596.
31. Sutton FM, Graham DY, Goodgame RW. Infectious esophagitis. *Gastrointest Endosc Clin N Am* 1994;4:713–729.
32. Fried RL, Brandt LJ, Kauvar D, Simon D. Esophageal motility in AIDS patients with symptomatic opportunistic infections of the esophagus. *Am J Gastroenterol* 1994;89:2003–2005.
33. Levine MS, Woldenberg R, Herlinger H, Laufer I. Opportunistic esophagitis in AIDS: radiographic diagnosis. *Radiology* 1987;165:815–820.
34. El-Serag HB, Johnston DE. *Mycobacterium avium* complex esophagitis. *Am J Gastroenterol* 1997;92:1561–1563.
35. Pursner M, Haller JO, Berdon WE. Imaging features of *Mycobacterium avium-intracellulare* complex (MAC) in children with AIDS. *Pediatr Radiol* 2000;30:426–429.
36. Laine L, Bonacini M, Sattler F, Young T, Sherrod A. Cytomegalovirus and *Candida* esophagitis in

patients with AIDS. *J Acquired Immune Defic Syndrome* 1992;5:605–609.
37. Monkemuller KE, Wilcox CM. Esophageal ulcer caused by cytomegalovirus: resolution during combination antiretroviral therapy for acquired immunodeficiency syndrome. *South Med J* 2000;93:818–820.
38. Wilcox CM, Straub RF, Schwartz DA. Cytomegalovirus esophagitis in AIDS: a prospective evaluation of clinical response to ganciclovir therapy, relapse rate, and long-term outcome. *Am J Med* 1995;98:169–176.
39. Balthazar EJ, Megibow AJ, Hulnick D, Cho KC, Beranbaum E. Cytomegalovirus esophagitis in AIDS: radiographic features in 16 patients. *Am J Roentgenol* 1987;149:919–923.
40. Balthazar EJ, Megibow AJ, Hulnick DH. Cytomegalovirus esophagitis and gastritis in AIDS. *AJR Am J Roentgenol* 1985;144:1201–1204.
41. Wilcox CM, Straub RF, Schwartz DA. Prospective endoscopic characterization of cytomegalovirus esophagitis in AIDS. *Gastrointest Endosc* 1994;40:481–484.
42. Genereau T, Lortholary O, Bouchaud O, et al. Herpes simplex esophagitis in patients with AIDS: report of 34 cases. The Cooperative Study Group on Herpetic Esophagitis in HIV Infection. *Clin Infect Dis* 1996;22:926–931.
43. Ruiz-Arguelles GJ, Ponce-De-Leon S, Soto-Priante H, Castellanos-Perez JM, Moreno-Ford V, Garces-Eisele J. Nodal radiotherapy in refractory tuberculosis in an AIDS patient. *Arch Med Res* 1996;27:93–95.
44. Sor S, Levine MS, Kowalski TE, Laufer I, Rubesin SE, Herlinger H. Giant ulcers of the esophagus in patients with human immunodeficiency virus: clinical, radiographic, and pathologic findings. *Radiology* 1995;194:447–451.
45. Frager D, Kotler DP, Baer J. Idiopathic esophageal ulceration in the acquired immunodeficiency syndrome: radiologic reappraisal in 10 patients. *Abdom Imaging* 1994;19:2–5.
46. Levine MS, Loercher G, Katzka DA, Herlinger H, Rubesin SE, Laufer I. Giant, human immunodeficiency virus-related ulcers in the esophagus. *Radiology* 1991;180:323–326.
47. Megibow AJ, Wall SD, Balthazar EJ, Ryback BJ. Gastrointestinal radiology in AIDS patients. In: Federle M, Megibow AJ, Naidich DP, eds. *Radiology of AIDS*. New York: Raven Press; 1988:77–105.
48. Wall SD, Howe JM, Sawhney R. Human immunodeficiency virus infection and hepatitis: biosafety in radiology. *Radiology* 1997;205:619–628.
49. Heller RM, Horev G, Kirchner SG, Schaffner W. AIDS awareness in the conduct of radiologic procedures: guidelines to safe practice. *Radiology* 1988;166:563–567.
50. Recommendations for prevention of HIV transmission in health-care settings. *MMWR Morb Mortal Wkly Rep* 1987;36(suppl 2):1S–18S.
51. Gerberding JL, Henderson DK. Design of rational infection control policies for human immunodeficiency virus infection. *J Infect Dis* 1987;156:861–864.

14
The Role of Radiology in Rehabilitation of Swallowing

JEFFREY B. PALMER AND EILEEN A. CARDEN

The preceding chapters have explored the contribution of imaging to the diagnostic evaluation of patients with impaired swallowing. Imaging also plays a vital role in their rehabilitation. Although a variety of imaging modalities are employed for diagnostic assessment, the videofluorographic swallowing study (VFSS) is the most useful for analyzing the character and degree of disability. The VFSS reveals the anatomical and functional status of individual components in the swallowing mechanism and the utility of specific therapeutic and compensatory techniques.

Patients with a wide spectrum of swallowing impairments may benefit from rehabilitation. A partial list includes neurogenic, myogenic, connective tissue, and developmental disorders affecting the oral cavity and pharynx, as well as structural deficits due to trauma or head and neck surgery. In fact, etiological diagnosis alone has little value in selecting patients for rehabilitation. Rather, the clinician must consider individually whether each patient can benefit from rehabilitation of swallowing (1).

This chapter will familiarize the reader with the principles of dysphagia rehabilitation. Concepts underlying the rehabilitation of swallowing are considered, and the method of examination is described. We present the physiological rationale for testing foods with a variety of physical characteristics and for selected therapeutic and compensatory techniques. By understanding and applying these principles, the reader can understand the role of the rehabilitation team.

Conceptual Framework for Rehabilitation of Swallowing

It is a truism that ingestion is important to human physiology. Less obvious is the enormous psychosocial importance of eating and swallowing. To a considerable extent, our society is structured around eating and drinking. The inability to eat a meal in the conventional manner creates a barrier to social interaction that may hinder essential relationships in the family, job, and community. For this reason, the evaluation of patients with impaired swallowing requires a holistic approach that considers psychology as well as physiology.

The rehabilitation approach emphasizes function. Rehabilitation is defined as "the process of helping a person to reach the fullest physical, psychological, social, vocational, avocational, and educational potential consistent with his or her physiologic or anatomic impairment, environmental limitations, and desires and life plans" (2, p. 3). The focus on function rather than pathology makes rehabilitation different from other aspects of medical practice. Thus, rehabilitation evaluation incorporates psychological adjustment, home situation, family support, and vocational and avocational pursuits, in addition to pathophysiology. Disorders of swallowing are amenable to this approach because of their impact on physiological, psychological, and social function.

The aim of dysphagia rehabilitation is to establish and maintain the circumstances of safe, efficient swallowing, toward the long-term goal of resuming premorbid roles in society. Imaging plays an essential role in determining the circumstances of safe swallowing, since clinical evaluation alone is of limited value in detecting pharyngeal events. With the VFSS, we test empirically the effects of various therapeutic techniques on each patient's ability to swallow. An axiom underlying this approach is that the best exercise for swallowing is swallowing itself. Thus, therapeutic feeding is the mainstay of therapy. A critical objective of videofluorography is to formulate a prescription for safe and efficient feeding and swallowing.

A single VFSS usually suffices for both diagnostic and rehabilitation purposes. However, it is occasionally desirable to perform a "two-stage" radiological evaluation. This entails performing a VFSS initially to answer diagnostic questions, followed later by a second VFSS study to deal with rehabilitation issues. Choosing between these approaches depends on availability of resources as well as the needs of the patient. Regardless of the approach, obtaining precise anatomical and pathophysiological data is essential; accurate diagnosis is the cornerstone of rehabilitation. Dynamic imaging of the foodway for diagnostic purposes has been discussed elsewhere in this book. In this chapter, we focus on the special aspects of videofluorography for rehabilitation that differentiate it from routine diagnostic imaging.

Method of Examination

The rehabilitation approach to the VFSS is to have the patient eat various foods combined with barium, using appropriate compensatory maneuvers, toward the goal of establishing a safe and efficient method of eating (2,3). The conditions of the VFSS should approximate as much as possible the typical circumstances of eating. Thus, the patient sits comfortably in a chair during the study. Palatable radiopaque foods are presented in a natural way, using conventional utensils. Therapeutic techniques are introduced systematically to assess their effects on the patient's swallowing, particularly the occurrence of tracheal aspiration or retention in the foodway after swallowing. These therapeutic techniques include varying the physical characteristics of the food or modifying the circumstances of feeding, including the manner of presenting the food, posture and position of the patient, and patient behaviors.

A thorough clinical evaluation before VFSS is necessary for **every patient**; the clinical evaluation includes determining the patient's ability to perform and utilize compensatory techniques (2,4,5). This examination is usually completed by the speech-language pathologist or occupational therapist. The clinical observations also contribute to planning the strategy for the videofluorographic study.

Use of standardized protocol for the VFSS and report generation can improve reliability and efficiency (3). This should include a list of radiographic views, food types, and methods of feeding that are tested on every patient. When abnormalities are detected, one can then vary the protocol, including additional modifications of food consistency and compensatory maneuvers as appropriate for the individual patient. Because patients vary greatly, the specific choice of food consistencies and compensatory maneuvers **cannot** be standardized. The flexibility to make crucial decisions "on line" is an essential aspect of videofluorography for rehabilitation. For these reasons and others, a clinician familiar with the patient should always be present during the VFSS. The examination team will often include the treating therapist (usually a speech pathologist or occupational therapist) and a physician (usually a radiologist or physiatrist). If respiratory sequelae are anticipated, it is prudent to include a respiratory therapist and/or a nurse familiar with the patient.

The VFSS is useful in a wide variety of structural and physiological disorders. Most commonly, these studies are undertaken because of complaints referable to pharyngeal and laryngeal dysfunction. However, it is not always possible to exclude esophageal pathology on the basis of history and physical examination; patients with esophageal or gastroesophageal sphincter dysfunction may present with pharyngeal complaints (6). Imaging of the esophagus should be performed in each patient, unless the patient is unable to cooperate.

Equipment

Videofluorography provides immediate playback; this is valuable for making decisions in the fluoroscopic suite and for educating the patient. Because studies may be lengthy, the low radiation exposure with videofluorography is also advantageous. The videocassette recorder should provide slow motion and still-frame capabilities with high image quality. Image quality is best with super-VHS tape. We recommend using a digital videotimer, such as Thalner Electronics Model VC 436. This device imprints the time (in hundredths of a second) on each frame of video, permitting precise timing of events.

Positioning System

The optimal system for positioning of the patient is highly flexible, permitting lateral or posteroanterior views of the pharynx and esophagus with the patient sitting upright or reclining. Ideally, the patient is transferred onto the fluoroscopy chair at the bedside, avoiding the need for transfers in the fluoroscopy suite. A high-backed chair with removable headrest is helpful in examining patients with poor head and neck control.

Observations

The spectrum of observations made during dynamic imaging of the foodway has been discussed in previous chapters and is not reviewed here. However, certain phenomena deserve special attention in videofluorography for rehabilitation, in keeping with the goal of safe and efficient feeding.

Safe swallowing refers to swallowing without jeopardizing airway integrity. To this end, it is essential to recognize occurrences of laryngeal penetration or aspiration (7). Noting the presence and effectiveness of airway protective responses is also vital. Aspiration of minute quantities of food is tolerated by most patients.

However, the failure to cough or clear the throat after aspirating (so-called silent aspiration) may lead to serious respiratory sequelae, such as aspiration pneumonia (8). If radiopaque material is aspirated during the study, the examiner should note whether there is spontaneous coughing or throat clearing, and whether the material is ejected from the airway. It is also important to note whether each episode of aspiration produces a change in voice quality, because this information may be helpful during later therapeutic feedings. If aspiration consistently changes voice quality, this change can serve as a clinical marker of aspiration during subsequent swallowing therapy.

The importance of observing retention in the foodway after swallowing is often overlooked. Food present in the pharynx after swallowing presents a constant danger of aspiration until it is removed. Airway obstruction can result, especially after inhalation of solid food.

Physical Characteristics of Food

Assessing the patient's ability to swallow foods with a variety of physical characteristics is a key component of the videofluorographic study. The ability of a dysphagic individual to swallow a food safely often depends on its physical characteristics (Table 14.1) (9).

Liquids

Liquids require no mastication, so they may be easier to handle than solid foods for individuals with dysfunction of the oral cavity. Liquids flow readily with minimal propulsive forces and are easily deformed. Thus, they present little danger of airway obstruction, are easily propelled by weak constrictor muscles, and easily pass through areas of anatomic or functional narrowing. On the other hand, their propensity to flow makes liquids difficult to contain. They may leak out of the oral cavity and into the pharynx involuntarily and prematurely. Liquids may penetrate the larynx and enter the trachea if brisk laryngeal closure does not occur. Thicker (i.e., more viscous) liquids are easier

TABLE 14.1. Characteristics of solids and liquids.

Characteristic	Liquids	Solids
Ease of deformation	High	Low
Tendency to flow	High	Low
Tendency to leak	High	Low
Passage through narrow passages	Easy	Difficult
Need for mastication	Little	Much
Risk of laryngeal penetration[a]	High[b]	Low
Risk of laryngeal obstruction[a]	High	Low
Risk of pharyngeal retention[a]	Low	High

[a] Characteristics greatly simplified to provide a frame of reference; not true in every case.
[b] The risk of laryngeal penetration is usually lower for thick than for thin liquids.

for many patients to control (10), since they are less readily deformed. Liquids should always be the first materials presented to the patient during a videofluorographic swallowing study, because they present little risk of airway obstruction.

We use three general categories of liquids in our studies, as shown in Table 14.2: thin, nectar-thick, and honey-thick liquids. Other liquids can be thickened to the desired consistency by using commercially available powdered thickening agents.

Solid Foods

Solid foods are less readily deformed. They are less readily propelled by weak oral and pharyngeal muscles, are difficult to push through narrow passages, and may be retained in the foodway after swallowing. They are easier to control and (for most patients) less likely to enter the larynx. On the other hand, penetration of the larynx or trachea by solid food may cause upper airway obstruction, with potentially fatal consequences. Solid boluses also may induce esophageal spasm. It is essential to test mastication and swallowing of solid food in the videofluorographic study to obtain a realistic picture of the patient's ability to consume food (4,5).

We use two categories of solid foods in our studies (Table 14.2). The first category includes foods that are homogeneous and readily change shape to form a bolus, but resist breakage into particles. These "purée consistency" solids include mashed potatoes, pudding, and puréed foods. We use a pudding as a purée during the VFSS. The second category is mechanical soft solid foods, such as fruit cocktail and scrambled eggs. These are less easily shaped and require more chewing. The last category is regular solid food. We use a shortbread cookie during the VFSS.

TABLE 14.2. Food categories.

Category	Examples[a]
Thin liquids	Apple juice, soda pop, water
Nectar-thick liquids	Tomato juice, fruit nectar, milk shakes
Honey-thick liquids	Made by adding thickening powder to any liquid
Puréed solids	Custard, yogurt, pudding, applesauce
Mechanical soft solids	Bananas, deviled chicken spread, fruit cocktail
Regular solids	Hamburger, crackers, cookies, salad

[a] The category of a particular food may vary depending on its manner of preparation.

TABLE 14.3. Therapeutic and compensatory techniques.

Head and neck position	Upright, flexed, extended, rotated
Trunk posture	Upright, reclined
Feeding devices	Spoon, cup, straw, syringe, fork
Bolus volume	Small (<5 mL) moderate (5–10 mL), large (>10 mL)
Respiratory and phonatory maneuvers	Throat clearing, supraglottic swallow, super supraglottic swallow
Clearance maneuvers	Multiple swallows, alternating consistencies, effortful swallow, Mendelsohn maneuver

Therapeutic and Compensatory Techniques (Table 14.3)

Head and Neck Position

Changing the position of the head and neck during the swallow changes the size and shape of the pharynx, resulting in altered bolus flow through the pharynx (11). In most individuals the anatomical reference position is natural for eating. It is comfortable for oral and pharyngeal motor function, permitting gravity to help in transporting the bolus and preventing aspiration or nasal regurgitation. **Flexing the neck** (tucking the chin) widens the valleculae and narrows the laryngeal vestibule, reducing laryngeal penetration and aspiration in many individuals (11–13) (Figure 14.1). It also facilitates pharyngeal clearance (reducing retention in valleculae) by positioning the base of the tongue posteriorly, closer to the pharyngeal wall. Surprisingly, **extending the neck** also has therapeutic utility in some patients. Since this movement allows gravity to help transport food from the oral cavity into the pharynx, it can help patients who have impaired oral bolus propulsion (11). However, neck extension also makes elevation of the pharynx and larynx more difficult, thereby hindering airway protection and pharyngeal clearance, and narrowing the lumen of the pharyngoesophageal segment.

Rotation of the neck (turning the head to one side) affects the mechanism of pharyngeal constriction in an asymmetrical fashion. It improves transport from the pharynx into the esophagus in some patients with unilateral pharyngeal weakness or paralysis by closing the affected side of the pharynx, and directing the bolus down the stronger side (Figure 14.2) (12,14). Tilting the head toward the stronger side can also be helpful if there is unilateral, oral, and pharyngeal weakness by allowing gravity to pull the bolus down the stronger side (12). These postural changes may be combined for patients who have complex deficits. For example, tucking the chin may be combined with rotating the head (15).

Body Position

Sitting upright is the typical position for eating and drinking in our society. This position permits gravity to assist esophageal transit. Patients with neurogenic disorders may have difficulty maintaining the upright posture. The **reclining position**, which may make it easier to maintain trunk control, simplifies positioning of the head in individuals with weak neck muscles. Reclining places the laryngeal aditus at a higher level relative to the hypopharynx; thus gravity pulls the food toward the posterior wall of the pharynx and away from the larynx, reducing the likelihood of laryngeal penetration and aspiration. This position allows gravity to assist oral food transport such as discussed for neck extension. Reclining may also facilitate laryngeal and pharyngeal elevation by reducing the opposing affect of gravity (via traction on the larynx, trachea, and lungs).

Respiratory and Phonatory Behaviors

The "**supraglottic swallow**" is a useful compensatory technique utilizing a learned voluntary alteration in respiration (11). The supraglottic swallow has three phases: taking a deep breath before swallowing, holding the breath during

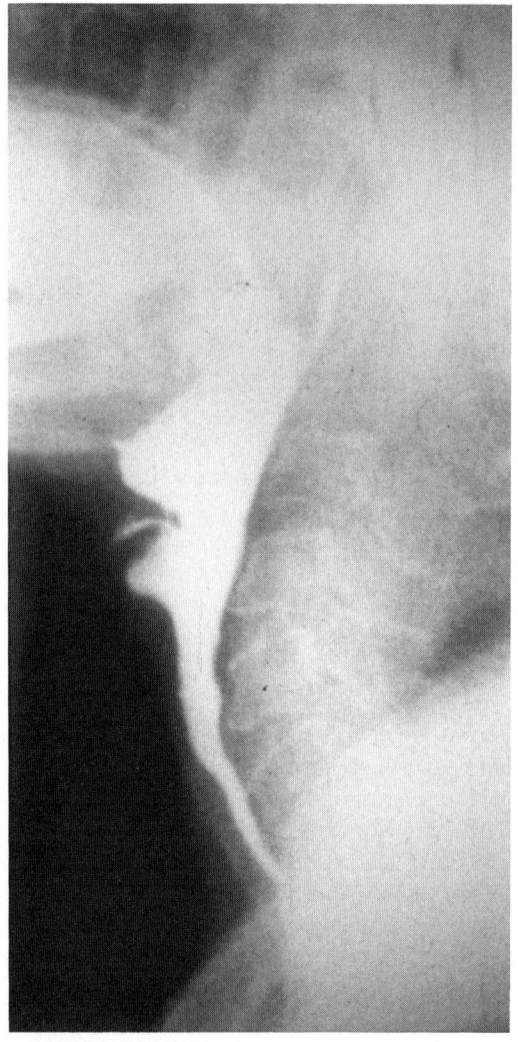 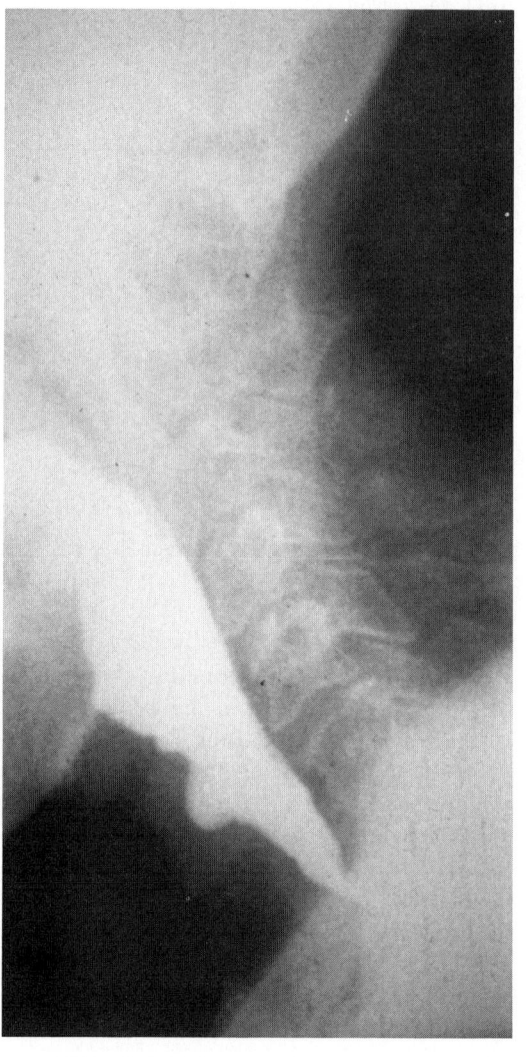

FIGURE 14.1. Effect of neck flexion. Flexing the cervical spine changes the relationship of the foodway to the pull of gravity. It narrows the laryngeal vestibule, reducing laryngeal penetration in many individuals. In contrast, extending the cervical spine makes closure of the larynx more difficult. These stop-frame prints from a pharyngogram show laryngeal penetration occurring during extension (A). Flexion prevented the penetration in this patient (B).

swallowing, and then exhaling after swallowing. This method may prevent aspiration before and during swallowing by producing volitional closure of the glottis before and during swallowing. This technique can be beneficial for the patient who exhibits decreased or delayed closure of the vocal folds or delayed onset of the swallow. The exhalation phase can prevent aspiration after the swallow by removing material from the laryngeal additus. The "**super-supraglottic swallow**" is a modification of this technique. It differs from the supraglottic swallow in that it adds a Valsalva maneuver. After taking the initial inhalation, the patient bears down to facilitate sealing of the vocal folds. The patient continues this until the completion of the swallow, whereupon he or she then exhales and gently coughs.

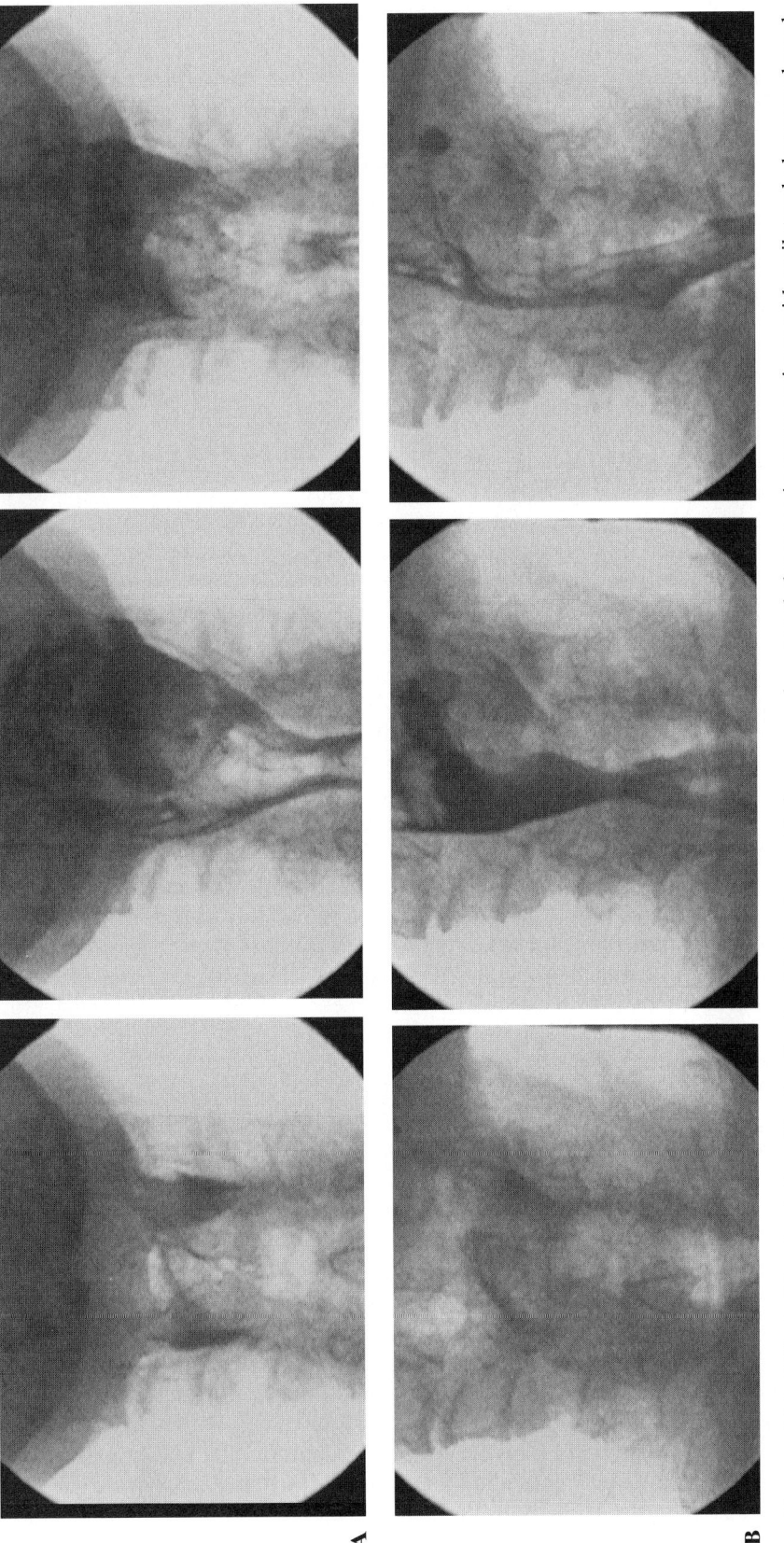

FIGURE 14.2. Effect of head rotation. Turning the head toward one side improves pharyngeal clearance in many patients with unilateral pharyngeal weakness. These are stop-frame prints from a videofluorographic swallowing study on a patient with lateral medullary infarction in posteroanterior projection. (A) Severe left-sided pharyngeal weakness with retention of a large amount of barium in the piriform sinuses after swallowing. (B) The same individual turns the head to the weak left side before swallowing, and the barium is deflected to the right (strong) side, with minimal retention after swallowing.

Pharyngeal Clearance Maneuvers (Table 14.3)

Several maneuvers are used to improve pharyngeal clearance, that is, to reduce retention of food in the pharyngeal recesses after swallowing. Simplest is **alternating food consistencies**. Drinking liquid after eating solid food, often washes retained material out of the pharynx. **Multiple swallows** (2–3 swallows per bolus) comprise another simple strategy to promote pharyngeal clearance if there is retained material in the valleculae and piriform sinuses. The patient is instructed to swallow two or three times instead of relying on the one swallow that would ordinarily have been sufficient. A third very simple technique is the **effortful swallow**. The patient is instructed to "swallow really hard," consciously squeezing the pharyngeal muscles tightly during the swallow. Although its precise mechanism is not yet clear, this technique can be beneficial in reducing pharyngeal retention after swallowing, and it appears to be particularly useful for individuals who have poor pharyngeal contraction during swallowing (15).

The **Mendelsohn maneuver** is used to improve opening of the upper esophageal sphincter. Although it does not actually increase the diameter of the sphincter, it can prolong the duration of sphincter opening (11,16). The patient is instructed to feel the upward movement of the larynx during swallowing by palpating the anterior neck. When this has been accomplished, the patient learns to "catch" the larynx in its elevated position and hold it there for several seconds by a voluntary contraction of the suprahyoid and thyrohyoid musculature. Although this technique is difficult for some individuals, it can usually be learned in just a few minutes and is sometimes very effective in improving pharyngeal clearance.

The use of these compensatory and therapeutic techniques is inextricably bound to the VFSS. Only with a VFSS can the examiner determine the precise pathophysiology of the swallowing impairment in a given individual, and so determine which of the techniques is likely to be effective. Furthermore, it is impossible to predict with certainty which maneuvers will be effective in the individual patient, even with a thorough understanding of the etiology and pathophysiology of the impairment. Each relevant therapeutic and compensatory technique must be tested individually during the VFSS to determine which ones are effective for each specific individual with impaired swallowing.

Devices for Feeding

The method for bringing a bolus of food to the oral cavity may affect the patient's ability to swallow it. The volume presented is particularly significant (10,17). With a smaller volume of material per ingestion, there is obviously less to control, and less that can penetrate the larynx or remain in the pharynx after swallowing. If tiny amounts are ingested with each swallow, however, eating a meal will take a very long time.

Larger volumes permit more rapid intake of a meal. They may also provide more stimulation to oral and pharyngeal sensory systems, facilitating the occurrence of the pharyngeal swallow in patients with disorders of initiation. However, large volumes may predispose the patient to laryngeal penetration or overflow phenomena, with involuntary spillage of material from the oral cavity into the pharynx or larynx.

The choice of utensils for presenting food deserves careful consideration. A **cup** provides rapid flow of liquid into the foodway, and is perceived as a normal way to drink. However, it is difficult to control flow rate and volume with a cup. A **spoon** limits volume and rate, but is extremely slow. It requires upper extremity dexterity, which may be a problem for disabled patients. A **straw** limits rate and volume to some degree, providing a more natural rate of ingestion. Unfortunately, using a straw demands of the oral cavity a degree of strength and coordination often lacking in patients with dysphagia due to neurogenic or structural disabilities.

Factors Affecting Patient Performance

Mental State

Central nervous system disorders frequently cause dysphagia. In patients with structural or physiological brain dysfunction, it is important to consider level of consciousness and cognitive function. These may vary over the course of weeks, days, hours, or even minutes, especially during the acute stages of illness. Lapses in concentration and attention may lead to difficulty following instructions, maintaining posture, or even remembering that there is food in the oral cavity. Mastication, oral food transport, and pharyngeal swallowing may be impaired, and airway protective reflexes may be suppressed. These deleterious effects often vary markedly over the course of a single day. This makes it difficult to get an accurate view of the patient's swallowing function during a comparatively brief videofluorographic study. In developing a plan for feeding the patient based on observations made in the fluoroscopy suite, it is essential to design a strategy for dealing with these variations in level of consciousness.

Effects of Fatigue

Fatigue may have an impact on swallowing. A complete videofluorographic swallowing study can be a long, tedious affair, exhausting for the patient. Peripheral and central types of fatigue should be distinguished. Peripheral fatigue refers to reduction in strength due to failure of the neuromuscular junction or the mechanism of muscle contraction. Central fatigue, which is caused by impaired brain arousal mechanisms, cardiopulmonary limitations, or sleep disturbance, occurs commonly in patients with brain disorders. Fatigue of this type may worsen a patient's level of consciousness, with effects on swallowing as described earlier. In either case, observing the phenomena with VFSS provides documentation of their effects on swallowing.

Medications

Medications may have beneficial or harmful effects on swallowing. Central nervous system (CNS) depressants, such as tranquilizers, narcotic analgesics, or barbiturates, may impair level of consciousness and suppress protective reflexes of the airway and foodway. Benzodiazepines, such as clonazepam or nitrazepam, can hamper the coordination of pharyngeal swallowing. Dopamine antagonists such as neuroleptics can cause involuntary movement disorders, which can cause difficulty with body position for eating or impair coordination of the oral and/or pharyngeal stages of the swallow. Medications that affect the peripheral nervous system and striated muscle include corticosteroids, lipid-lowering agents, and colchicine. Anticholinergic drugs, such as tricyclic antidepressants or propantheline, may reduce production of saliva and also worsen esophageal motility. Stopping these drugs may result in a rapid improvement in swallowing (18).

On the other hand, some medications may have beneficial effects on swallowing. Cholinergic drugs (such as bethanechol) may enhance esophageal motility and gastroesophageal sphincter activity. Acetylcholinesterase inhibitors, such as physostigmine or edrophonium, may ameliorate neuromuscular fatigue in patients with myasthenia gravis, improving both oral and pharyngeal swallowing. Appropriate pharmacotherapy of Parkinson's disease may improve swallowing. These drug effects must be considered thoughtfully in interpreting videofluorographic observations.

Dysphagic individuals may be unable to swallow pills. Pills may be retained in the foodway after swallowing, with potential adverse effects including aspiration or medication-induced esophagitis. These patients may require an alternative pharmaceutical preparation or route of administration. In some cases, it is advisable to administer a barium tablet during videofluorography to assess the ability to swallow pills. This may uncover a subtle stricture or spasm induced by the solid bolus.

Generating a Report

At our institution, the report is generated jointly by the clinicians performing the study. It includes a brief discussion of medical history, clinical findings (especially speech production, language skills, and cognitive function), a summary of videofluorographic findings, an assessment, and recommendations. The summary of videofluorographic findings lists the views obtained, position of the patient, foods presented, and therapeutic techniques tested, as well as the actual observations. Occurrences of aspiration, laryngeal penetration, and retention of food in the foodway after swallowing are described. The effects of varying posture, the physical characteristics of the food, head and neck position, and other therapeutic techniques are discussed in detail, particularly their utility in preventing laryngeal penetration or retention of food after swallowing (3).

The assessment and recommendations should state clearly whether the patient is capable of safe and efficient swallowing. If the patient is capable of swallowing safely, the preferred method of feeding is described. Restrictions based on consistency of the food, control of the environment, patient behavior, or need for supervision are specified. Different purposes for oral feeding may be considered. These include hydration, alimentation, therapeutic feeding, and hedonic feeding. (Hedonic feeding refers to eating or drinking purely for the pleasure of the experience, but not for alimentation or hydration.) One or more of these may be appropriate for a given patient. Formulating a useful prescription for safe swallowing requires a knowledge of not only the patient's oral, pharyngeal, laryngeal, and esophageal function, but also cognitive ability, family support system, home and work environments, and motor function of the limbs and trunk (4,5).

Pharyngeal Bypass Procedures (Table 14.4)

Procedures for bypassing the pharyngeal foodway are recommended for certain patients (e.g., those with severe swallowing disorders who cannot safely consume adequate fluid or nutrients by mouth). Behavioral or cognitive deficits may also affect a person's ability to maintain substantial nutrition (4,5). A patient who is able to swallow specific consistencies safely may have fluctuating alertness or be unable to carry over the strategies necessary to allow for safe swallowing because of a cognitive impairment. Under these circumstances the patient may be a good candidate for pharyngeal bypass procedure. For short-term nutrition and hydration, a nasogastric (NG) tube feeding may be beneficial. This can be used with, for example, an acute stroke patient, since although swallowing may be unsafe in the acute stage, there is good potential for a quick recovery to the point that the patient will be able to take a modified diet. The NG tube is not recommended for long-term feeding because it is often uncomfortable and cosmetically unacceptable. Gastrostomy tube feeding, particularly the percutaneous endoscopic gastrostomy (PEG) tube is primarily used for long-term pharyngeal bypass. This can be very beneficial to the dysphagic patient who is unable to swallow safely or cannot fully maintain adequate nutrition and hydration through oral intake alone. While the patient is receiving the tube feeds as the main source of nutrition, he or she can work on the rehabilitation of the swallow through therapeutic feeds. A therapeutic feeding program is formulated by the speech-language pathologist who determines, through analysis of the videofluorographic swallow study, what textures are safely swallowed, with the ultimate goal of resuming oral intake for alimentation. Gastroesophageal reflux disease is a major concern when naso-

TABLE 14.4. Pharyngeal bypass procedures.

Nonsurgical	Surgical
Nasogastric tube	Esophagostomy
Nasoenteric tube	Gastrostomy
Orogastric tube	Jejunostomy
Percutaneous endoscopic gastrostomy	
Fluoroscopically guided gastrostomy	
Gastrojejunostomy	

gastric and gastrostomy tube feeding is used because the patient is at risk for regurgitation and possible aspiration of stomach contents. Jejunostomy or gastrojejunostomy tube feeding is usually recommended for patients with severe gastroesophageal reflux disease, since the tube inserts into the jejunum, where the pyloric sphincter helps to prevent reflux. Videofluorography may contribute to selecting among bypass procedures by demonstrating gastroesophageal reflux.

Case Studies

Two case studies show how the principles just discussed were applied to actual patients. Each case illustrates the interaction of the physical characteristics of the food with the patient's ability to swallow, and the utility of varying head and neck positioning to reduce laryngeal penetration and improve pharyngeal clearance. Other issues bearing on these cases are the effects of varying bolus volume, the method of presenting the food, the importance of monitoring voice quality during feeding, the use of therapeutic feeding, and the value of feeding gastrostomy for alimentation and hydration. Each case demonstrates that the ability to swallow can change over time and may require serial evaluations.

Case 1

A 38-year-old white male was admitted to the hospital with complaints of vertigo, numbness of the arm, and dysphagia. There was significant difficulty with management of oral secretions. A magnetic resonance imaging scan of the brain revealed infarction of the left brain stem and cerebellum. A speech-language pathologist was consulted on day 3. A clinical bedside swallow evaluation revealed impaired respiratory support for speech with a hoarse, wet, breathy voice quality. Articulation was mildly imprecise; however, speech was 100% intelligible at the conversational level. Both volitional and reflex coughing were weak, and had a wet quality. Velopharyngeal incompetence was noted, and the velum was asymmetrical on inspection, with deviation to the right during phonation. Food with a purée consistency was presented at the bedside, and there was an immediate cough response with regurgitation of the bolus. It was recommended that the patient take nothing through the mouth (NPO) until completion of a VFSS. A PEG tube was placed prior to the VFSS because the attending physician felt it was necessary for adequate nutrition and hydration.

The VFSS was completed 4 days after the initial assessment. The patient was given only thin liquids during the study and was found to have severe pharyngeal dysphagia with retention of liquid in the pharynx after swallowing due to paresis of the left hemipharynx. Aspiration of barium was noted, with prompt reflexive cough. A paralysis of the left vocal fold was also observed. Rotating the head to the left side before swallowing reduced both the pharyngeal retention and the aspiration. It was recommended that the patient continue NPO except for thin liquids under direct supervision of the speech-language pathologist. A therapeutic feeding program was established incorporating the use of head rotation to the left while drinking thin liquids.

The patient was discharged home about a week later and continued to receive alternate means of nutrition and hydration via the PEG tube, but he was taking small amounts of water using head rotation. Swallowing therapy continued at home.

One month later, a follow-up VFSS revealed significantly improved pharyngeal function. Pharyngeal retention was rated as minimal for liquids and moderate for solids. There was laryngeal penetration with thin and thick liquids but no aspiration through the vocal folds. A supraglottic swallow maneuver was attempted but was not effective. However, the patient did benefit from alternating solids and liquids to clear residue in the pharynx. He was discharged from our care on a regular diet including thin liquids, using the compensatory strategy of alternating solids and liquids.

Case 2

Another 38-year-old male presented with C3 complete tetraplegia due to a gunshot wound to the neck. He developed acute respiratory failure and underwent tracheostomy and PEG placement during acute hospitalization. Mechanical ventilation was necessary, but he was successfully weaned from the ventilator prior to transfer to the rehabilitation hospital. The patient, who was eating a mechanical soft diet with nectar-thick liquids for several days prior to transfer, had intermittent fevers. A clinical bedside assessment revealed intact oral-motor and velopharyngeal function. At the time the patient had a #4 plastic tracheostomy tube with the cuff deflated. He was using a unidirectional tracheostomy speaking valve to aid oral communication. Vocal quality was hoarse and breathy, and the right vocal fold was immobile. Reflexive and volitional coughing were weak, and there was poor management of secretions, requiring frequent deep tracheal suctioning. A volitional swallow was possible, but laryngeal excursion was reduced. A modified Evans blue dye test was conducted by the speech-language pathologist, using mechanical soft solids and nectar-thick liquids. During the test, there was infrequent, weak coughing. Tracheal suction immediately after the meal revealed a moderate amount of blue dye in the tracheal secretions. These findings indicated aspiration with inadequate cough response. A VFSS was scheduled to investigate the mechanism of swallowing dysfunction. All oral intake was discontinued, except for trial swallows supervised by the speech-language pathologist.

The VFSS revealed pharyngeal dysfunction with silent aspiration. Imaging in the lateral projection revealed that laryngeal excursion and epiglottic tilt were reduced, and pharyngeal contraction was impaired, resulting in minimal retention of thick liquids and moderate retention of chewed solid foods in the pharynx. (The retention cleared after three swallows per bolus.) Nectar- and honey-thick liquids were presented by teaspoon, and each produced silent aspiration. Compensatory strategies were tested to reduce aspiration. When the supraglottic swallow was used, honey-thick liquids were swallowed without aspiration. Neck flexion could not be tested because of the recent spinal injury. On the posterior-anterior view, paralysis of the right vocal fold was appreciated, as was paresis of the right hemipharynx. Compensatory head and neck postures could not be used because of the cervical spine injury.

A therapeutic feeding program was established by the speech-language pathologist based on the VFSS. The patient was started on a diet of puréed solids using multiple swallows per bolus, as well as honey-thick liquids using the supraglottic swallow, all under direct supervision of the speech-language pathologist. Additionally, the patient was given therapeutic exercises to improve respiratory support and encourage laryngeal adduction.

A repeat VFSS one month later revealed significantly improved pharyngeal function. Laryngeal penetration was noted with nectar-thick and thin liquids, but no aspiration using the supraglottic swallow. Minimal pharyngeal retention was noted with solids, and cleared with a second swallow; there was no retention with liquids. The patient was advanced to a mechanical soft diet, using the supraglottic swallow with thin liquids and multiple swallows with solids. The diet was tolerated without difficulty. A third VFSS 3 weeks later revealed further improvement, and the patient was discharged on a regular diet including thin liquids.

Acknowledgments. We are grateful to the late Drs. Arthur Siebens and Martin Donner and to members of the Johns Hopkins University–Good Samaritan Hospital Swallowing Rehabilitation Program, who shared in developing the methods and concepts presented here. Supported in part by an award (DC02123) from the National Institutes of Health–National Institute on Deafness and Other Communicative Disorders.

References

1. Palmer JB. Evaluation of Swallowing Disorders. In: Grabois M, Garrison SJ, Hart KA, Lehmkuhl LD, eds. *Physical Medicine and Rehabilitation: The Complete Approach.* Malden, MA: Blackwell; 1999:277–290.
2. DeLisa JA, Currie DM, Martin GM. Rehabilitation medicine: past, present and future. In:

DeLisa JA, Gans BM, Bockenek WL, et al., eds. *Rehabilitation Medicine: Principles and Practice.* 3rd ed. Philadelphia: Lippincott-Raven; 1998: 3–32.
3. Palmer JB, Kuhlemeier KV, Tippett DC, Lynch C. A protocol for the videofluorographic swallowing study. *Dysphagia* 1993;8:209–214.
4. Palmer JB, DuChane AS. Rehabilitation of swallowing disorders due to stroke. *Phys Med Rehabil Clin North Am* 1991;2:529–546.
5. Palmer JB, DuChane AS. Rehabilitation of swallowing disorders in the elderly. In: Felsenthal G, Garrison SJ, Steinberg FU, eds. *Rehabilitation of the Aging and Older Patient.* Baltimore: Williams & Wilkins; 1994:275–287.
6. Jones B, Ravich WJ, Donner MW, Kramer SS, Hendrix TR. Pharyngo-esophageal interrelationships: observations and working concepts. *Gastrointest Radiol* 1985;10:225–233.
7. Teasell RW, McRae M, Marchuk Y, Finestone HM. Pneumonia associated with aspiration following stroke. *Arch Phys Med Rehabil* 1996;77:707–709.
8. Horner J, Massey EW. Silent aspiration following stroke. *Neurology* 1988;38:317–319.
9. Coster S, Schwarz W. Rheology and the swallow-safe bolus. *Dysphagia* 1987;1:113–118.
10. Bisch EM, Logemann JA, Rademaker AW, Kahrilas PJ, Lazarus CL. Pharyngeal effects of bolus volume, viscosity, and temperature in patients with dysphagia resulting from neurologic impairment and in normal subjects. *J Speech Hear Res* 1994;37:1041–1059.
11. Logemann JA. Behavioral management for oropharyngeal dysphagia. *Folia Phoniatr Logop* 1999;51:199–212.
12. Logemann JA, Rademaker AW, Pauloski BR, Kahrilas PJ. Effects of postural change on aspiration in head and neck surgical patients. *Otolaryngol Head Neck Surg* 1994;110:222–227.
13. Shanahan TK, Logemann JA, Rademaker AW, Pauloski BR, Kahrilas PJ. Chin-down posture effect on aspiration in dysphagic patients. *Arch Phys Med Rehabil* 1993;74:736–739.
14. Logemann JA, Kahrilas PJ, Kobara M, Vakil NB. The benefit of head rotation on pharyngoesophageal dysphagia. *Arch Phys Med Rehabil* 1989;70:767–771.
15. Poertner LC, Coleman RF. Swallowing therapy in adults. *Otolaryngol Clin North Am* 1998;31:561–579.
16. Kahrilas PJ, Logemann JA, Krugler C, Flanagan E. Volitional augmentation of upper esophageal sphincter opening during swallowing. *Am J Physiol* 1991;260(*Gastrointest Liver Physiol* 23):G450–G456.
17. Ekberg O, Olsson R, Sundgren-Borgstrom P. Relation of bolus size to pharyngeal swallow. *Dysphagia* 1988;3:69–72.
18. Buchholz DW. Oropharyngeal dysphagia due to iatrogenic neurological dysfunction. *Dysphagia* 1995;10:248–254.

Conclusion
What Does the Future Hold?

BRONWYN JONES

Diagnosis and therapy must proceed hand in hand. At present practitioners in the field believe that we are affecting the outcome of our patients' illness, but is that indeed true? We need carefully controlled randomized clinical trials to study outcome measures in patients with dysphagia. End points of disease must be expanded. For example, the prevention of or development of aspiration pneumonia would seem to be too extreme an outcome measure for aspiration-related disease. Perhaps measures such as change in total lung capacity or in forced expiratory volume over time would predict a poor prognosis before the patient develops a full-blown aspiration pneumonia and perhaps dies. Prognostic factors need to be defined: for example, why do some patients aspirate only a small amount and die of pneumonia and others aspirate large volumes and live out a full life span without disease related to the copious aspiration?

Advances in Imaging

Improvement in imaging techniques is expected to allow better resolution of the structures involved in swallowing. Such techniques include high-resolution, fast fluorocomputed tomography and cine–magnetic resonance imaging. The improvement of resolution in three-dimensional imaging, especially 3D ultrasound, 3D computed tomography, and 3D MRI, hopefully will show in exquisite detail the movements of the individual muscles, not just the external or internal structures. Movements that at present are inferred by shape and position of the bolus in future can be confirmed. Computer modeling may prove to be vital also in this understanding.

Joint Studies

More studies using simultaneous joint technology such as videofluorography and electromyography, or videofluorography and manometry, are needed to expand our understanding of the interaction of forces and pressure on the bolus.

Mapping of the Swallowing Process

The areas in the brain that affect certain aspects of the swallow need to be accurately mapped. This kind of correlative study of deficits resulting from diseases, such as those following cerebrovascular accidents, must be matched with abnormalities of swallow diagnosed, for example, by videofluorography.

There exist many areas of ignorance in the field of dysphagia toward which future research should be directed. For example, much needs to be learned about the neuroregulation of the airway-foodway interchange, about sensory feedback mechanisms, and about the effects of pharmacological agents on swallowing. Other areas still to be explored in more depth include the effects of bolus size, consistency, and texture on swallowing performance, and the timing of normal swallowing as well as timing deviations in neurologically impaired patients.

More precise anatomical and physiological information will lead to improved patient management. Elucidation of postoperative dysphagia may result in modification of surgical techniques with better restoration of swallowing performance.

Summary

Based on the experience of multidisciplinary swallowing teams in recent years, interspecialty collaboration, both clinically and in research, is optimal. Collaboration of a multidisciplinary team in which the radiologist is an integral part has proved effective in dealing with difficult problems in diagnosis and therapy. In patient management, radiography techniques are needed to assess the results of surgical intervention and/or to work with swallowing therapists in swallowing rehabilitation to tailor maneuvers that will compensate for deficits. In these efforts the radiologist supports the speech-language pathologist in finding the most opportune patient position, breathing and feeding maneuvers, and bolus size and consistencies. Clinicians involved in the diagnosis and treatment of swallowing impairment, working together and with basic scientists in physiology, pharmacology, and engineering (to mention just a few), are likely to improve the quality of life of such patients in the future.

Glossary

Aspiration	Entry of liquid or food below the vocal cords. This may occur prior to swallow, during swallow or after swallow.
Dysphagia	Difficulty in swallowing, often implying a sense of food or liquids sticking—can be further classified symptomatically by area, namely, oral, pharyngeal, or esophageal.
Laryngeal penetration	Entry of swallowed material into the laryngeal aditus during swallowing. This may be further categorized by whether it is or is not extruded during laryngeal elevation and closure.
Pharyngoesophageal segment (P-E segment)	Junction of pharynx and esophagus, which includes the cricopharyngeal sphincter, the closed portion of the hypopharynx between swallows. This corresponds in usage to the upper esophageal sphincter.
Premature leakage	Incompetence of soft palate—tongue blade seal, allowing spillage from the mouth into the pharynx prior to swallow.
Reflux	Gastroesophageal reflux, that is, retrograde movement of gastric contents into the esophagus.
Regurgitation	Retrograde movement within the esophagus, the extreme of which is esophagopharyngeal regurgitation, through the P-E segment into the pharynx, mouth, and/or larynx.
Retention	Residual bolus remaining in the valleculae and/or piriform sinuses after the bolus has passed from the pharynx into the esophagus.
Upper esophageal sphincter	Defined manometrically as a resting zone of high pressure between swallows thought to result from the action of the cricopharyngeus, thyropharyngeus, and proximal circular muscle of the esophagus. The main contribution is thought to come from the cricopharyngeus muscle, hence the term, "cricopharyngeal sphincter." Radiographically, an indentation posteriorly at about the C5-6 disk corresponds to the level of the cricopharyngeus muscle.

Index

A

Abnormalities
  of the oral phase, 61–63
  of the swallowing function, 211–220
Acetylcholinesterase inhibitors, effects of, on swallowing, 269
Achalasia
  clinical studies of, 95–98
  computed tomography scan of the esophagus to evaluate, 156–157
  cricopharyngeal, 72–73
Acid barium swallow test, 46
Acquired immunodeficiency syndrome (AIDS), dysphagia in, 243–259
Acquired immunodeficiency syndrome-related lymphomas (ARL), 246–247
Acyclovir, for treating herpes simplex infection, 255
Adaptation, defined, for the normal swallow, 83
Adenoma, pleomorphic, computed tomography scan of, 152
Adults, ultrasound imaging applications, 125–126
Aging
  defined, 227
  and neurological disease, 227–242
Airway protection, reflexes involved in, 91–100
Amyloidosis, tongue in, 75–76
Amyotrophic lateral sclerosis (ALS)
  and aging, 227
  decompensation in, 238
  impairments associated with, 234–236
Anatomy
  age-related, and swallowing function, 209–211
  of the cranial nerves, 160
  of the masticator space, 152
  of the mediastinum, 155–156
  of the parapharyngeal space, 150–151
  radiographic, and analysis of function, 55
  of swallowing, 11–34
    cross-sectional imaging to evaluate, 140–151
  ultrasound, normal, 124–125
Angiography, for differentiating vascular lesions, 146
Anticholinergic drugs, effects of, on swallowing, 269
Aperistalsis, with chilled barium, 46
Aphagia, following acute lateral medullary infarction, 234
Arteries, right subclavian, aberrant, cross-sectional imaging of, 157–159
Aspiration
  assessing during a rehabilitation study, 263
  after glossectomy, 190
  versus laryngeal penetration, 218–219
  oral stage dysfunction in, 73–74
  protection from, 69–71
Asthma, late-onset adult, caused by gastroesophageal reflux, 93
Atherosclerosis, acceleration of, with radiation therapy, 196
Atrophy, soft palate, after radiation therapy, 200

B

Benzothiaprine, association with dysphagia, 239
Biphasic study, routine sequence for, 41
B-mode ultrasound display, 122
Bolus
  compression of, 87
  compression and propulsion of, 64–71
  consistency of
    initial, for radiographic examination, 36
    varying in an examination, 45–46
  examining the pattern of, for functional abnormalities, 55–71
Bones, roles of, in swallowing, 11
Brain, mapping of, to understand swallowing, 274–275
Bulbar palsy, 160

C

Cancer
  childhood, risk from maternal radiation exposure during pregnancy, 4
  esophageal, computed tomography for evaluation of, 157–158
  laryngeal, reflux as factor in development of, 93
  mortality rate from, increase due to radiation exposure, 3
  See also Carcinoma; Squamous cell carcinoma
Candida infection, esophagitis due to, 249–253
Carcinoma
  association with Plummer-Vinson syndrome, 105–106
  esophageal, risk of, following squamous cell carcinoma of the head and neck, 111
  gastric, presenting as dysphagia, 41
  metastatic small-cell, magnetic resonance image, 154
  mimicking esophagitis, association with acquired immunodeficiency syndrome, 247–251
  pharyngeal, 111
  of the tongue, 75–76
    magnetic resonance imaging of, 146
  See also Cancer; Squamous cell carcinoma
Cardiorespiratory changes, gastroesophageal reflux-induced, 93–94
Cardiovascular supply, to the oropharyngeal region, Doppler ultrasound imaging studies, 123–124
Cartilage, roles of, in swallowing, 11
Case studies, of rehabilitation of swallowing, 271–272
Centers for Disease Control, recommendations to radiology departments about HIV infection, 257
Cerebrovascular accident/disease, 160–161
  dysphagia resulting from, 233–234
Cervical nodes, 155
Chemicals, damage from ingestion of, 115–116
Children
  older, feeding in, 210–211
  swallowing in, 205–226
Chipmunk swallow, defined, 61
Cholinergic drugs, effects of, on swallowing, 269
Cinefluorography, comparison with videofluorography (VTF), 1
Cinepharyngoesophagogram
  showing a late-emptying pouch, 107
  showing the components of the oropharyngeal phase of swallowing, 22–25
Cinepharyngogram, of a normal swallow, 62
Cineradiogram, cephalad movement of the posterior pharynx during deglutition, 23–26
Clinical assessment
  of dysfunctional feeding, 205–207
  prior to videofluorographic swallowing study, 262
Color Doppler flow (CDF), 123–124
Compensation
  defined, for swallowing, 83–90
  motions of tongue and hyoid in, 128
  in rehabilitation of swallowing, 265–268
Complications
  after a glossectomy, 190
  of a jejunal free graft, 180
  of neck dissection, related to anatomy, 182–183
  after supraglottic laryngectomy, 185
  after surgical treatment of Zenker's diverticulum, 195–196
  after total laryngectomy
    common, 173–177
    uncommon, 177–178
Computed tomography (CT)
  description of, 140
  for evaluating lesions of the pharyngeal space, 149
  for evaluating the mediastinum, 155–156
  for imaging conditions resulting in dysphagia, 139
Congenital anomalies, dysphagia associated with, 141, 146, 157–158. *See also* Genetic syndromes
Contrast media, for pharyngography, 169–170
Cordectomy and laryngofissure, 185
Coronal view, normal ultrasound imaging, 125
Cough reflex, sensitivity of, and aging, 230
Cranial nerves, anatomy of, 160
Cricopharyngeal area, 71–73
Cricopharyngeal prominence, 71–72
  esophageal findings on cineradiography, 94–95
Cricopharyngeal segment, voluntary opening of, 84
Cricopharyngeus (CP)
  abnormalities of, in children, 219
  and gastroesophageal reflux, manometric data, 91–92
  histopathology of, experimental studies, 93
  premature closure of, 95
Cross-sectional imaging, techniques for, 139–140
Cytomegalovirus, infection by, accompanying acquired immunodeficiency syndrome, 253–254

D

Decompensation
  in amyotrophic lateral sclerosis, 238
  examples of, 85
  neurological diseases indicated by, 231–233
  oral versus pharyngeal, 73–74
  in Parkinson's disease, 234–235
Degenerative diseases, association of dysphagia with, 163–164

Deglutition, laryngeal airway during, 215
Depressants, effects of, on swallowing, 269
Development, intrauterine, of swallowing, ultrasound observation of, 131–132
Developmental history, of children with feeding problems, 206
Diagnosis, failure of, reasons for, 40
Dipper swallow, defined, 61
Distance, from x-ray tubes, and radiation exposure, 7
Diverticulum. See Zenker's diverticulum
Dohlman's operation, for treating Zenker's diverticulum, 192–195
Doppler ultrasound imaging, 123–124
Dorsal medullary pathways, in control of the pharyngeal and esophageal phases of swallowing, 28–29
Double-contrast radiography
  biphasic examination including, 38–41
  to differentiate fungal from viral esophagitis, 253
  to evaluate ulceration in the hypopharynx and esophagus, 254
  to identify pharyngeal carcinomas, 111
Down's syndrome, accelerated aging in, 227
Duke University, 135
Duplex ultrasound, 123
Dynamic imaging
  analysis of, 64
  value of, 40
Dysphagia
  causes of, 35
  cross sectional imaging in, 139–166
  after glossectomy, 190
  in neurologic disease, 231–233
  oropharyngeal, 91–98
  postoperative, surgical technique modification to manage, 275
  pre-pharyngeal, in Parkinson's disease, 235
  after radiation therapy, 196–198
  after total laryngectomy, 175–177
Dysphagia (journal), 227

E

Eaton-Lambert myasthenic-myopathic syndrome, 236–239
Edema, after radiation therapy, significance of, 199–200
Electromyographic activity, of the muscles of deglutition, 21
Electromyography (EMG), submental surface, synchronization with ultrasound imaging, 133
Electron microscopy, for identifying esophageal ulcers with human immunodeficiency virus infection, 256
Embryos, effects of radiation exposure on, 4
Endoscopic dilatation, for treating Zenker's diverticulum, 192
Endoscopy
  damage during, 114
  web rupture during, 103
Epiglottic tilt, 68–69
Equipment, for videofluorography, 263
Erythema, from radiation, 3
Esophageal disorders
  in human immunodeficiency virus-infected patients, 243–246
  presentation with pharyngeal symptoms, 97–98
Esophageal phase of swallowing, 27–29
  abnormalities of, in children, 219–220
Esophageal speech, after total laryngectomy, 180–181
Esophagitis
  Candida causing, in acquired immunodeficiency syndrome, 249–253
  contrast-enhanced spiral computed tomography scan in, 156
  due to cytomegalovirus infection, with acquired immunodeficiency syndrome, 253–254
  diagnosis of, in children, 222
  due to herpes simplex virus infection, in acquired immunodeficiency syndrome, 254–255
  from radiation damage, 113
  response to acid reflux in, 92
  tuberculous, accompanying acquired immunodeficiency virus syndrome, 255–256
Esophagoglottal closure reflex, experimental studies of, 93
Esophagogram, tube, 48–49, 52
Esophagus
  abnormalities of
    association with pharyngeal abnormalities, 95
    association with Zenker's diverticulum, 95
    in oculopharyngeal muscular dystrophy, 239
  cervical, ultrasound imaging of infants, 131
  changes in, with aging, 230–231
  pneumatic rupture of, 114
Evaluation, of surgery for Zenker's diverticulum, 194–195
Examination, tailored, 35–53
Experimental studies
  of reflexes involved in airway protection, 91–98
  of swallowing in the elderly, 228
Eyes, protecting from radiation exposure, 8

F

Facial nerve (cranial nerve VII), 159–160
Fatigue, effect of, on swallowing, 269
Fetus, effects of radiation exposure on, 4

Fiberoptic endoscopy, for swallowing evaluation in children, 222
Films, spot, of the pharynx, 48
Fisted tongue, 76
Fistula
  carotid sheath, 194–195
  formation after radiation therapy for laryngeal carcinoma, 199
  orocutaneous, 193
Fluoroscopy, videorecorded, radiation in, 1–9
Food/feeding
  problems with
    in children, 205
    in children, managing, 222–223
    devices for managing, 268
    rehabilitation study review of, 263–264
  therapeutic, in rehabilitation of swallowing, 262, 270–271
Foreign bodies
  intraluminal, experimental studies of, 91
  trauma from ingestion of, 116
Functional aspects of swallowing, analysis of, 55–71
Future, expectations for therapy, 274–275

G
Gancyclovir, for treating cytomegalovirus esophagitis, 256
Gastroesophageal reflux (GAR)
  in children, 220, 223
  experimental studies of, 93–94
  manometric data, 91–92
  observing in a biphasic examination, 41
  relationship with Zenker's diverticulum, 110
  risk of, in nasogastric or gastrostomy tube feeding, 270–271
  upper esophageal sphincter response to, 92
Gastrointestinal tract, opportunistic disorders targeting, in acquired immunodeficiency syndrome, 243

Gastrojejunostomy tube feeding, 271
Gastrostomy, for tube feeding, 270
Genetic syndromes, accelerated aging accompanying, 227
Globus hystericus, 95–98
Glossary, 277
Glossectomy
  partial, orocutaneous fistula after, 193
  for treating cancer, 188–192
Glossopharyngeal nerve (cranial nerve IX), 160
Gray (Gy), defined, 2

H
Hemilaryngectomy, vertical, 187–188
Herpes simplex virus (HSV), infection by, accompanying acquired immunodeficiency syndrome, 254–255
History, medical, for children with feeding problems, 206
Human immunodeficiency virus (HIV) disease
  dysphagia in, 243
  esophageal ulcers in, 256
Hyoid bone
  action during swallow, 66–67
  ultrasound scan, 127–128
  movement of
    in a normal swallow, 23
    ultrasound scan, 123–124
  preservation of, in supraglottic laryngectomy, 183–184
Hypoglossal nerve (cranial nerve XII), 160
  damage to, after total laryngectomy, 177
Hypopharyngeal diverticulum. See Zenker's diverticulum
Hypopharynx, defined, 79–80
  Kaposi's sarcoma in, demonstrating, 245–247

I
Imaging, advances in, expectations for, 274

Immunodeficiency syndromes, lymphoid enlargement in the pharynx accompanying, 149
Infant, anatomy and swallowing function in, 209–210
Infections
  of the nervous system, dysphagia due to, 235–236
  of the oral cavity, computed tomography for evaluating, 146–147
Inflammatory processes, magnetic resonance imaging for evaluating, 164
In situ hybridization, for identifying esophageal ulcers with human immunodeficiency virus infection, 256
Insufflation, to reveal abnormalities, 44, 48
Interpretation, of radiographic studies, 55–82
Intubation, emergency endotracheal, trauma during, 114
Iron-deficiency anemia, relationship with webs, 103–104
Ischemic infarction, cerebral, cross-sectional imaging to evaluate, 160–162

J
Jejunal free flap, for repair after total laryngectomy, 179–182
Jejunostomy tube feeding, 271
Jet effect, in luminal narrowing, 103–105
Johns Hopkins Swallowing Center, 94
  study of psychogenic dysphagia, 95–96
Joint studies, simultaneous techniques for observing swallowing, 274
Junctional nodes, lymphatic system, 155

Index

K
Kaposi's sarcoma, diagnosis of, in human immunodeficiency virus infection, 244–250
Killian's triangle
  as the site of a Zenker's diverticulum, 106

L
Laimer's triangle, as the site of a Zenker's diverticulum, 106
Laryngeal action, during swallowing, 66–67
Laryngeal airway, during deglutition, 215
Laryngeal penetration
  versus aspiration, 218–219
  bolus-specific, 47
  defective, in the aging, 230
Laryngectomy
  horizontal (supraglottic), 183–185
  total, 171–181
  vertical partial, 185–187
Laryngofissure and cordectomy, 185
Larynx
  closure of, 87
  lesions of, associated with gastroesophageal reflux, 93
  movement of, in a normal swallow, 23
  surgical procedures for removal of, 170–181
  transverse ultrasound scanning of, 125–126
Lesions
  causing dysphagia, 35
  laryngeal, associated with gastroesophageal reflux, 93
  mucosal, double-contrast technique for identifying, 38
  neural, 160–164
  oropharyngeal, malignant, 190–191
  of the oropharynx, malignant, 190–194
  structural, 103–118
  See also Ulcers
Localization, of obstructing lesions, 36–37

Lumen, at the cricopharyngeal level, opening of, 71
Lungs, effects of gastroesophageal reflux on, 93
Lymphatic system, of the cervical region, 155
Lymphoma, association with acquired immunodeficiency syndrome, 246–248

M
Magnetic resonance imaging (MRI), 140
  in cerebrovascular disease, 160–161
  for imaging conditions resulting in dysphagia, 139
  of lesions of the parapharyngeal space, 151
  of lesions of the pharyngeal space, 149
  of venous malformations, 141, 146
Manofluoroscopy, of the pharyngeal phase of swallowing, 21–22
Manometric study
  in children, 222
  of globus pharyngeus, 97–98
  of oculopharyngeal muscular dystrophy, 239
Masticator space, anatomy and pathology of, 152–154
Mealtimes, work of, modifying for children, 223–224
Mediastinum, anatomy and pathology of, 155–159
Medications
  effects of
    in myasthenia gravis, 239
    on swallowing evaluation, 269
    esophageal ulcerations associated with, 254
Mendelsohn maneuver, to hold the esophageal sphincter open, 268
Mental state, affecting dysphagia, 269
M-mode ultrasound display, 122–123

Motor dysfunction, oral, in feeding difficulties, 216
Mouth
  abnormalities of, 75
  aging, changes in, 228
  junction with the pharynx, control of, 86
Multidetector computed tomography (MDCT), 140
Multi-instrumental applications, 132–133
Multiple sclerosis (MS)
  cross-sectional imaging to evaluate, 163–164
  impairments in, 234
Muscles
  cricopharyngeus, 71
  longitudinal layer of the pharynx, 80
  oral phase use of, 11–17
  pharyngeal phase use of, 14–21
Mutations, resulting from radiation exposure, 4
Myasthenia gravis, 236–239
Mycobacterium avium-intracellulare, esophageal ulceration due to infection by, 256
Mycobacterium tuberculosis, accompanying acquired immunodeficiency virus syndrome, 255–256
Myoneuronal junction disorders, 236–239
Myopathy, causes of, 239
Myotomy, cricopharyngeal
  for neuromuscular disorders, 196
  in Parkinson's disease, 235
  in patients with high intrabolus pressure, 95, 110
  in supraglottic laryngectomy, 183
  to treat Zenker's diverticulum, 194–195
Myotonic dystrophy, tongue in, 76

N
Nasogastric (NG) tube feeding, 270
Nasopharyngeal reflux, in children, 217–218

Nasopharyngeal regurgitation, 64–66
Nasopharynx, defined, 79
National Council on Radiation Protection (NCRP), recommendation on radiation dose during pregnancy, 4
National Dysphagia Diet Project, 46
Neck
 dissection of, 181–183
  in treating malignant oropharyngeal lesions, 190
 radiation to, malignancy and dysfunction due to, 112
Neopharynx, hirsute, 182
Neoplasms, intracranial, differential diagnosis of, 161–163
Neural control
 of the esophageal phase of swallowing, 28–29
 of the oral phase of swallowing, 17–18
 of the pharyngeal phase of swallowing, 27
Neurodegenerative disorders, 234–235
 associated with dysphagia in the elderly, 232–233
Neurogenic dysphagia, study of, 97–98
Neuroleptics, effects of on swallowing, 269
Neurological diseases, 233–234
 and the pharynx, 231–233
Neurological impairment
 dysphagia caused by, 159–160
 swallowing patterns in, ultrasound evaluation of, 128
Neuroma, carotid sheath sympathetic, magnetic resonance image, 153
Neuromuscular disorders
 causing dysphagia, 35
 cricopharyngeal myotomy for managing, 196
Neuromuscular transmission, medications interfering with, 239
Non-Hodgkin's lymphoma, pharyngeal, 148–150

Nonstochastic effects, of radiation, 2–3
Normal swallow, line drawing of, 60
Nuclear medicine studies, in children, 221

O
Oculopharyngeal muscular dystrophy (OMD), studies of, 239
Odynophagia
 accompanying acquired immunodeficiency syndrome, 243
 after radiation therapy, 196–198
Operator, protection of, during videofluorography, 7–8
Oral cavity, anatomy of, 141–145
Oral health, in the aging, longitudinal study of, 228
Oral-motor function, optimizing, 223
Oral phase of swallowing, 11–17, 61
 abnormalities of, in children, 215–216
 dysfunction of, as a cause of aspiration in the elderly, 73–74
Oropharyngeal compensation, signs of, 88–89
Oropharyngeal dysphagia, 91–98
Oropharyngeal swallow, study of, age and gender related observations, 230
Oropharynx
 defined, 79
 integrated movements of, in infants, 131
 ultrasound imaging of, 119–120
Oropharynx, malignant lesions of, 190–194

P
Palatopharyngeal isthmus, closure of, during swallowing, 86
Palatopharyngeus muscle, 80
Pallidotomy, in Parkinson's disease, 235

Paragangliomas (glomus tumors), magnetic resonance imaging of, 152–153
Paralysis, of the pharynx, 65–67
Parapharyngeal space, 150–152
Parathyroid glands, damage to, in total laryngectomy, 178
Paravertebral space, anatomy and pathology of, 154
Paresis, pharyngeal, after radiation therapy, 196–198
Parkinson's disease (PD)
 dysphagia associated with, 234–235
 pre-pharyngeal dysphagia identified with, 73, 235
Parotid tumors
 cross-sectional imaging to evaluate, 151
 risk of, following radiotherapy, 111
Paterson-Kelly syndrome, 103
Pathology
 of the masticator space, 154
 of the mediastinum, 156–159
 of the oral cavity, 141, 146–147
 of the parapharyngeal space, 151–152
 of the pharyngeal space, cross-sectional imaging of, 148–150
Patient
 preparation of, for postoperative videopharyngoesophagography, 167–168
 protecting from radiation exposure, 6
Pediatrics, ultrasound imaging applications for, 129–132
Percutaneous endoscopic gastrostomy (PEG) tube, 270
Perioral muscles, use in the oral phase, 11–17
Peristalsis
 assessing
  in infants using ultrasound, 131
  position for, 38
 changes in, with aging, 230
 esophageal, analysis of, 75

Index

pharyngeal, dynamic imaging of, 66
roles of the vagus nerve and intrinsic esophageal neurons in, 27
Phagophobia, in psychogenic dysphagia, 73
Pharyngeal bypass, for feeding, 270–271
Pharyngeal clearance, compensatory maneuvers for, 268
Pharyngeal constrictors, identifying weakness in, importance of position, 44–45
Pharyngeal dysphagia, studies of, 95
Pharyngeal phase of swallowing
abnormalities of, in children, 216–219
description of, 18–26
muscles involved in, 14–21
Pharyngeal pouches, lateral, 106–111
surgery for, 192–196
Pharyngeal space, anatomy of, cross-sectional imaging, 147–148
Pharyngeal symptomatology, in gastroesophageal reflux, 94
Pharyngeal wall, lateral, ultrasound scan during swallowing, 129–130
Pharyngoesophageal interrelationships, 91–100
Pharyngoesophageal junction, diverticula at, 110–111, 194
Pharyngoesophageal segment, 87
Pharyngoglotttal adduction reflex, experimental studies of, 93
Pharyngography
for screening, in patients with human immunodeficiency virus disease, 246
after surgery, 167–203
Pharyngolaryngectomy, 178–179
Pharynx, 78–80
abnormalities of, in oculopharyngeal muscular dystrophy, 239
anatomy and pathology of, 147–155
changes in, with aging, 228–230
coronal view of, 58–59
lateral sagittal views of, 56–57
and neurological diseases, 231–233
paresis/paralysis of, 65–67
pneumatic rupture of, 114
severe compromise of, tube esophagogram in, 48–49, 52
stimulation of, response of the upper esophageal sphincter, 92
Phases, of swallowing, 61
Phonation
comparison of the pharynx and surroundings during, with the same structures at rest, 42
compensatory, in rehabilitation of swallowing, 265–266
value in diagnosis, 48–51
pH probe study, in children with swallowing impairment, 222
Physiatrist, role in videofluorographic swallowing studies, 262
Physical examination
for children with feeding difficulties, 206–207
routine, suggested sequence for, 40
Physiology, of swallowing, 11–34
Pierre-Robin syndrome, feeding difficulties associated with, 216–217
Piriform sinuses, 80
lateral, weblike defect in, 103
Platysma muscles, use in the oral phase, 11–17
Plummer-Vinson syndrome, 103–105
Poliomyelitis, dysphagia in, 235–236
Positions
of the body, for swallowing, 265
for feeding, 223
for fluoroscopic examination erect and recumbent, 38
in rehabilitation assessment, 263
of the head and neck, for swallowing, 265–267
patient, for videopharyngoesophagography, 168–169
for stressing patients to reveal subtle abnormalities, 41–45
Postcricoid impression, 103
Postpolio syndrome (PPS)
aging of motoneurons in, 227
differentiating from progressive postpolio muscular atrophy, 235–236
Pouches. See Zenker's diverticulum
Power Doppler flow (PDF), 123–124
Pregnancy, protection of operators from radiation during, 7–8
Premature leakage
in abnormal tongue-palate seal, 64–65
supine fluoroscopic assessment to identify, 41
Pre-pharyngeal dysphagia, in Parkinson's disease, 73
Presbyesophagus, 230–231
Presbyphagia, 227
Pressure recordings, during sucking, coordination with ultrasound imaging, 135
Prevalence, of dysphagia, in hospitals and nursing homes, 228
Progeria, 227
Progressive postpolio muscular atrophy (PPMA), differentiating from postpolio syndrome, 235–236
Progressive supranuclear palsy (PSP), dysphagia in, 235
Pseudobulbar palsy, 160
Pseudoepiglottis, formation in total laryngectomy, 173
Psychogenic dysphagia, 73, 95–98
Pterygoid muscles, use in the oral phase, 11–17

R

Radiation
  avoiding with ultrasound imaging, 119
  effective dose, in videofluoroscopy, 4
  effects of, stochastic and nonstochastic, 2–3
  monitor badge placement for operators, 7–8
  risks of, 111–113
    estimating, 4–6
  in videorecorded fluoroscopy, 1–9
Radiation absorbed dose (Gray), defined, 2
Radiation dose equivalence (Sievert), defined, 2
Radiation therapy, 196–200
Radiological examination
  centering the initial swallow, diagnostic considerations, 36
  of children with feeding difficulties, 207–220
Radiology, role in rehabilitation of swallowing, 261–273
Radionuclide scintigraphy, 49
Real-time ultrasound, three-dimensional imaging, 135
Reconstructive ultrasound, three-dimensional imaging, 135
Regurgitation, nasal, supine fluoroscopic assessment to identify, 41
Rehabilitation
  defined, 261
  of swallowing, radiology's role in, 261–273
Reporting, of a videofluorographic swallowing study, 270
Respiration
  compensatory behaviors in, in rehabilitation of swallowing, 265–266
  coordination with sucking and swallowing in infants and children, 135
Respiratory compromise, interference with feeding, 223
Respiratory therapist, role in videofluorographic swallowing studies, 262
Retropharyngeal space, anatomy and pathology of, 154–156
Risk factors
  in human immunodeficiency virus infection, 256–257
  of radiation
    in therapy, 196
    in videofluorography, 2

S

Sagittal view, normal ultrasound, 124–125
Saliva, roles of, 75
Salivary glands, roles of, in swallowing, 11
Salpingopharyngeus muscle, 80
Schatzki's ring, 37–38
  position of the patient to reveal, 39
Shielding, from radiation exposure, 7
Sialolithiasis, computed tomography image, 147
Sideropenic dysphagia, 103
Sievert (Sv), defined, 2
Sinuses, piriform, 80, 103
Sjögren's syndrome, dysphagia in, 75
Small-cell carcinoma, metastatic, magnetic resonance image, 154
Soft palate
  abnormalities of, 75–77
  atrophy of, after radiation therapy, 200
Soft palatectomy, partial, 194
Soft palate—Passavant's cushion seal, normal, 64
Spasm, solid-induced, identifying, 46
Sphincter, accessory, 71
Sphinx view, for evaluating velopharyngeal portal closure, 78
Spiral computed tomography, 140
Split-screen duplex ultrasound imaging, 129
Squamous cell carcinoma
  of the esophagus, accompanying acquired immunodeficiency syndrome, 251
  of the head and neck, radiation therapy for, 196
  of the oral cavity, 147
  oropharyngeal, soft palate partial removal in, 190
  of the pharyngeal space, 148–150
  of the pharynx, 111
  recurrent
    after radiation therapy, 198–199
    after total laryngectomy, 179
    after tongue and retromolar trigone surgery, 193
Steroids, for treating human immunodeficiency virus-related ulcers, 256
Stochastic effects, of radiation, 2–3
Stomach, examining, in a biphasic examination, 41
Storage, of ultrasound data, 122
Stress, using during an examination to reveal subtle abnormalities, 41–48, 90
Structure, analysis of, 75–78
Stylopharyngeus muscle, 80
Sucking physiology, ultrasound studies of, 129–133, 135
Suckle feeding, patterns of, 209–210, 212–215
Supersupraglottic swallow, compensatory, 266
Supraglottic laryngectomy, voice-preserving, 183–185
Supraglottic swallow, compensatory, 265–266
Surgical procedures, voice-preserving, 183–188
Swallow, stages of, 85, 90
Systemic disorders, causing dysphagia, 35

T

Tardive dyskinesia, relationship with choking episodes, 239
Team approach, to videopharyngoesophagography, 168
Therapeutic techniques, in rehabilitation of swallowing, 265–268
Therapists, for rehabilitation of swallowing, 262
Therapy, for children with feeding deficits, 215

Index

Three-dimensional imaging
  real-time ultrasound, 135
  reconstructive ultrasound, 135
Thyroglossal duct cyst, computed tomography image, 146
Thyroid gland
  carcinoma of, risk following radiotherapy, 111
  damage to, after total laryngectomy, 177
  shields to limit operator's radiation exposure, 7
Time
  duration of fluoroscopy, and radiation exposure, 6–7
  duration of the pharyngeal state of swallowing, 21
Tipper swallow, defined, 61
Tongue
  abnormalities of, 75
    and feeding difficulties in children, 216
  cancers of, surgery for, 188–190
  changes in, with aging, 228
  coronal section through, 19
  ultrasound scan
    coronal, 125
    midline sagittal, 121
    during swallowing, 126–128
Tongue-palate seal, normal and abnormal, analysis of, 61–64
Tracheal cartilage, movement of, in a normal swallow, 23
Tracheoesophageal fistula, 40
  esophageal tube technique for identifying, 49
Tracheostomy, 191–192
Tranquilizers, dysphagia associated with, 239
Transducer, characteristics and placement of, ultrasound imaging, 121–122
Transverse view, larynx in, normal ultrasound imaging, 125–126
Trauma, closed, 113–116
Trigeminal nerve (cranial nerve V), 159
Tube feeding, 270–271
  gastrojejunostomy for, 271

U
Ulcers, evaluating
  in cytomegalovirus infection, 253–254
  in human immunodeficiency virus infection, 256
  See also Lesions
Ultrasound imaging, 119–138
  advanced technologies for, 135
  in children, 222
Units of radiation, 2
Upper esophageal sphincter (UES), 71
  response to acid reflux, 92
Upper gastrointestinal (UGI) series, in children, 220–221

V
Vagus nerve (cranial nerve X), 160
  innervation of the esophagus by, and referred reflexes, 27
Valleculae, defined, 80
Valsalva maneuver, comparison of the pharynx and surroundings during, with the same structures at rest, 43
Vascular disorders, dysphagia associated with, in the elderly, 232–233
Velopharyngeal closure, in infants, ultrasound evaluation of, 131
Videofluorographic swallowing study (VFSS)
  for analyzing impaired swallowing, and therapeutic possibilities, 261
  for assessing compensatory techniques for rehabilitation, 268
  negative, interpreting, 74, 98
Videofluorography (VTF)
  biphasic examination including cinefluorography, 38–41
  comparison with cinefluorography, 1
  time range of radiation exposure in, 4
Videofluoroscopy, radiation effective dose in, 4
Videopharyngoesophagography
  components of the examination, 169
  postoperative, 167–170
  preoperative, 167
Videopharynography, advantages and disadvantages of, 139–166
Videorecording
  analysis of, for the functional aspects of swallowing, 55–71
  fluoroscopic, radiation exposure in, 1–9
  specifications for videofluorography, 1–2
Vocal fold, ultrasound imaging of, 128–129
Voice preservation, surgical procedures for, 183–188

W
Waldeyer's ring, 155
Wallenberg's syndrome, 234
Webs, 103–106
  weblike structure after total laryngectomy, 175–176

X
Xerostomia (salivary hypofunction)
  following radiotherapy, and esophageal acid clearance, 75
  swallowing patterns in, ultrasound evaluation of, 128

Z
Zenker's diverticulum, 106–110
  histopathology of the cricopharyngeus muscle accompanying, 93, 95–97
  surgery for, 192–196